Social and Cultural Contributions to
Health, Difference, and Inequality

THE
SOCIAL
MEDICINE
READER

Second edition

VOLUME II   Social and Cultural
Contributions to
Health, Difference,
and Inequality

GAIL E. HENDERSON

SUE E. ESTROFF

LARRY R. CHURCHILL

NANCY M. P. KING

JONATHAN OBERLANDER

RONALD P. STRAUSS

editors

DUKE UNIVERSITY PRESS
Durham and London 2005

© 2005 Duke University Press • All rights reserved
Printed in the United States of America on acid-free paper ∞
Typeset in Trump Mediaeval by Keystone Typesetting, Inc.
Library of Congress Cataloging-in-Publication Data
appear on the last printed page of this book.

Contents

Preface to the Second Edition

Of the six editors of this second edition of the *Social Medicine Reader*, five are current members and one a former member of the Department of Social Medicine, University of North Carolina at Chapel Hill School of Medicine. Founded in 1977, the Department of Social Medicine includes scholars in medicine, the social sciences, the humanities, and public health. Its mission is to inform the work and thought of researchers, teachers, and practitioners on the social conditions and characteristics of patients, causes of illness, and barriers to effective care; and the responsibilities of the medical profession and other medical institutions.

This reader is based on the syllabus of a year-long, required, interdisciplinary course, Medicine and Society, which has been taught to first-year students at the University of North Carolina at Chapel Hill School of Medicine since 1978. The goal of the course since its inception has been to demonstrate that medicine and medical practice have a profound influence on—and are influenced by—social, cultural, political, and economic forces. Teaching this perspective requires integrating medical and nonmedical materials and viewpoints. This reader, therefore, arises not from one or two academic disciplines, but from many fields within medicine, the social sciences, and humanities.

With health care and health so central to the political, personal, and financial discourse of the day, this reader provides a starting point for informed, critical analysis. The three volumes of the *Social Medicine Reader* represent the most engaging, provocative, and informative materials and issues we have traversed with our students. While the origin of these volumes lies in the teaching of medical students, the selections were deliberately made with an eye toward engaging nonmedical readers, both from the interested public and from students in the arts and sciences.

The selections challenge standard ways of thinking about medical categories of disease, social categories of risk, and the types of moral reasoning on which much of the field of bioethics has been based. Their many voices include individual narratives of illness experience, commentaries by physicians, debate about complex medical cases, and conceptually and empirically based writings by scholars in medicine, the social sciences, and humanities. These are readings with the literary and scholarly power to convey the complicated relationships between medicine, health, and society. They do not resolve the most vexing contemporary issues, but illuminate them.

Medicine's impact on society is multidimensional. Biomedical technology and practice, including its latest expression, genomic medicine, have profoundly affected our institutions and our social relations. Medicine has affected how we think about the most fundamental, enduring human experiences—conception, birth, maturation, sickness, suffering, healing, aging, and death—and it has shaped the metaphors we use to express our deepest concerns. Medical practices and our responses to them have helped to redefine the meaning of age, race, and gender. Technological advances in medicine have produced ethical dilemmas expressed in new vocabularies of science and economics, as well as in the familiar languages of morality and human relationships.

Social influences on medicine are apparent in several ways. First, modern science presumes that the pursuit of knowledge can and should be conducted with an unwavering adherence to neutral, objective observation and experimentation. Yet medical knowledge and practice, like all knowledge and practice, is shaped by political, cultural, and economic forces, within which doctors' ideas about disease—in fact their very definitions of disease—depend on the roles science and scientists play in particular cultures, as well as on the cultures of laboratory and clinical science. Medicine tends to reduce the world to a vocabulary of its own, one that seems immune to the vagaries and vicissitudes of culture. But diseases are not immutable; they are shaped by person, time, and place, and are identified and endowed with significance only within social and cultural contexts.

Despite the power of the biomedical model of disease and the increasing specificity of molecular and genetic knowledge, social factors have always influenced the occurrence and course of most diseases. And once disease has occurred, the power of medicine to alter its course is constrained by the larger social and economic context. Beyond these problems, many medical interventions are themselves of contested or unclear value. Spending on health care in the United States has long outstripped that of other industrialized nations, but that spending has not resulted in a healthier population. What does our medicine produce? Who benefits from these enormous expenditures of resources?

Repeatedly, the readings throughout these three volumes make clear that much of what we encounter in science, in society, and in everyday and extraordinary lives is indeterminate, ambiguous, complex, and contradictory. And because of this inherent ambiguity, the interwoven selections highlight conflicts—conflict about power and authority, autonomy and choice, security and risk. By critically analyzing these and many other related issues, we can open up possibilities, change what seems inevitable, and practice medical education and doctoring with an increased capacity for reflection and self-examination. The goal is to ignite and to fuel the inner voices of social, human, and moral analysis among health care professionals, and among us all.

Any collection of readings like the three volumes that make up the *Social Medicine Reader* is open to challenges about what has been included and what has been left out. This collection is no exception. The study of medicine and society is dynamic, with large and ever expanding bodies of new literature from which to draw. We have omitted some readings widely considered "classics" and included some readings that are classic only in our experience. We have chosen to include material with literary and scholarly merit and that has worked well in the classroom, provoking discussion and engaging readers' imaginations. These readings invite self-conscious, multilevel, critical examination, a work of reading and discussion that is inherently difficult but educationally rewarding.

The first edition of the *Social Medicine Reader* was a single volume. We decided to make the second edition three volumes to facilitate use by different audiences with different interests; however the three volumes also function as an integrated whole. Volume I, *Patients, Doctors, and Illness*, examines the experience of illness, the roles and training of health care professionals and their relationships with patients, ethics in health care, and experiences and decisions at the end of life. It includes fiction and nonfiction narratives and poetry; definitions and case-based discussions of moral precepts in health care, such as truth telling, informed consent, privacy, autonomy, and beneficence; and scholarly readings providing legal, ethical, and practical perspectives on many familiar but persistent ethical and social questions raised by illness and health care. Volume II, *Social and Cultural Contributions to Health, Difference, and Inequality*, explores health and illness, focusing on how difference and disability are defined and experienced in contemporary America and how the social categories commonly used to predict disease outcomes—gender, race/ ethnicity, and social class—have become contested terrain. Narratives and essays feature individuals managing illness in daily life, and families both coping with and contributing to the challenges of ill health. Social epidemiological categories are examined empirically and critically. Volume III, *Health Policy, Markets, and Medicine,* examines issues and controversies in health policy. Essays analyze a broad spectrum of topics, from the historical forces that shaped development of the American health system to contemporary reform debates over controlling medical care spending and covering the uninsured. International health systems, medical care rationing, and emerging policy issues—including the rise of consumer-driven insurance and population aging—are also explored.

We thank our teaching colleagues who helped create and refine both the first and the second editions of this reader. These colleagues have come over the years from both within and outside the Department of Social Medicine and the University of North Carolina at Chapel Hill. Equal gratitude goes to our students, whose criticism and enthusiasm over two decades have improved our teaching and have influenced us greatly in making the selections for the reader. The leadership of Department of Social Medicine chairs and course directors since 1978 has also been invaluable. We thank the Department's faculty and staff, past and present; we especially thank Judy Benoit, for many years the Medicine and Society course coordinator, and Jeff Kim, our student research assistant. In addition, Larry Churchill thanks the faculty who have taught with him in the Ecology of Health Care course at Vanderbilt School of Medicine during 2002 and 2003 for their many ideas for improving the second edition of the reader. Jon Oberlander gratefully acknowledges the support of the Greenwall Foundation and its Faculty Scholars Program in Bioethics. The editors gratefully acknowledge support from the Department of Social Medicine, University of North Carolina at Chapel Hill School of Medicine, and the Center for Clinical and Research Ethics, Vanderbilt University.

**Social and Cultural Contributions to
Health, Difference, and Inequality**

Introduction

The selections that comprise Volume II of the *Social Medicine Reader* introduce fundamental dimensions of health inequality and difference. These include social and cultural shaping of the meaning of health, disease, and illness, and various explanations for why some groups within and across societies experience a disproportionate burden of disease and unequal access to health care. Disease is a pathological event that occurs within a body; yet an individual always defines illness and disability within a cultural milieu, in which the experience may have both universal components and features that are unique to a particular time and place.

Similarly, when individuals who belong to certain social groups, such as people who are impoverished or who belong to racial and ethnic minorities, have higher rates of disease, epidemiologists seek to explain these variations by identifying risk factors that can account for the disparities. Yet concepts of disease and risk factors themselves reflect deeply held assumptions about the meanings of illness and causation, and about the validity and significance of group labels based on ethnicity and race. Just as the experience of illness must be understood in terms of both individuals and their society and culture, explaining the occurrence of disease by individual risk factors is of most value when combined with a broad examination of the influences of family, community, and the social environment.

To examine these factors, this volume takes a multidimensional perspective that draws on the frameworks and findings of a variety of academic disciplines. The most prominent of these are sociocultural and medical anthropology, sociology, and social history and the history of medicine and science. As in volumes I and III of the *Social Medicine Reader*, the six editors have assembled a diverse collection of essays in this volume to illustrate these themes. The selections consist of empirical, conceptual, and narrative materials about sociocultural markers such as gender, race, ethnicity, and social status, and difference and inequality in health. Most of the selections have been used successfully in medical school curricula and in undergraduate and graduate courses, and can be adapted to fit a variety of formats and perspectives for courses and students in social science, science, and the humanities.

The readings in part I of this volume explore how difference and disability are defined and experienced in contemporary America. We begin with two readings that feature the revolutionizing prism of genetics, a historical essay on eugenics and an ethnographic description of some contemporary experiences of expectant parents receiving the diagnosis of Down syndrome for their fetus. The next readings introduce three people who live with multiple sclerosis, spasticity, and paraplegia respectively, and do so with humor, rage, confidence, self-loathing, and a memorable array of other entirely recognizable styles and characteristics. These vivid narratives of managing illness in daily life and disablement in a lifetime contribute to a textured, biographical understanding of the individuals whose experiences with illness and disability are as varied as they are powerful. These accounts also challenge presumptions of sameness among people who are profoundly different and presumptions of difference between the disabled and the "temporarily abled" by bringing to the foreground unrecognized commonalities.

Part II covers the broad territory of social and cultural inequalities in health. The essays examine how gender, race/ethnicity, and social class are predictors of disease outcomes, in global and local contexts. At the same time, they demonstrate how the categories themselves have become problematic, contested terrain. Readers are invited into the current complex debates carried out in popular media and academic journals. Is race a valid and/or biological category, or is it socially and culturally defined? What does gender mean in the context of increasingly fluid definitions of male and female? What implications do these debates have for how we understand differences in health and illness? Using the lens of now familiar diseases like AIDS and breast cancer, as well as newly emerging ones such as male "andropause," the readings highlight social and cultural forces that determine not only who gets these diseases, but also how both patients and health care professionals define and accommodate to them.

Finally, this volume turns attention to families, the critical social unit through which individuals experience their own and family members' illnesses, and that may provide either a buffer against or a vulnerability to inequalities in health and health care. The essays in this final part document the important care-giving roles that relatives and loved ones fill, but also convey graphically the depletion of emotional and financial resources of families least able to provide needed care, and the consequent tension between family members' rights and responsibilities.

Social and Cultural Contributions to Health, Difference, and Inequality
Sue E. Estroff and Gail E. Henderson

Once the purview of laboratory scientists and clinicians in white coats, the domains of disease and health, birth and death, bodily suffering and debilitation are now inhabited also by scholars from the social sciences and humanities. Their contributions provide tools for understanding the experiences and meaning of illness, and the social as well as biological causes of disease. In this essay, we introduce the basic concepts and perspectives of social and cultural approaches to health and illness and provide examples from recent scholarship in the fields of medical sociology and anthropology, public health, and health services research. Our respective anthropological and sociological vantage points are sometimes divergent but more often complementary or shared.

The key shared concepts include the mutual molding of culture, biology, and illness; the distinction between disease as a pathological event and illness as a lived experience; the impact of role expectations on how sick people are seen and see themselves; and the ways that gender, social class, race, and ethnicity are associated with disease and are also indicators of broader economic, political, and cultural forces that influence a person's health status and exposure to or protection from illness and injury. Two central concerns of our scholarship are the experiences of difference engendered by labels of disability and disease, and inequality in health status and health care related to social identities such as gender and race. It is in these areas that sociocultural influences on health and illness are perhaps the most prominent and observable.

Basic Concepts

The terms "social" and "cultural" are often used together, interchangeably, or combined into a single word "sociocultural." These two words actually represent different disciplinary perspectives and reflect varied definitions, questions, and approaches to research. Despite divergent vocabularies and interests, much recent social science scholarship on health and illness integrates qualitative and quantitative methods and analytic techniques from a variety of disciplines.

As used in this essay, the term "social" encompasses selected characteristics of a defined, organized group that can range in size from a family unit to a nation. The characteristics of interest include social institutions like families, schools, hospitals, and prisons; local and national political institutions; and systems of production, such as private or public ownership, manufacturing, agriculture, and the like. These social institutions and economic systems structure social roles and opportunities that affect health and health care for individual citizens, and provide both obstacles and assistance to those unable to carry out normal functions due to disease or disability. Individuals are also part of social groups, such as race, gender, or religion, woven together by systems that reflect differential or hierarchical access to resources of wealth, power, and social status. Social groups may overlap with cultural groups, and many of these categories have developed fuzzy edges under scrutiny. For example, Hispanics are often considered a social group in health research, and for administrative and political purposes. But the grouping is based largely on language or surnames, and masks dozens of cultural and ethnic differences. Still, there are undeniable differences in disease frequencies and health outcomes between (and within) social groups, however contested the definitions and however complex the reasons for these differences may be.

Culture can be viewed as an evolving collective product, a negotiable and negotiated template for leading and making sense of daily life. The properties of culture are values, rules, prohibitions, preferences, symbols, meanings, language, and practices that guide how everyday life is lived and how extraordinary events are understood. Culture includes definitions of health and illness, responses to disease and injury, and how pain, discomfort, and disfigurement are experienced. These components are shared among a group of people, despite variations among them in interpretation of principles or in practices. Finally, culture is enduring at a fundamental level but also changing in form and content over time, produced and reproduced by those who learn the rules and apply them in daily living.

The idea of culture, as Comaroff and Comaroff (2004, p. 188) observe, has taken on increasing power and application as "peoples across the planet have taken to invoking it, to signifying themselves with reference to it, to investing it with an authority, a determinacy" that some scholars would dispute. Investing culture with such power can lead to stereotyping, or a cookie cutter view of culture—that it produces identical people with identical beliefs within particular groups. For example, race and gender-based stereotypes presume that one characteristic, such as darker skin color or being male, play the lead role in defining anyone with that characteristic. Variation and individuality become "exceptions." In a clinical setting, stereotypes can be convenient, but are often inaccurate and can be mistakenly deployed as a form of cultural competence.

Instead, culture is better understood as "less a sign of racial marking or an alibi for difference than as . . . a description of a more or less open repertoire of styles, a mode of conduct, a set of programmatic values always under (re)construction . . . [as] a thoroughgoing qualification to everyday life" (Comaroff & Comaroff 2004, p. 198). It is helpful to think of culture as agreed upon enough to contribute to and to sanction recognizably patterned ideas about social categories like gender, age, and social status, and responses to disease, disability, or death.

Culture in Biology, Biology in Culture

Biology and culture do not stand in opposition, the one fixed and the other malleable. The biological, social, and cultural realms are profoundly intertwined. The claim is not that culture includes everything, but that nearly every part of biological and social life is culturally influenced, that life is "cultured." In any locale, for example, the plants that are used for healing, the kind of crops that are grown, and the climate help to shape local customs and beliefs. In turn, these customs and beliefs interpret or give symbolic meaning to the weather or to food. Further, social hierarchies often determine how protein is distributed within a group—who gets what kind and amount of food—which may then influence patterns of disease.

Illness is sensate. It is felt in the body through pain, discomfort, and loss or change of function. Illness and injury are embodied—seen, displayed, apparent to self and to others. How we feel, what we feel, what we identify as pain and discomfort and disfigurement are all learned and shaped in cultural context. Expected and ideal bodies are imagined within cultural parameters that in turn shape and are shaped by new medical technologies. The availability of new technologies for replacing body parts, for example, creates the expectation, not just the possibility, of playing tennis at age 70, or replacing a diseased kidney with a donated or purchased organ. Cosmetic surgery and botox injections to rid the face of wrinkles, or liposuction to remove body fat, become the means to maintain or achieve new bodily shape and function over a lifetime. At the same time, the availability and intense marketing of these and numerous other body-enhancing procedures help to create evolving ideals about physical form. This interplay between medical technology and bodily expectations is an important arena for the mutual molding of culture and medicine (Rothman and Rothman 2000).

Margaret Lock's (1994) work on aging and menopause in Japan and North America illustrates the intimate interactions between biology and culture. Lock finds that Japanese women physically experience menopause differently from American women. They do not report the hot flashes and emotional liability that Americans do. Rather, their primary sensations include aching joints and other bodily pains. Likewise, Japanese and American physicians differ widely in how they approach menopause. Their relationships with patients are embedded in cultural contexts with differing ideas about gender, authority, female biology, and aging. How can it be that Japanese women experiencing menopause actually feel differently from American women? Their aching shoulders are as culturally influenced and as real as are American and Canadian hot flashes, but all the women are going through the same biological process. Or are they?

The recognition of cultural influences on bodily experience is not confined to the social sciences. An investigator in a large clinical trial studying the impact of hormone replacement therapies on cognitive function (Espeland et al., 2004) was quoted as saying, "The true interpretation of menopause is cessation of menses from decreased production of female hormones. . . . And while, in our culture, it's often associated with hot flashes and other symptoms, in some other cultures women breeze right through it. There may be lots of factors here. . . . It's not my area of specialty. . . . It's been debated considerably" (Shamp, 2004). The inclusion of sociocultural influences on biological events by researchers outside the social sciences demonstrates the expanding application of interdisciplinary findings and perspectives to medicine.

Disease and Illness

Culture and social relationships are deeply implicated in the recognition, experience, and treatment of disease. Social scientists have found it useful to make a distinction between "disease" as a pathological process and biological condition, and "illness" as the personal, socially, and culturally influenced experience of impairment or pathology (Fabrega, 1974; Young, 1982). Within this framework, multiple sclerosis is the disease, and feeling tired, or unable to climb steps, as well as being treated as an object of pity, curiosity, or suspicion, and facing discrimination in employment, all constitute the illness. While the disease-illness distinction calls attention to the concurrent processes of personal experience and pathophysiology, if applied simplistically, it runs the risk of reinforcing a separation of biology from culture and of body from person (Taussig, 1980).

Illness has multiple narrators (Hawkins, 1993). Many are clinicians and physicians, who through scholarly publication (Decker, 1998), or literary rendering (Williams, 1936), have written about disease and illness in general and spoken for and about specific patients. This tradition continues (Quill, 1991; Groopman, 2000; Gawande, 2002) in the scientific and literary world and has spawned various efforts to apply the resulting insights to clinical practice and doctor-patient relations (Kleinman, Eisenberg, and Good, 1978; Charon, 2004; Fadiman, 1997). Descriptive, biographical, and ethnographic accounts of illness and healing also have an established place in medical anthropology and sociology (Charmaz, 1991; Liebow, 1993; Frank, 2000). These third-person, scholarly or medical expert storytellers have been joined by a substantial chorus of first-person reports and reflections (Styron, 1990; Mairs, 1996; Grealy, 1994; Zola, 1982) and accounts written by relatives of people who have various debilitating or fatal conditions (Bayley, 1999; Neugeboren, 1997). What this tells us is that the experiences of injury, illness, treatment, birth, death, and not-so-everyday life give rise to multiple versions. There is no undisputed sole authority—only the collective experiences, recollections, sensations, and points of focus among the participants.

Culture, Health, and Illness

Demographers predict that between 2000 and 2050, white people of European descent will decline from 69.4% of the total population to 50.1% (U.S. Census, 2004). Soon thereafter whites will be a numerical minority again for the first time since the colonization of the North American continent. America will be an increasingly mixed society, with social identities and cultural backgrounds that are more accurately described as multiracial and multicultural. The social and cultural worlds of the 21st-century United States, its language, music, food, and political figures and forces, are profoundly different from just half a century ago when the idea of an "American culture," or a dominant white Anglo-Saxon tradition, was accepted by many as both accurate and desirable.

Members of a dominant culture are inclined to view their own ways as logical and natural, to see "culture" as something that others have. *We* have values or principles; *they* have beliefs and customs. *We* have science and knowledge; *they* have traditions and myths. Yet Western history, the social history of science and medicine, and the cultural study of health and illness challenge these dichotomies.

The United States has always been a culturally diverse society, home to Anglo-Saxon, Slavic, African, Asian, and Mediterranean groups with clear linguistic and cultural boundaries. Ethnicity and cultural diversity, which faded literally and figuratively from view for many decades, are now center stage in the politics, economy, social life and health care of the 21st-century United States. For example, Rayna Rapp (1993) demonstrates how the ethnic diversity of both the producers and receivers of biomedical information influences their responses to it: patients "have culture," but so do lab technicians, geneticists, and perinatologists. She shows how people from profoundly diverse cultural worlds come into contact during the laboratory procedure of amniocentesis and that the ways they determine, communicate, and receive the findings are not predictable with a deterministic, or stereotypic view of culture. The reemerging multicultural and ethnically diverse society of this century adds to the importance of understanding health, illness, and medical practice as both product and producer of larger social and cultural domains.

As much as change is anticipated and often lauded, each age and era develops a sense of inevitability about itself, about its ways and ideas. And so we have about ours, particularly in the ways that we regard knowledge in science and medicine as immutable. Yet illness and disease categories both lay and scientific, are, at base, cultural categories and as such change over time. For example, historian Michael MacDonald (1989) describes how in 16th- and early 17th-century England suicide shifted from a "heinous crime . . . a kind of murder committed at the instigation of the devil" to a secularized and medical condition. He argues that physicians had little to do with the evolution of concepts of suicide; rather, philosophers, laymen, and particularly coroners' juries led the way within a context of increasing secularization in other social realms.

Examining illness and disease categories as evolving cultural constructs

9

leads us to investigate how new diagnoses emerge, expand, or gain unprecedented prominence among the public or within medicine. For example, the development of Prozac and other psychotropic drugs offered the opportunity and demand for enhanced or elevated moods and increased happiness in life. The possibilities for increasing well-being courtesy of Prozac changed our view of sadness and melancholy as part of daily living. Familiar emotions, the blues, and distress have been redefined as diseases in order to "treat" them with this and other drugs. This process is called medicalization. The direct marketing of prescription drugs to consumers also influences what gets defined as pathological, problematic, and treatable. There are, for example, incessant media invitations to ease the heretofore "normal" aches and pains of aging by renaming them osteoarthritis—which can be controlled by a variety of drugs. A medical vocabulary replaces social terminology. A similar dynamic is apparent in the defining and redefining of so-called attention deficits and hyperactivity disorders, but this phenomenon occurs primarily in clinical and educational settings (Lakoff, 2000). Did school-age children have such disorders 40 years ago? Does the availability and widespread use of drugs to treat attention disorders influence their identification? What role might increased class size and a shortage of teachers in primary schools play in the definition of problem behaviors among students? Finally, the recent rise in interest in Asperger's syndrome, a cluster of behaviors and cognitive styles similar to autism but much less debilitating, is further illustrative of medicalization. There are increasing accounts of people who suddenly "recognize themselves" when reading about the disorder, having found a medical term for their social awkwardness, multiple rituals, intense focus on a particular topic, and inability to tolerate intimacy (Harmon, 2004).

The process of defining something heretofore unlabeled, or known by a secular term, as a disease or medical problem reflects ongoing ambiguity and disagreement about the role of will and personal responsibility in preventing dysfunction or maintaining health. Deeply rooted Western ideologies about independence, individualism, and mastery over nature also underlie many of the moral conflicts that arise in and from medicalization. The conflicting cultural logic is as follows: On the one hand, if a drug can treat or alleviate a problem, then it must be biologically based, and therefore not attributable to personal failure. On the other hand, many treatable, verified diseases and injuries may result from voluntary behaviors such as smoking, drinking, downhill skiing, or playing professional basketball.

The widely varied conceptions and representations of HIV/AIDS through-out its brief history also reveal the signature of culture, politics, and social forces. HIV/AIDS has evoked a mixture of moral, spiritual, virological, neu-rological, and social explanations. Paul Farmer's (1992) study of Haitian understandings of HIV/AIDS describes the centrality of blame and accusa-tion in American and Haitian views, constituting the "third epidemic"—worse than the disease. Accusations of sorcery arose in a Haitian village to account for the disease. The American public feared that the virus was introduced by infected Haitian immigrants. Haitians countered with con-spiratorial ideas about U.S. motivations to weaken or defame impover-ished black immigrants who would carry the affliction home. Fears of contagion and pollution by outsiders or malevolent others were shared by Americans and Haitians alike. Like homelessness and poverty, HIV/AIDS now infects more women and children of color than persons who are homosexual in the United States, yet HIV/AIDS bears the mark of sinfulness for some because of the first people who were infected.

In Africa, HIV/AIDS has always been a " 'heterosexual" disease, but be-cause of its spread by prostitutes, it has acquired yet another moral va-lence. In fact, the sensitivities associated with the main routes of HIV/AIDS transmission—risky sexual behaviors and the use of illegal drugs—coupled with the deadly nature of the disease, have created one of the most power-ful examples of stigma and discrimination in the history of human disease. Ominous diseases like HIV/AIDS provide both a window and a mirror into deeply held values, ideas about order, and about good and bad.

The reciprocal influence of cultural conceptions, social sentiment and policy, and medical practice is also well demonstrated by remarkable changes during the past three decades in the care and treatment of persons with severe physical and mental disabilities (Grob, 1991). Institutions for mentally retarded and mentally ill persons have been all but emptied, and even the most seriously impaired individuals now live and receive treat-ment in community settings. Several governors have publicly apologized to the thousands of mentally retarded people in their states who were sterilized without consent until the mid-1970s. These changes took place because of a confluence of forces: the development of effective drugs and treatment modalities, civil rights litigation and resulting rights to "least restrictive" treatment, the fiscal motivations of public mental health au-thorities, and self-advocacy and advocacy from relatives of severely dis-abled persons. People with disabilities now have a larger presence in the media, the workplace, and in the overall consciousness of society at large.

Just as important, clinical practice and the medical assessment of their abilities have changed dramatically as a result of changes brought about in part by social forces. Had these individuals remained confined in institutions, their capacities to work or to navigate public transportation systems, for example, might have remained undiscovered.

The efforts of advocates to alter public and scientific conceptions of problems like alcoholism and mental disorder do not always work the same cultural territory. For example, self-advocacy among persons with psychiatric diagnoses emphasizes their civil rights and defines themselves as a minority group that is subject to discrimination, for example, in the workplace. Activist relatives of individuals with psychiatric disorders like schizophrenia seek to normalize mental illness by medicalization, more precisely by locating these disorders in the brain. Promotional materials declare schizophrenia to be a "no-fault brain disease." Some advocates wish to replace the term mental illness with "neurobiological disorder" or NBD, and have succeeded in what for them was a vital symbolic move—the National Institutes of Mental Health were administratively joined with the National Institutes of Health. Recent public opinion research reveals that most Americans now view depression and schizophrenia as biologically based diseases, though there is much confusion about what kind of disease and what mechanisms are at work.

The Sick Role and Illness Behaviors

How people who are sick and those around them respond to illness and disease is part of a cultural code and social roles that are learned, often without noticing. The most enduring articulation of this perspective is sociologist Talcott Parsons's (1951) idea of the sick role. Parsons described expectations for people who are ill that are based on American values of responsibility, independence, and productivity. First, if the illness is severe enough, a person is excused from normal social role responsibilities. People are allowed to stay home from school or work if ill, for example. The second component of the sick role is that a person who is ill deserves to be taken care of, by either family or social institutions, in order to get well.

Third, people who are infirm are expected to consider illness as undesirable and are obligated to try to get well—to seek treatment, to change diet, quit smoking, or to follow doctor's orders. Violating this expectation— refusing treatment for drug addiction, for example—may lead to loss of the deserving-of-help status. In 1994 federal legislation was passed that strictly limited disability income support for people with substance abuse disorders and revoked the benefit for those who did not comply with treatment. In 1995 persons with substance abuse disorders were excluded from eligibility for disability benefits altogether. Here, the emphatic medicalization of addictions within biomedical practice did not influence public sentiment or policy regarding the moral status of addicted persons. Cultural ideas about responsibility and will overrode the medical mantle of deservedness via disease.

Similarly, exemption from responsibilities because of illness is hotly contested in the case of mental illness. In the realm of criminal law, "diminished capacity" and "not guilty by reason of insanity" are legal concepts that express the cultural exemption from full responsibility if a person is sick. Yet recent U.S. history is filled with controversial examples, from John Hinckley to Jeffrey Dahmer, that demonstrate clearly the social and cultural influences on this intersection of medical and legal concepts. Increasingly, states are replacing their "not guilty by reason of insanity" statutes with "guilty and mentally ill" legislation. This may represent a shift in basic cultural frameworks about illness and responsibility, and about the notion that punitive and therapeutic practices cannot be combined.

People who have other chronic and disabling conditions encounter difficulties when they "try to get well" but cannot. Their inabilities often become the object of intense scrutiny, for example, when they seek public assistance or require substantial resources to attend school, because of an underlying cultural formulation about legitimate need and deservedness. The formula derives from the sick role. Those who cannot get well or who need assistance because of medically determined pathologies are deemed deserving. When there is a possibility that lack of will is involved, that a person will not try to improve or become more productive, public benevolence is held in abeyance.

No matter what kind of healing system prevails, there are well-understood codes of conduct for "illness behaviors," another informative concept (Mechanic, 1962). Illness behaviors are those practices that accompany disease and dysfunction—from eating chicken soup to chanting all night to appease an offended spirit. Illness behaviors are learned, and although they change over time, American illness behaviors still reflect ancient humoral medicine principles of balance, of hot and cold, and wet and dry. Thus many Americans explain the onset of an upper respiratory

13

infection with a story of getting overtired, getting wet and cold, not eating enough—not keeping the balance—even though they understand the viral nature of most colds.

It is important to remember that while the reach of biomedicine is global, a minority of the world's population relies solely or even primarily on biomedical care or adheres to ancient Greek humoral beliefs about disease. Ayurvedic, traditional Chinese, and spiritist medical traditions— to name only the most prominent—are also used along with biomedicine by a large proportion of the world population. So-called alternative or complementary medicine, often consisting of techniques borrowed from these traditions, is increasingly popular among Americans. The repertoire of sick roles and resulting illness behaviors varies both within and across social and cultural groups, and will undoubtedly reflect the increasingly multicultural nature of the U.S. population.

Gender, Health, and Illness

Gender encompasses both sociocultural and biological processes. Gender differences in disease rates, the experiences of illness, medical treatment, and health outcomes are common in all cultures, but the specifics of those differences vary considerably. In developing nations, where the leading causes of sickness and death are infectious diseases like AIDS, tuberculosis, and malaria, striking gender differences are found in literacy, political rights, family roles, and economic resources, all of which are related to access to health services and to health outcomes (World Bank, 2004). Studies in the United States and other industrialized countries focus on why women report higher levels of illness and use health care services more frequently, even when reproduction-related conditions are excluded, while men seek health care less frequently, and often in later stages of disease (Gijsbers van Wijk et al., 1992; Lorber, 1995; Doyal, 2001). In developed nations, women live longer than men; and men have higher mortality rates for all major causes of death—heart disease, cancer, infectious and parasitic diseases, and accidents, poisonings, and violence (Waldron, 1990; Verbrugge and Wingard, 1987; Wingard et al., 1989).

Explanations for these gender differences in morbidity, mortality, and use of health care include biological, social, and cultural factors. The earlier onset of coronary heart disease for men, for example, is often attributed to the protective effect of estrogen in premenopausal women, and different complications for women are associated with later onset of the disease. Studies have also examined variation in individual behaviors such as smoking (Waldron, 1990), personality traits, different degrees of social connectedness (Kaplan et al., 1988; Lasker et al., 1994), and whether systematic biases in diagnosis, referral, and treatment might explain different health outcomes. In the case of heart disease, most studies of referral and treatment have shown that when potential confounders are taken into account, gender differences are not significant. On the other hand, Bickell and colleagues (1992) demonstrated that when admitted to hospitals with less serious heart disease or less certainty in recommended treatment regimen, women underwent fewer procedures. What is not clear, however, is whether they received less appropriate care or whether men were overtreated.

There is strong evidence that different rates of mortality and morbidity, and use of health care services, are related to cultural expectations about appropriate social roles for men and women (Horton, 1984; Lorber, 1995; Ratcliff, 2002). These social roles often dictate diet, smoking behavior, alcohol and drug use, and exposure to occupational and environmental hazards (Verbrugge and Wingard, 1987; Verbrugge, 1989; Waldron, 1990). Different socialization of men and women—particularly in the United States with its "rugged individualist" role model for young men—is associated with differences in risk-taking behaviors and integration into social networks, which has been shown to provide a buffer against illness (Berkman and Syme, 1978). Early childhood socialization also produces different illness behaviors. For example, going to the doctor may be a sign of weakness for many men, while for women, seeking help is more acceptable. Many of these factors combine to affect disease rates in complex and interesting ways; however it is also important not to oversimplify the relationship between gender and health, nor to stereotype gender roles and socialization processes, either within one society or in comparison to other sociocultural conceptions of gender.

Gender has traditionally been viewed as a basic social category, clearly determinable and obviously immutable. Yet the category of gender is increasingly fluid, challenged by an enlarging and energetic presence of various sexualities in the social and political landscape. People who consider themselves to be transgendered or transsexual do not fit conventional social categories of gender, nor have same-sex couples had access to traditional social institutions such as marriage and parenthood. Nonetheless, medical technology via assisted reproduction such as artificial insemination, and hormonal and surgical alteration of primary and secondary sex characteristics, has challenged these conventions and blurred the lines around gender. As ideas about and the enactment of gender continue to expand, this mainstay category will continue to be challenged (Fausto-Sterling, 1985). As the socialization of men and women changes over time, and as cultural conceptions of maleness and femaleness evolve and expand—compare the "metrosexual" male to the rugged cowboy—it will be important to determine whether there are accompanying shifts in health status and illness behaviors.

Social Factors and Inequality

Over time, different religions, cultures, and scientific and other academic disciplines have taken varying approaches to defining the causes of disease and examining why some people or groups tend to be burdened more than others (Rosenberg, 1962; Brandt, 1985; McKeown, 1976). Epidemiologists describe the frequency and distribution of disease in a population and focus on immediate risk factors that predict disease occurrence. The logic of this perspective is that the more closely related a risk factor is to the biological mechanism of disease, the more likely it is to account for the occurrence of that disease, and the more useful it will be in developing an effective intervention. Classic causal pairs include mosquito bites and malaria, walking barefoot in snail-infested waters and schistosomiasis, and living in close quarters with TB-infected people and tuberculosis. Some of the foundational work in epidemiology (Cassel, 1976) features the importance of cultural influences on such behaviors. In addition, epidemiological perspectives on chronic conditions involve more complex webs of explanatory factors than are required to explain infectious diseases (Kreiger, 1994). Nevertheless, the principal focus of epidemiology remains the immediate determinants of disease.

In contrast, sociologists and other social scientists focus on the structure and social processes of societies and find that rates of disease can be predicted by knowing the characteristics of a society's class structure (Townsend and Davidson, 1982; Navarro, 1990), its rate of social change (Durkheim, 1951; Cassel, 1976), and group characteristics within a society, such as race, ethnicity, gender, and age (Dressler, 1993; Kreiger and Bassett, 1993; Kreiger et al., 1993; Verbrugge, 1989; Waldron, 1990; Estes and Binney, 1989). Cultural influences are integrated into this view at both societal and individual levels. For more than a decade, scholars also have debated whether the degree of income inequality that characterizes a society as a whole exerts an independent effect on individual health out-comes, perhaps through increased social disruption or crime (Kawachi, Kennedy, and Wilkinson, 1999), though recent evidence has demonstrated no independent effect (Mackenbach, 2002).

In this broader view of disease causation, differential exposures to bio-logical risks are seen as determined by one's position in society, and dif-ferential responses to biological risks are affected by the overall social and economic environment, which in turn influences the health care environ-ment. As early as 1910, a local government board in England pronounced: "No fact is better established than that the death rate, and especially the death rate among children, is high in inverse proportion to the so-cial status of the population" (Antonovosky and Bernstein, 1977, p. 453). Numerous studies since then have confirmed the relationship between socioeconomic status and health outcomes, finding that every step up the social class ladder is accompanied by an incremental increase in health status as well (McKeown, 1976; Marmot et al., 1987; Kitagawa and Hauser, 1973; Pappas et al., 1993; Mechanic, 2000). As a result, social scientists increasingly define social conditions as "fundamental causes" of disease, observing that they persist in being linked to morbidity and mortality even as the actual diseases that people suffer change over time (Link and Phelan, 1995).

Scholars who focus on the role of inequality in health often adopt a case-based approach in their work. Paul Farmer's writing on HIV/AIDS in Haiti (1992) and infectious diseases in developing countries (1999) draws readers in through vivid personal illness stories and then moves to broader political critiques of global poverty and limited access to needed drugs. In her book *Mama Might Be Better Off Dead*, journalist Laurie Abraham (1993) chronicles the life histories of an inner-city African American fam-ily to demonstrate how individual outcomes are inextricably linked to family, neighborhood, community, and to inadequate government pro-grams. Similarly, Eric Klinenberg (2002) undertakes a "social autopsy" to explain the unprecedented death toll of 700 people in Chicago's 1995 heat wave, examining how the social isolation of the urban elderly combined with other place-specific risk factors like high crime levels and poor hous-ing to produce heightened vulnerability during the disaster. In the best of these accounts, individual experiences with disability and disease are de-fined on multiple levels, locating personal events within their broader social and cultural contexts.

Although debates about the nature and causes of illness and health may seem academic, there are real political consequences. Individuals are members of social classes, races, ethnicities, genders, and age groups, all of which entail differential risk of illness and mortality, and directly increase or decrease their chances of suffering illness or premature death. When differences in individual behavior are linked to these group characteristics and used to explain higher risks for morbidity and mortality, the tendency is to conclude that people have or get the health they deserve. Research that takes a broader approach, focusing on the structure of society and the health risks of living in poverty and of being a racial or ethnic minority in America, demonstrates that health is not solely the result of individual initiative or failure. Rather, it is also the product of society, and society's economic and cultural forces.

Special Problems of Race and Ethnicity in the United States

Because most health statistics in the United States are collected by race and ethnic group categories, much of the current debate about health inequalities has been framed by examination of disparities between different racial and ethnic groups. Yet just as the biological category of gender has been contested, the use of race and ethnic group categories in studies of health and illness has been the subject of ongoing controversy. The view of race as a biologically based and meaningful category has been challenged by social science critiques that recast race categories as fluid and socially constructed, varying across time and place as a function of historical circumstance, and created to establish and reinforce social hierarchies (American Anthropological Association, 1998; Lee et al., 2001). For example, Dressler (1993) argues that race as defined by skin color actually determines or defines one's social class position in America. Health differences between whites and minorities in the United States are thus seen as an expression of the pervasive health disadvantage that always accompanies being in the lower social classes, where a disproportionate number of minorities find themselves. It is not surprising, then, that medical researchers often think of those categories as shorthand terms or proxies for social class—despite contradictory findings such as the "Hispanic paradox" of better than predicted infant mortality rates for Hispanics than for other minority groups with similar income levels (Scriber, 1996).

At the same time, medical texts, clinical literature, and research routinely use race and ethnicity categories without definition or explanation, and when health differences are documented, race is often understood or implied as a biological rather than social or cultural variable (Schwartz, 2001). This is further complicated by the increasingly common application of race to genetic and pharmacogenomic research, reifying already problematic categories (Lee et al., 2001; Duster, 2003).

How, then, should race and ethnicity be defined and used? Much scholarship since the 1990s (LaVeist, 1994; LaVeist and Gibbons, 2001; Williams, 1999; van Ryn, 2002) has been devoted to identifying the sociocultural and biological factors that race and ethnicity do represent, and advocates that researchers adopt more specific measures in studies of health disparities. When factors such as individual lifestyle and behaviors, cultural beliefs, physiologic measures, geographical location, insurance coverage, education, and income are included in studies, the remaining health differences may be attributed to the effects of racial bias or discrimination (Cooper-Patrick et al., 1999; Jones, 2001). Research has shown that compared to whites, minorities perceive higher levels of racial discrimination in medical care and research settings and express greater mistrust of physicians and medical research (Corbie-Smith et al., 2002; Lillie-Blanton et al., 2000). Estimating how and to what extent bias and discrimination is implicated in health disparities outcomes is both challenging and complex. Increasingly, researchers are undertaking systematic studies of the doctor-patient encounter to delineate the nature and scope of intended and unintended bias (Roter and Hall, 1992; van Ryn, 2002).

The importance of this research is reinforced by a recent Institute of Medicine report, *Unequal Treatment: Confronting Racial and Ethnic Disparities in Healthcare* (Smedley, Stith, and Nelson, 2003), which found consistent evidence of disparities in health care in a remarkable range of illnesses and services, and demonstrated that when social and economic factors are accounted for, there are still significant health differences between minorities and whites. These differences occur in the context of broader historic and contemporary social and economic inequality and provide evidence of persistent racial and ethnic discrimination in many sectors of American life.

Conclusion

Health inequalities both reflect and reflect on the societies within which they exist. They may be seen as morally problematic; or they may be seen as unfortunate, but not necessarily unfair. Some identify inequality, itself, as a pathology (Kawachi, Kennedy, and Wilkinson 1999) or what Paul Farmer (1999) refers to as our "modern plague," and advocate greater economic equality as a pathway to improved health. Regardless of the moral stance one takes about health inequality, it is likely to be a focus of ongoing attention in the near future, both in the United States and worldwide.

Global health inequalities between wealthy countries and resource-poor nations have long been seen as unchangeable facts of life. Spurred by recent controversies in the field of HIV/AIDS, however, this view has begun to change. The enormous disparities created by the HIV/AIDS epidemic in sub-Saharan Africa, where life expectancy in some nations is less than 40, has generated pressure for higher standards of justice, in the form of new international funding sources and reduced prices for needed drugs (De Cock and Janssen, 2002; Farmer, 1999). Recent debates over the ethical conduct of clinical research in international HIV/AIDS trials have also contributed to this perspective shift: research in the context of extreme poverty and lack of access to life-saving drugs came to be seen as potentially exploitative (Benatar, 2001, 2002; participants in the 2001 Conference on Ethical Aspects of Research in Developing Countries, 2002; Arras, 2004). The SARS epidemic in 2003 provided further momentum for the emerging view of an interdependent global population. Together, HIV/AIDS and SARS have demonstrated how connected and vulnerable the world's people are when confronted with a deadly infectious pathogen.

While progress has been made in advocating for global justice in the context of HIV/AIDS, there are many areas in which health and health care inequalities remain unchallenged. The global trade in transplantable organs is one example (Rothman, 2002). Currently, the flow of transplant organs is overwhelmingly from impoverished donors to wealthy recipients, and from developing to developed countries (Scheper-Hughes, 2000). While some view organs as private property and therefore marketable, most analysts observe that informed, voluntary donating or selling is questionable in circumstances of economic deprivation (Goyal et al., 2002). Until the underlying inequalities are reduced, however, such activities are unlikely to be restricted.

Here at home, the contradictions between the American ethic of equality and the substantial and growing inequities in access to health insurance and health care also await resolution. (See *Health Policy, Medicine and Markets*, volume III of *The Social Medicine Reader*, for extensive treatment of these issues.) Social science critiques focus on individual

experiences of difference and disability, and social conditions that underlie disparate health outcomes for population groups. But researchers and
their approaches to science are also situated in the same societies that
produce the inequalities, and as we have argued, sometimes reproduce
these same inequalities. For example, anthropology developed and flourished in the era of social Darwinism, and initially promoted a hierarchical
view of cultures—from primitive to civilized. Often based on measurement of brain size, the dogma of that period reified and reinforced the
position of Western cultures at the evolutionary apex (Gould, 1996). Similarly, but much more recently, some practitioners of sociobiology have
returned to the theme of inherent difference in cognitive ability and capacity based on race (Jensen, 2000; Wilson, 2000).

The view that science is morally neutral and should be free of political
constraint is challenged by other deeply held, if sometimes contested,
beliefs about privacy, autonomy, and the sanctity of life. New possibilities
to make choices about life and death, and about altering bodies, come at
a rapid pace courtesy of medical technologies. Each innovation spawns
more possibilities, and often as much controversy. Then the social fabric
and cultural frameworks among us serve as reference points. Yet they
shift because we do. Can social arrangements and cultural conceptions
keep pace with medical science and practice?

Recent developments in genetics and the Human Genome Project (HGP)
illustrate this question. Originally, the HGP promoted the "sameness" of
human beings, emphasizing that we all share 99.9% percent of the same
sequences of DNA. However, geneticists have now turned to investigations of "difference," relying upon roadmaps within the human genome to
identify patterns of genetic variation linked to common diseases. As Troy
Duster observed, "Suddenly the realization of a considerable amount of
differentiation between individuals is the new perspective—and lurking
in the corridors of computer-generated correlations and patterns, there
will be the inevitable shift to a concern for differences between population groups" (2003, p. 147). The renewed legitimacy of assessing individual and group difference, particularly regarding genetically linked risk and
vulnerability, raises additional concerns when this genetic variation is
linked to race groups (Duster 2003, p. 148; Lee et al., 2001). What impact
will these new scientific and technological forces have on the contested
category of race? How can we avoid reinforcing a prior ideology about
human difference and avert the use of science and medicine to divide,
rank and control people? (American Anthropological Association, 1998,

pp. 2–3). Will countervailing science and a new willingness to confront the broader, societal sources of health disparities in the U.S. (Smedley, Stith, and Nelson, 2003) construct a new dialog about race?

The relationships between medicine and society have created, and will continue to create, intellectual and moral challenges that require physicians, patients, and medical, social science, and humanities scholars whose understandings and training are both broad and deep. Continued improvement of the health of individuals, groups, and nations rests in large part on multidisciplinary, multidimensional research and practice. One of the best allies we have in facing the perils and enticements ahead is the ability to view medicine in society, and society in medicine, and to continually reflect critically on the meaning of both.

References

Abraham, L. K. 1993. *Mama Might Be Better Off Dead: The Failure of Health Care in America.* Chicago: University of Chicago Press.

American Anthropological Association. 1998. Statement on "Race." From *http://www.aaanet. org/stmts/racepp.htm.*

Antonovsky, A., and Bernstein, J. 1977. Social class and infant mortality. *Social Science and Medicine 11,* 453–470.

Arras, J. D. 2004. Fair benefits in international medical research. *Hastings Center Report 343,* 3.

Bayley, J. 1999. *Elegy for Iris.* New York: Picador USA.

Benatar, S. R. 2001. Commentary: justice and medical research: A global perspective. *Bioethics 154,* 333–340.

———. 2002. Reflections and recommendations on research ethics in developing countries. *Social Science and Medicine 547,* 1131–1141.

Berkman, L. F., and Syme, S. L. 1979. Social networks, host resistance, and mortality: A nine-year follow-up study of Alameda County residents. *American Journal of Epidemiology 109,* 186–204.

Bickell, N., et al. 1992. Referral patterns for coronary artery disease treatment: Gender bias or good clinical judgment? *Annals of Internal Medicine 116,* 791–797.

Brandt, A. 1985. *No Magic Bullet: A Social History of Venereal Disease in the United States since 1800.* Oxford: Oxford University Press.

Cassel, J. 1976. The contribution of the social environment to host resistance: The fourth Wade Hampton Frost lecture. *American Journal of Epidemiology 104,* 107–123.

Charmaz, K. 1991. Good days, bad days: The self in chronic illness and time. New Brunswick, NJ: Rutgers University Press.

Charon, R. 2004. Narrative and medicine. *New England Journal of Medicine 3509,* 862–864.

Comaroff, J. L., and Comaroff, J. 2004. Criminal justice, cultural justice: The limits of liberalism and the pragmatics of difference in the new South Africa. *American Ethnologist 313,* 188–204.

Cooper-Patrick, L., Gallo J. J., Gonzales J. J., Vu, H. T., Powe, N. R., Nelson, C., and Ford, D. E. 1999. Race, gender, and partnership in the patient-physician relationship. *Journal of the American Medical Association 2826*, 583–589.

Corbie-Smith, G., Thomas, S. B., and George, D. M. 2002. Distrust, race, and research. *Archives of Internal Medicine 16221*, 2458–2463.

De Cock, K. M., and Janssen, R. S. 2002. An unequal epidemic in an unequal world. *Journal of the American Medical Association 2882*, 236–238.

Decker, H. S. 1998. Freud's Dora. *Journal of the History of the Behavioral Sciences 342*: 213–215.

Doyal, L. 2001. Sex, gender, and health. *British Medical Journal 323*, 34–38.

Dressler, W. W. 1993. Health in the African American community: Accounting for health inequalities. *Medical Anthropology Quarterly 7*, 325–345.

Durkheim, E. 1951. *Suicide: A Study in Sociology*, J. A. Spaulding and G. Simpson, trans. Glencoe, IL.: Free Press.

Duster, T. 2003. *Backdoor to Eugenics*, 2nd ed. New York: Routledge.

Espeland, M. A., et al., for the Women's Health Initiative Memory Study. 2004. Conjugated equine estrogens and global cognitive function in postmenopausal women: Women's Health Initiative Memory Study. *Journal of the American Medical Association 291*, 2959–2968.

Estes, C. L., and Binney, E. A. 1989. The biomedicalization of aging: Dangers and dilemmas. *The Gerontologist 29*, 587–596.

Fabrega, H. 1974. *Disease and Social Behavior*. Cambridge, MA: MIT Press.

Fadiman, A. 1997. *The Spirit Catches You and You Fall Down: A Hmong Child, Her American Doctors, and the Collision of Two Cultures*. New York: Farrar, Straus and Giroux.

Farmer, P. 1992. *AIDS and Accusation*. Berkeley: University of California Press.

——. 1999. *Infections and Inequalities: The Modern Plagues*. Berkeley: University of California Press.

Fausto-Sterling, A. 1985. *Myths of Gender: Biological Theories about Women and Men*. New York: Basic Books.

Frank, G. 2000. *Venus on wheels: Two decades of dialogue on disability, biography, and being female in America*. Berkeley: University of California Press.

Gawande, A. 2002. *Complications: A Surgeon's Notes on an Imperfect Science*. New York: Metropolitan Books.

Gijsbers van Wijk, C. M. T., et al. 1992. Male and female morbidity in general practice: The nature of sex differences. *Social Science and Medicine 35*, 665–678.

Gould, S. J. 1996. *The Mismeasure of Man*. New York: Norton.

Goyal, M., Mehta, R. L., Schneiderman, L. J., and Sehgal, A. R. 2002. Economic and health consequences of selling a kidney in India. *Journal of the American Medical Association 28813*, 1589–1593.

Grealy, L. 1994. *Autobiography of a Face*. New York: Houghton Mifflin.

Grob, G. N. 1991. *From Asylum to Community: Mental Health Policy in America*. Princeton, NJ: Princeton University Press.

Groopman, J. E. 2000. *Second Opinions: Stories of Intuition and Choice in the Changing World of Medicine*. New York: Viking Press.

Harmon, A. 2004. Finding out: Adults and autism. *New York Times*, April 29, 2004, p. A1.

Hawkins, A. H. 1993. *Reconstructing Illness: Studies in Pathography*. West Lafayette, IN: Purdue University Press.

Horton, C. F. 1984. Women have headaches, men have backaches: Patterns of illness in an Appalachian community. *Social Science and Medicine 19*, 647–654.

James, S. 1994. John Henryism and the health of African-Americans. *Culture, Medicine, and Psychiatry 18*, 163–182.

Jensen, A. 2000. *Intelligence, Race, and Genetics.* New York: Westview.

Jones, C. P. 2001. Invited commentary: "Race," racism, and the practice of epidemiology. *American Journal of Epidemiology 1544*, 299–304.

Kaplan, G. A., et al. 1988. Social connections and mortality from all causes and from cardiovascular disease: Prospective evidence from Eastern Finland. *American Journal of Epidemiology 128*, 370–380.

Kawachi, I., Kennedy, B. P., and Wilkinson, R. G., eds. 1999. *The Society and Population Health Reader*, vol. 1, *Income Inequality and Health.* New York: New Press.

Kitagawa, E. M., and Hauser, P. M. 1973. *Differential Mortality in the United States: A Study in Socioeconomic Epidemiology.* Cambridge, MA: Harvard University Press.

Kleinman, A. 1988. *The Illness Narratives.* New York: Free Press.

Kleinman, A., Eisenberg, L., and Good, B. 1978. Culture, illness, and care: Clinical lessons from anthropologic and cross-cultural research. *Annals of Internal Medicine 88*, 83–93.

Klinenberg, E. 2002. *Heat Wave: A Social Autopsy of Disaster in Chicago.* Chicago: University of Chicago Press.

Kreiger, N. 1994. Epidemiology and the web of causation: Has anyone seen the spider? *Social Science and Medicine 39*, 887–903.

Kreiger, N., and Bassett, M. 1993. The health of black folk: Disease, class and ideology in science. In S. Harding, ed., *The "Racial" Economy of Science: Toward a Democratic Future.* Bloomington: University of Indiana Press.

Kreiger, N., et al. 1993. Racism, sexism, and social class: Implications for the study of health, disease, and well-being. *American Journal of Preventive Medicine 9* Suppl. 2, 81–122.

Lakoff, A. 2000. Adaptive will: The evolution of attention deficit disorder. *Journal of the History of the Behavioral Sciences 362*, 149–169.

Lasker, J. N., Egolf, B. P., and Wolf, S. 1994. Community social change and mortality. *Social Science and Medicine 39*, 53–62.

LaVeist, T. A. 1994. Beyond dummy variables and sample selection: What health services researchers ought to know about race as a variable. *Health Services Research 1*, 1–16.

LaVeist, T. A., and Gibbons, M. C. 2001. Measuring racial and ethnic discrimination in the U.S. health care setting: A review of the literature and suggestions for a monitoring program. Final report to U.S. DHHS, April 12, 2001.

Lee, S. S., Mountain, J., and Koenig, B. A. 2001. The meanings of 'race' in the new genomics: Implications for health disparities research. *Yale Journal of Health Policy, Law, and Ethics 12*, 15:33–75.

Liebow, E. 1993. *Tell Them Who I Am.* New York: Free Press.

Lillie-Blanton, M., Brodie, M., Roland, D., Altman, D., and McIntosh, M. 2000. Race, ethnicity, and the health care system: Public perceptions and experiences. *Medical Care Research Review 57* Suppl. 1, 218–235.

Link, B., and Phelan, J. 1995. Social conditions as a fundamental cause of disease. *Journal of Health and Social Behavior* Extra Issue, 80–94.

Lock, M. 1994. *Encounters with Aging.* Berkeley: University of California Press.

Lorber, J. 1995. *Gender and the Social Construction of Illness.* New York: AltaMira Press.

MacDonald, M. 1989. The medicalization of suicide in England: Laymen, physicians, and cultural change, 1500–1870. *Milbank Quarterly 67* Suppl. 1, 69–91.

Macintyre, S., Hunt, K., and Sweeting, H. 1996. Gender differences in health: Are things really as simple as they seem? *Social Science and Medicine 42* 4, 617–624.

Mackenbach, J. P. 2002. Income inequality and population health. *British Medical Journal 324*, 1–2.

Mairs, N. 1996. *Waist High in the World.* Boston: Beacon Press.

Marmot, M. G., Kogevinas, M., and Elston, M. A. 1987. Social/economic status and disease. *Annual Reviews of Public Health 8*, 111–135.

McKeown, T. R. 1976. *The Role of Medicine: Dream, Mirage, or Nemesis.* London: Nuffield Provincial Hospitals Trust.

Mechanic, D. 1962. The concept of illness behavior. *Journal of Chronic Disease 15*, 189–195.

——. 2000. Rediscovering the social determinants of health. *Health Affairs* May–June 2000, 269–276.

Mosely, W. H., and Chen, L. C. 1984. An analytical framework for the study of child survival in developing countries. In Mosely and Chen, eds., *Child Survival: Strategies for Research.* Cambridge: Cambridge University Press.

Navarro, V. 1990. Race or class versus race and class: Mortality differentials in the United States. *The Lancet 336*, 1238–1240.

Neugeboren, J. 1997. *Imagining Robert: My Brother, Madness, and Survival.* New York: William Morrow.

Pappas, G., et al. 1993. The increasing disparity in mortality between socioeconomic groups in the United States, 1960 and 1986. *New England Journal of Medicine 329*, 103–109.

Parsons, T. 1951. *The Social System.* New York: Free Press.

Participants in the 2001 Conference on Ethical Aspects of Research in Developing Countries. 2002. Fair benefits for research in developing countries. *Science 298*, 2133–2134.

Quill, T. E. 1991. Death and dignity: A case of individual decision making. *New England Journal of Medicine 32410*, 691–694.

Rapp, Rayna. 1993. Accounting for amniocentesis. In *Knowledge, Power, Practice.* In S. Lindenbaum and M. Locke, eds. Berkeley: University of California Press.

Ratcliff, K. S. 2002. *Women and Health: Power, Technology, Inequality, and Conflict in a Gendered World.* Boston: Allyn and Bacon.

Rosenberg, C. 1962. *The Cholera Years: The United States in 1832, 1849, and 1866.* Chicago: University of Chicago Press.

Roter, D. L., and Hall, J. A. 1992. *Doctors Talking with Patients, Patients Talking with Doctors: Improving Communication in Medical Visits.* Westport, CT: Auburn House.

Rothman, D. J. 2002. Ethical and social consequences of selling a kidney. *Journal of the American Medical Association 28813*, 1640–1641.

Rothman, S., and Rothman, D. 2003. *The Pursuit of Perfection.* New York: Pantheon Books.

Scheper-Hughes, N. 2000. The global traffic in human organs. *Current Anthropology 41*, 192–224.

Schwartz, R. S. 2001. Racial profiling in medical research. *New England Journal of Medicine 344*, no. 18, 1392–1393.

Scriber, R. 1996. Paradox as paradigm—The health outcomes of Mexican Americans. *American Journal of Public Health 86*, 303–304.

Shamp, J. 2004. Study: Estrogen pills may cause dementia. *Durham Herald-Sun* June 23, 2004, p. A2.

Smedley, B. D., Stith, A. Y., and Nelson, A. R., eds., Committee on Understanding and Eliminating Racial and Ethnic Disparities in Health Care; Board on Health Sciences Policy, Institute of Medicine. 2003. *Unequal Treatment: Confronting Racial and Ethnic Disparities in Healthcare.* Washington, DC: National Academies Press.

Styron, W. 1990. *Darkness Visible: A Memoir of Madness.* New York: Random House.

Taussig, M. 1980. Reification and the consciousness of the patient. *Social Science and Medicine 14 B,* 3–13.

Townsend, P., and Davidson, N. 1982. *Inequalities in Health: The Black Report.* New York: Penguin Books.

U.S. Census Bureau. 2004. U.S. interim projections by age, sex, and Hispanic origin. Retrieved from http://www.census.gov/ipc/www/uninterimproj/, on March 18, 2004.

van Ryn, M. 2002. Research on the provider contribution to race/ethnicity disparities in medical care. *Medical Care 40* Suppl. 1, I-140–I-151.

Verbrugge, L. M. 1989. The twain meet: Empirical explanations of sex differences and mortality. *Journal of Health and Social Behavior 30,* 282–304.

Verbrugge, L. M., and Wingard, D. L. 1987. Sex differentials in health and mortality. *Women and Health 12,* 103–146.

Waldron, I. 1990. What do we know about causes of sex differences in mortality? A review of the literature. In P. Conrad and R. Kern, eds., *The Sociology of Health and Illness.* New York: St. Martin's Press.

Wingard, D. L., et al. 1989. Sex differentials in morbidity and mortality risks examined by age and cause in the same cohort. *American Journal of Epidemiology 130,* 601–605.

Williams, D. R. 1999. Race, socioeconomic status, and health: The added effects of racism and discrimination. *Annals of the New York Academy of Sciences 896,* 173–188.

Williams, W. C. 1936. *The Doctor Stories.* New York: New Directions.

Wilson, E. O. 2000. *Sociobiology: The New Synthesis.* 25th anniversary ed. Cambridge, MA: Belknap Press of Harvard University Press.

World Bank 2004. Gendernet. Cite on gender and health. Retrieved from http://www.world bank.org/gender/new on June 19, 2004.

Young, A. 1982. The anthropology of sickness and illness. *Annual Review of Anthropology 11,* 257–285.

———. 1995. *The Harmony of Illusions.* Princeton, NJ: Princeton University Press.

Zola, I. K. 1982. *Missing Pieces: A Chronicle of Living with a Disability.* Philadelphia: Temple University Press.

PART I

Defining and Experiencing Difference

Defining the Defective: Eugenics, Aesthetics, and Mass Culture in Early 20th-Century America
Martin S. Pernick

From 1915 to 1918 Chicago surgeon Harry Haiselden electrified the nation by allowing the deaths of at least six infants he diagnosed as "defectives."[1] Seeking publicity for his efforts to eliminate those he considered "unfit," he displayed the dying infants to journalists and wrote a book-length series about them for the Hearst newspapers. His campaign was front-page news for weeks at a time.[2] He also wrote and starred in a feature motion picture, *The Black Stork*, a fictionalized account of his cases.[3]

In the unprecedented debate prompted by Haiselden's actions, hundreds of Americans took a public stand. A majority of those quoted in the press *opposed* preserving the lives of "defectives." They included public health nurse Lillian Wald, family law pioneer Judge Ben Lindsey, civil rights lawyer Clarence Darrow, historian Charles A. Beard,[4] even the blind and deaf reformer Helen Keller.[5]

Yet despite these dramatic events, media coverage of the issue faded rapidly during the 1920s. By the time similar proposals surfaced again in the mid-1930s, Haiselden and his actions appeared to have been almost totally forgotten.[6]

This story is important, not just for its novelty and drama but because it vividly demonstrates the crucial though little-recognized role played by mass culture in constructing both the meanings and the memory of the early 20th-century movement for hereditary improvement known as "eugenics." (The term "mass culture" includes any productions made for a mass audience, whether or not they were demonstrably "popular" in origin.)

Martin S. Pernick, "Defining the Defective: Eugenics, Aesthetics, and Mass Culture in Early 20th-Century America," from *The Body and Physical Differences: Discourses of Disability*, ed. David T. Mitchell and Sharon L. Snyder, 89–110. © 1997 by University of Michigan Press. Reprinted by permission of the publisher.

Eugenics leaders frequently attacked mass culture for what they considered its vulgar distortion of scientific ideas. The Yale professor Irving Fisher complained, "Eugenics is one of the few cases in which a scientific term has come into popular use, but it is subject to a great deal of misconception."[7]

Historians of eugenics focus on the movement's professional leadership, and many have implicitly adopted the leaders' views of mass culture. But I will argue that such an approach misses the vital role of mass culture as a battleground on which scientists, physicians, popularizers, journalists, censors, and audiences struggle to shape the meanings of "eugenics" and "heredity."[8]

The passage of time makes it easier to see the aesthetic, epistemological, and ethical values inherent in early 20th-century eugenics. But that should not be taken to mean that eugenics was either *uniquely* value laden or peculiarly influenced by mass culture. Nor am I arguing that mass culture corrupted "pure" genetic science by infecting it with "extraneous" aesthetic and moral concerns. Rather, I believe the history of eugenics is valuable because it makes so dramatically visible the cultural value judgments that are inevitably part of defining any human difference as a disease or a disability and identifying any specific factors as "the" cause.[9]

The role of aesthetic judgments in the definition of disease and disability is still a highly controversial issue today. Should laws protecting the disabled against discrimination apply to those who are simply judged unattractive? Should health insurance cover "cosmetic" surgery?[10] Do aesthetic values create disability in the same way that high stairs and other physical barriers do? Could changing such values create a more accessible culture? I believe that the history of eugenics shows the futility of trying to answer such questions by seeking a sharp line between "objective" physical diseases and "subjective" values. Any time a culture defines disease or causation, it is making a partly subjective, value-based judgment. Greater awareness of the inevitability of the value-based component of these debates might or might not help in reaching more satisfactory decisions. But pretending that such decisions can ever be made without values only delegitimates and prevents the necessary critical analysis of the implicit values at stake.

The American eugenics movement supported a very diverse range of activities, including advanced statistical analyses of human pedigrees, "better baby contests" modeled on rural livestock shows, compulsory sterilization of criminals and the retarded, and selective ethnic restrictions on immigration.[11] These efforts all were seen as "eugenic" because they all aimed at "improving human heredity." But the meanings of eugenics also depended on the answers to at least four related but separate and distinct questions.

1. What does "improvement" mean?
2. What does "heredity" mean?
3. By what methods should heredity be improved?
4. Who has the authority to answer questions 1–3?

This essay examines the role of mass culture in defining eugenics by providing one illustrative example of how that culture served as a battleground for competing answers to each of these key questions. In the first section, mass culture's representations of beauty and ugliness illustrate the construction of what counted as "improvement." The second example explores why in mass culture the meaning of "heredity" was not limited to traits caused by genes. The final section traces the debate over whether eugenic methods included death for those judged defective, and the ironic role of the mass media in creating a professional monopoly over such decisions.

In its heyday during the 1910s and 1920s, eugenics was widely accepted as being an objective science, and when I use words like "defective" and "unfit," I am quoting what eugenicists believed to be purely technical terms. But while eugenics claimed to be purely objective, this essay will show that subjective values, such as aesthetic standards of beauty and ugliness and moral attributions of responsibility, were central to eugenic constructions of hereditary disease and disability.

What Traits Are Good? Eugenics and Aesthetics

Aesthetic values played a critical though little-known role in eugenic constructions of fitness and defectiveness. Eugenics promised to make humanity not just strong and smart but beautiful as well.

Efforts by leading scientists to explain the evolutionary role of beauty began in 1871 with Darwin's analysis of sex selection in *The Descent of Man*. Darwin's cousin Francis Galton, who coined the term "eugenics," began his scientific career by compiling a "beauty map" of Britain, for which he calculated the ratio of attractive to plain and ugly women he encountered at various locations.[12]

But while these and other evolutionary scientists studied the aesthetic component of eugenic "fitness," aesthetic concerns appeared more frequently in the mass media.[13] One major eugenic popularizer, Albert Wiggam, saw an attractive appearance as the *best* external indicator of overall hereditary fitness. He regarded health, intellect, morality, and beauty as "different phases of the same inner . . . forces." "Good-looking people are better morally, on the average, than ugly people." Thus he concluded, "If men and women should select mates solely for beauty, it would increase all the other good qualities of the race." In the most extreme version of this view, aesthetic preferences were simply Nature's instinctive guide to finding the fittest mate, a view both Wiggam and Haiselden sometimes explicitly endorsed.[14]

But both eugenics leaders and popularizers were skeptical that truly healthy beauty could be recognized by the untrained eye. Scientists since Darwin found beauty problematic precisely because aesthetic preferences in choosing a mate often did *not* seem to favor other adaptive traits.[15] Thus eugenicists did not simply endorse existing cultural preferences but actively attempted to "improve" current standards. Fisher explained that careful propaganda was needed to "unconsciously favorably modif[y] the individual taste . . . in mate-choosing." Wiggam agreed: "If their ideals of human beauty are properly *trained*," young people will "unconsciously reject the ugly" and will "fill their homes with beautiful wives and handsome husbands."[16]

To illustrate the content of this aesthetic propaganda, I will focus on the only two surviving proeugenic full-length American motion pictures of the 1910s and 1920s: *The Black Stork*, a feature film that dramatized Dr. Haiselden's crusade against saving impaired newborns, and the pioneering government-produced health education series *The Science of Life*, a twelve-reel survey of high school biology, distributed by the U.S. Public Health Service from 1922 to 1937.[17] In *The Black Stork*, Claude, who has an unnamed inherited disease, ignores graphic warnings from his doctor, played by Haiselden, and marries Anne. Their baby is born "defective" and needs immediate surgery to save its life, but the doctor refuses to operate. After God provides a horrific vision of the child's future of misery and crime, Anne agrees to withhold treatment, and the baby's soul leaps into the arms of a waiting Jesus.

Both films equated beauty with fitness. "An attractive appearance goes hand in hand with health," explained *The Science of Life*.[18] And both attempted to influence audience concepts of beauty. But each presented internally conflicting aesthetic standards, an ambivalent mix of modernism and romanticism.

The Science of Life emphasized stark mechanical images. It urged "The Woman of Tomorrow" to develop strength and beauty through vigorous exercises, demonstrated by a short-haired woman whose hard, flat body was accentuated by stark black tights and knee-level photography. An attractive body also was explicitly equated with a sleek, streamlined locomotive, whose beauty became manifest in powerful motion and efficient function. Photographed in a low-angle tilt shot that swept upward from wheel level, the engine's sharp clean lines and powerful mass appeared starkly silhouetted against the sky. Motion pictures first made it possible to display the beauty of bodily action. The desire to depict the poetry and science of motion contributed to the development of cinema, while the use of film helped reshape modern beauty in terms of physiology, not anatomy, as active function, not just static form.[19]

But *The Science of Life* also promoted older romantic concepts of beauty. Intercut with the starkly modern images were scenes in which health and fitness were represented by a long-haired, round-cheeked, young woman in calm repose, photographed in gauzy soft focus as glowing with cleanliness and natural sunlight.[20]

The Black Stork emphasized the more naturalistic modernism of Thomas Eakins. Beauty was illustrated by athletic adolescents in outdoor settings: five naked boys diving into a swimming hole, a woman in a swimsuit doing handstands on the beach. The 1916 edition of *The Black Stork* explicitly *attacked* mechanical standards of beauty, using a speeding motorcar to represent not modern aesthetics but the false allure of the "fast" life. Yet, when the film was rereleased in 1927, industrial modernism dominated. The sequence linking fast cars to loose living was deleted, while lengthy new scenes portrayed beauty as a massive new automobile, owned by a "professor of heredity."

This ambivalent aesthetic vision exemplified what Thomas Mann called "a highly technological romanticism." Eugenics promised to create a romantic utopia by means of modern science, and its aesthetic propaganda reflected this uneasy mix of goals.[21]

If eugenics equated fitness with beauty, it labeled ugliness a disability. "It was terribly ugly," Haiselden wrote of one baby. Such ugliness was not "light or superficial"; it was a true "handicap."[22] Both films selectively highlighted the repulsive ugliness of the "unfit," as in several scenes comparing them to cattle.[23] Again echoing Thomas Eakins, Haiselden described the case on which *The Black Stork* was based as "not a pretty one. It mars the pages of this book—as I intended it should mar them. It is better that the deformities of this tiny castaway should sear themselves into the minds of thinking men."[24]

Eugenics popularizers promoted definitions of ugliness that reinforced their judgments on other human differences, including gender, class, race, and nationality. Wiggam lamented: "We want ugly women in America and we are getting them in millions. . . . [T]hree or four shiploads have been landing at Ellis Island every week. . . . I have studied thousands of them. . . . They are broad-hipped, short, stout-legged with big feet; . . . flat-chested . . . and with faces expressionless and devoid of beauty. These 'draft horses' were rapidly replacing 'the beautiful women of the old American stocks, the Daughters of the Revolution.' "[25]

Both films linked aesthetics, disability, and race. The only identifiable blacks in each were photographed as repulsive defectives, and Haiselden repeatedly linked "blackness" with "ugliness."[26] Like race, economics also shaped the aesthetic distinctions between the fit and the defective. *The Science of Life* promised that both "health and success" awaited the visually attractive, and in both films, couples who illustrate "wise mating" wear tastefully conservative but up-to-date business suits and dresses on their prosperously stout bodies. Portraying "others" as ugly was central to labeling them defective, while diagnosing "others" as diseased reinforced the perception of them as repulsive.

Eugenicists insisted that their diagnoses were based entirely on objective science. Even Helen Keller, the famed reformer who had become blind and deaf in childhood, believed that objective science could determine which mentally impaired infants should be eliminated. "A jury of physicians considering the case of an idiot would be exact and scientific. Their findings would be free from the prejudice and inaccuracy of untrained observation."[27]

Many eugenicists admitted that the distinction between "fit" and "defective" relied on aesthetic values, yet they denied that such classifications were therefore subjective or unscientific. They did not claim to be "value-free" but rather that their aesthetic values had been validated by objective scientific methods.[28]

Eugenic aesthetic judgments were based on broad cultural values that were not unique to eugenicists. But eugenics did not simply reflect cultural values indiscriminately. The movement's technocratic utopianism attracted mostly middle-class, native born segments of the population who brought with them a specific set of values shared with others of their background, including their ambivalent romantic-modern aesthetic, and these selected preferences in turn shaped eugenic representations of beauty and ugliness.

Thus, eugenics popularizers promised to make people more attractive while they intervened in mass culture to selectively enhance the attractiveness of what they considered beautiful. They offered to eliminate ugliness while depicting as ugly everything they wished to eliminate. Their media efforts reveal the internal tensions and circular logic that characterized their constructions of the "fit" and the "defective."

These contradictions were heightened by the ease with which viewers found alternative meanings in such propaganda. For example, many reviewers of *The Black Stork* reported that the film's exhibition of deformed bodies evoked pity, or even fascination, rather than disgust. Disregarding the titles that labeled Claude and Anne's son an "abyss of abnormality" filled with "criminal desires," critics consistently praised the actor for making this character appealing, even noble.[29]

Others found that scenes intended to make disabled people look repulsive instead made the film itself "repellent" and "revolting." These critics often praised the film's educational and social value, but they found it aesthetically unacceptable: "grim," "depressing and unpleasant,"[30] "repulsive."[31] Louella Parsons complained that it was "neither a pretty nor a pleasant picture," because "it shows poor, misshapen bodies of miserable little children." Rival critic Kitty Kelly called it the "most repellent picture" she had ever seen.[32] Such reviewers concluded that anyone who wanted to see such films must be sick, suffering from a "morbid" perversion of the aesthetic senses.[33]

These unintended aesthetic responses were one important reason why films about eugenics were often banned.[34] Film censors went far beyond policing sexual morality, to include what I term "aesthetic censorship," much of which was aimed at eliminating unpleasant medical topics from entertainment films.[35] From the perspective of such aesthetic censors, both pro- and antieugenics films were unacceptably ugly. The powerful New York state film board banned both *The Black Stork* and *Tomorrow's Children*, a 1934 antieugenic melodrama, because eugenics was too "disgusting" a topic. They rejected *The Black Stork* in April 1923, not only for its "inhuman" position on euthanasia but for its "most unpleasant," "very distressing," "most revolting" depictions of disease. About *Tomorrow's Children* they concluded, "The sterilization of human beings is not a decent subject for public entertainment."[36]

Film censors shared the eugenicists' desire to pathologize and eradicate ugliness. They sought to ban the cinematic reproduction of ugly people, while eugenicists sought to ban their biological reproduction. But while eugenic publicists believed filming ugliness could help inoculate audiences against it, the censors feared that displaying ugly diseases would disseminate them, creating ugly-minded, diseased audiences. The attempt to make the disabled look ugly made eugenics seem repulsive as well.

What Is Heredity? Eugenics and Moral Responsibility

Between the 1880s and 1910s, scientific concepts of heredity changed dramatically. The 19th-century "Lamarckian" view that environmentally caused changes in individuals could be passed on to their offspring was gradually supplanted by August Weismann's doctrine that individual heredity was permanent and unaffected by environmental forces.[37]

Yet in mass culture, the terms "heredity" and "eugenics" continued to be applied to traits that most scientists now attributed to environmental causes, from infections like tuberculosis and syphilis to bad prenatal care and malnutrition. For example, the only movie made by the "Eugenic Film Company," the 1917 film *Birth*, never mentioned genetics but simply provided detailed pregnancy and child care advice.[38] A 1917 feature, *Parentage*, was advertised as strongly "eugenic." It contrasted the families raised by good and by bad parents, explicitly conflating the effects of genetics and environment.[39]

Historians of eugenics usually attribute such examples to mass culture's scientific illiteracy.[40] But in doing so they miss a complex interplay among scientists, popularizers, and the public in defining "heredity." First, many scientists argued that Weismann's theory left room for environmental contributions to genetic disease; such views were neither unscientific nor limited to mass culture.[41]

Second, and most significantly, in mass culture and occasionally in the scientific literature, the term "hereditary" was not limited to genetics but meant that you "got it from your parents," regardless of whether "it" was transmitted by genes, germs, precepts, or probate. Thus *The Science of Life* defined a man's heredity as "what he receives from his ancestors."

Such definitions were not based on wrong science but on a different set of concerns. On this view, what defined "heredity" was the parents' moral responsibility for causing the trait, not the technical mechanism through which parental causation was transmitted. By this definition of "heredity," "eugenics" meant not just having good genes but being a good parent.[42]

Mass culture hardly ignored Weismann's science. At least a dozen films of the 1910s dichotomized heredity and environment, usually by portraying the life of a child whose foster parents differed radically from the biologic parents. Most such films concluded that key human differences were caused by environment, not heredity (at least for girls), but almost all presumed Weismann's radical disjuncture between nurture and nature.[43] Thus mass culture clearly reflected scientific concepts of heredity.

But in turn, leading scientists sometimes used "heredity" to mean "parental responsibility." The eminent British statistical geneticist R. A. Fisher argued that syphilis was a eugenic concern because it ran in families. "There may be something very much like inheritance [of syphilis], in the practical sense. Whether there is inheritance in the biological sense is not the only matter. We are anxious to make a more perfect mankind and we are interested in the practical side."

Even eugenics leaders who limited "heredity" to biological inheritance defined their movement as seeking good parenting, not simply good genes. New Jersey physician Theodore Robie declared at the Third International Eugenics Congress in 1932 that "it would . . . be conducive to racial improvement to sterilize even those feeble minded who do not necessarily fall in the hereditary group," since *mental defectives tend to maintain inferior homes in inferior environments, and they quite generally rear their children in an inferior manner.*[44] Whether or not all traits caused by parents were labeled "hereditary," any trait caused by parents was part of "eugenics." Identifying the parents as the cause made the parents morally as well as medically responsible.[45]

How to Eliminate the Unfit: Euthanasia and Eugenics

A few prominent scientists like German zoologist Ernst Haeckel favored death for the unfit as early as 1868, but prior to Dr. Haiselden's cases such ideas rarely won public endorsement from eugenics leaders.[46] Most advocated selective breeding, not the death of those already born with defects.

Charles Davenport, perhaps the foremost American eugenics researcher of the period, insisted in 1911 that eugenics did "not imply the destruction of the unfit either before or after birth." Irving Fisher echoed Karl Pearson's "fundamental doctrine . . . that everyone, being born, has the right to live" but not the right "to reproduce his kind."[47]

Yet when Haiselden moved the issue from theory to practice, these same leaders proclaimed him a eugenics pioneer. Fisher now wrote to "emphatically approve" Haiselden's action. "I hope the time may come when it will be a commonplace that . . . defective babies be allowed to die." Davenport likewise now urged doctors not to "unduly restrict the operation of what is one of Nature's greatest racial blessings—death." If medicine prevented the death of defectives, "it may conceivably destroy the race."[48]

Haiselden's attention-grabbing actions were a calculated effort to radicalize the eugenics leadership, a strategy anarchists of the time popularized as "propaganda of the deed." "Eugenics had a million theories. . . . But it lacked drive," he explained. "The times were crying for some one central deed—some decisive action that would draw together all these theories . . . into one definite crusade."[49] Haiselden was only one doctor, but by gaining extensive media coverage of his dramatic acts, he was able to reshape the leadership's definition of eugenic methods.

Ironically, while mass culture provided a key battleground on which competing groups struggled to define eugenics, many powerful figures in the film and journalism industries opposed public involvement in making these life-and-death decisions. The *New York Times* demanded that the power to selectively withhold treatment from impaired infants be "kept strictly within professional circles," free from "unenlightened sentimentality."[50] One common suggestion was to create special medical committees, what Helen Keller called "physicians' juries for defective babies." Mass culture thus played an important role in promoting the expansion of professional power.[51]

This media deference to professional expertise in turn contributed to the rapid decline in coverage of Haiselden's crusade and its erasure from public memory. Even people who demanded the death of the unfit opposed publicizing the issue. "I think all monstrosities should be permitted to die," wrote university president Frank H. H. Roberts, "but I do condemn the physician for making such a public ado about the matter." In an editorial entitled "He Forgets Silence Is Golden," the *New York Times* endorsed Haiselden's right to let infants die but denounced his use of media publicity. "If he is wise, as most doctors are, he settles the question for himself . . . and the incident does not become a subject of public discussion."[52]

This growing support for professional power and secrecy combined with the growth of aesthetic objections to eugenics-related subjects drastically curtailed media coverage of Haiselden's activities. By 1918, Haiselden's last reported euthanasia case received only a single column inch buried deep inside the *Chicago Tribune*, a paper that had supported him editorially and given front-page coverage to all his previous cases. Mass media preoccupation with novelty and impatience with complex issues clearly played a role in this change, as did the altered agenda of wartime and postwar politics. But in part, the disappearance of public debate appears to reflect a deliberate decision that the topic itself was unfit to discuss in public.[53]

And, as soon as the media attention flagged, eugenics leaders resumed their prior assertions that they opposed euthanasia, as if Haiselden had never existed. Irving Fisher started to distance himself as early as 1917, reiterating his earlier view that "eugenics does not require the old Spartan practise of infanticide" while simply ignoring his recent accolades for Haiselden.[54]

Thus, by 1930, Haiselden and his cases were not simply forgotten but intentionally erased from the history of eugenics. Both the immediate success and the eventual erasure of his efforts were the sometimes ironic product of the struggle to shape how mass culture portrayed the meanings of eugenics.

Conclusions

Mass culture was a battleground on which elite and other concepts of eugenics competed and interacted. Aesthetic and moral values played a key role in eugenic constructions of the hereditarily "fit" and the "defective," and these values were products of complex struggles to impose meaning on mass culture. Eugenics popularizers tried to use mass culture to promote their complex and circular aesthetic vision, but their efforts often had unintended consequences. The scientists' focus on the genetic mechanisms of heredity coexisted in uneasy tension with a broader, explicitly moral language in which hereditary causation meant parental responsibility. And while mass culture revealed wide support for empowering doctors to let the unfit die, it provoked even stronger opposition to talking about it in public.

Notes

1   I am grateful to Peter Laipson for his many insightful contributions and to David Scobey for his helpful comments on the final draft. Marie Deveney's perceptive comments greatly helped sharpen my arguments. This essay is based on material from my book *The Black Stork: Eugenics and the Death of "Defective" Babies in American Medicine and Motion Pictures since 1915* (New York: Oxford University Press, 1996), used with the permission of Oxford University Press.

2   For easily accessible and/or unique accounts see the following. Bollinger case: *New York Medical Journal* 102 (4 December 1915): 1132. Meter case: *New York Times* (hereafter *NYT*), 25 July 1917, 11; *Chicago American* (hereafter *CA*), 24 July 1917, afternoon edition; *Medical Review of Reviews* (hereafter *MRR*), 23 (1917): 697–98; Werder case: *CA*, 8 December 1915, afternoon edition; Grimshaw case: *CA*, 28 December 1915, magazine page; *New York Call* (hereafter *Call*), 13 December 1915; Hodzima case: *CA*, 13 November 1917; *New York Sun* (hereafter *NYS*), 13 November 1917; *NYT*, 16 November 1917, 4; *Chicago Herald* (hereafter *CH*), 20 November 1917; Stanke case: *NYT*, 28 January 1918, 6. For cases prior to 1915, see *CA*, November 1915, 3.

   Extensive coverage may be found in newspapers nationwide, especially in the Midwest and East, for 12 November–30 December 1915; 5–7 February and 14–16 March 1916 (Bollinger, Roberts, Werder, and Grimshaw cases); 22–27 July and 12–20 November 1917 (Meter and Hodzima cases); 25–30 January 1918 (Stanke case); and 18–20 June 1919 (obituaries). *Note:* Unless otherwise stated all cited newspaper articles begin on page 1.

3   I found and restored the only viewable print, of the 1927 version. It is available for research use at the University of Michigan Historical Health Film Collection. An unprojectable fragmentary paper print of the 1916 version is at the Library of Congress Motion Picture, Broadcasting and Recorded Sound Division, Washington, DC (hereafter LC-MBRS), LU-9978, Box 110.

4   For Wald, see *Independent*, 3 January 1916, 25; for Lindsey, *CH*, 18 November 1915; Darrow, *Washington Post* (hereafter *WP*), 18 November 1915; Beard, *NYT*, 18 November 1915, 4. Darrow later repudiated eugenics in "The Eugenics Cult," *American Mercury* 8 (June 1926): 129–37.

   I have identified 333 individuals who were quoted in the mass media on this issue. Of these, 167 (51%) opposed treating at least some types of impaired newborns, including 14 advocates of active killing. Another 32 favored leaving the choice up to the doctor, without saying what they thought the doctor should do. Only 116 (35%) said doctors should try to save all infants. Of course, this was not a scientific public opinion sample, but it does reflect the image of public opinion that was presented by the press (Pernick, *Black Stork*, p. 31, table 1).

5   Keller, in *The New Republic* (hereafter *TNR*), 18 December 1915, 173–74; and *Call*, 26 November 1915. Haiselden's critics initially cited her case to prove the social utility of preserving the lives of those with disabilities, for example, *WP*, 18 November 1915, 6; *NYS*,

18 November 1915; but Keller strongly supported Haiselden; so did at least one other spokesperson for the disabled, see *Detroit News* (hereafter *DN*), 18 November 1915, 25.

6   I could find only three references to Haiselden in the *NYT* and *Chicago Tribune* (hereafter *CT*) between 1920 and 1960.

7   Fisher, in National Conference on Race Betterment, *Proceedings* 2 (1915): 64. Irving Fisher and Eugene Lyman Fisk, *How to Live*, 12th ed. (New York: Funk & Wagnalls, 1917), 294.

For many similar comments see Mrs. Melvil Dewey, National Conference on Race Betterment, *Proceedings* 1 (1914): 349; Michael Guyer, *Being Well-Born: An Introduction to Heredity and Eugenics* (Indianapolis, IN: Bobbs-Merrill 1927), 426; S. J. Holmes, "Misconceptions of Eugenics," *Atlantic*, February 1915, 222–27; Daniel Kevles, *In the Name of Eugenics: Genetics and the Uses of Human Heredity* (Berkeley: University of California Press, 1985), esp. 58; William J. Robinson, *Eugenics, Marriage and Birth Control*, 2d ed. (New York: Critic & Guide, 1922), 91–93; *Fourth Annual Report of the State Charities Commission [Illinois], Institution Quarterly* 5 (June 1914): 65, as quoted in Patrick Almond Curtis, "Eugenic Reformers, Cultural Perceptions of Dependent Populations, and the Care of the Feebleminded in Illinois, 1909–1920" (Ph.D. diss., University of Illinois at Chicago, 1983), 91.

For the occasional less hostile view of mass cultural meanings see National Conference on Race Betterment, *Proceedings* 1 (1914): 272; *Good Health Magazine* 50 (1915): 485–88, and 51 (1916): 594–95.

8   For a few important exceptions see Mary Bogin, "The Meaning of Heredity in American Medicine and Popular Health Advice, 1771–1860" (Ph.D. diss., Cornell University, 1990); Robert W. Rydell, "Eugenics Hits the Road: The Popularization of Eugenics at American Fairs and Museums between the World Wars" (paper presented to the annual meeting of the History of Science Society, Chicago, December 1984); Dorothy Nelkin and M. Susan Lindee, *The DNA Mystique* (New York: W. H. Freeman, 1995); and the work in progress on eugenics in mass circulation magazines by Juan Leon.

9   Peter Steinfels, introduction in issue on "The Concept of Health," *Hastings Center Studies* 1 (1973): 3–88; Charles Rosenberg, "Framing Disease," in *Framing Disease*, ed. Charles Rosenberg and Janet Golden (New Brunswick, NJ: Rutgers University Press, 1992), pp. xiii–xxvi; H. Tristram Engelhardt, "The Concepts of Health and Disease," *Evaluation and Explanation in the Biomedical Sciences* (Dordrecht: D. Reidel, 1975), 125–41; Sander Gilman, *Difference and Pathology* (Ithaca, NY: Cornell University Press, 1985). Pioneering work on these issues was done by Robert Veatch and Thomas Kuhn.

10   See, for example, T.R.B., "The Tyranny of Beauty," *TNR*, 12 October 1987, 4.

11   The literature on eugenics is vast. For an introduction to American eugenics, see Diane Paul, *Controlling Human Heredity 1865 to the Present* (Atlantic Highlands, NJ: Humanities Press, 1995); Kenneth L. Ludmerer, *Genetics and American Society* (Baltimore, MD: Johns Hopkins University Press, 1972); Mark Haller, *Eugenics* (New Brunswick, NJ: Rutgers University Press, 1963); Philip Reilly, *Genetics, Law, and Social Policy* (Cambridge, MA: Harvard University Press, 1977); Barry Alan Mehler, "A History of the American Eugenics Society, 1921–1940" (Ph.D. diss., University of Illinois, 1988).

To place the United States in comparative context, see Kevles, *In the Name of Eugenics*; Mark Adams, ed., *The Wellborn Science: Eugenics in Germany, France, Brazil, and Russia* (Oxford: Oxford University Press, 1989); Gar Allen, "Genetics, Eugenics, and Class Struggle," *Genetics* 79, suppl. (June 1975): 29–45; Jan Sapp, "The Struggle for Authority in the

Field of Heredity, 1900–1932: New Perspectives on the Rise of Genetics," *Journal of the History of Biology* 16 (1983): 311–42.

12 Cynthia Eagle Russett, *Sexual Science* (Cambridge, MA: Harvard University Press, 1989), 78–92; for Galton's "beauty map," see Kevles, *Name of Eugenics*, 12; Albert E. Wiggam, *The Fruit of the Family Tree* (Garden City, NY: Garden City Publishing, 1924); "Jackie Swims to Increase Beauty," *Call*, 24 November 1915, 5.

See also Lawrence Birken, *Consuming Desire: Sexual Science and the Emergence of a Culture of Abundance 1871–1914* (Ithaca, NY: Cornell University Press, 1989); Stephen Trombley, *The Right to Reproduce: A History of Coercive Sterilization* (London: Weidenfeld and Nicolson, 1988), 79; and H. G. Wells, *Modern Utopia* (London: Chapman & Hall, 1905).

13 Thus the aesthetic dimension of eugenics has often been overlooked. In addition, eugenicists' insistence on the objectivity of their science also made the movement seem hostile to emotions and art. Such was the view of James Joyce's Steven Daedalus, who contrasted "eugenics" and "esthetics" and accused eugenics of trying to reduce beauty to its biological functions. (James Joyce, *Portrait of the Artist as a Young Man* [1916; reprinted 1966, New York: Viking Press], quoted, in Kevles, *Name of Eugenics*, 119.)

Historians of Germany pioneered the recognition of the aesthetic dimension of eugenics, especially Sander L. Gilman, *Picturing Health and Illness* (Baltimore, MD: Johns Hopkins University Press, 1995); George Mosse, *Toward the Final Solution: A History of European Racism* (London: J. M. Dent, 1978), 2; George Mosse, *Nationalism and Sexuality* (New York: H. Fertig, 1985); Paul Weindling, *Health, Race and German Politics between National Unification and Nazism, 1870–1945* (Cambridge: Cambridge University Press, 1989); Willibald Saürländer, "The Nazis' Theater of Seduction," *New York Review of Books*, 21 April 1994, 16–19; Hillel Tryster, "The Art and Science of Pure Racism," *Jerusalem Post International*, 17 August 1991, 13.

14 Wiggam, *Fruit of the Family Tree*, 272, 279. For Haiselden, see *CA*, 2 December 1915, 2.

This view still surfaces in media accounts of modern evolutionary studies. Natalie Angier, "Why Birds and Bees, Too, Like Good Looks," and "Not Just a Beauty Contest," *NYT*, 8 February 1994, B5, B8; Jane Brody, "Ideals of Beauty Seen as Innate," *NYT*, 21 March 1994, A6.

For more sophisticated current theories on the evolution of beauty, see David M. Buss, *The Evolution of Desire* (New York: Basic Books, 1994); R. W. Smuts, "Fat, Sex, Class, Adaptive Flexibility, and Cultural Change," *Ethology and Sociobiology* 13 (1993), 523–42. I thank Bob Smuts for discussing these works with me and the research of his colleagues Richard Alexander and Robert Trivers and for saving me from my initial misrepresentation of Darwin's views.

15 Helena Cronin, *The Ant and the Peacock: Altruism and Sexual Selection from Darwin to Today* (New York: Cambridge University Press, 1992); Stephen Jay Gould, "The Great Seal Principle," in *Eight Little Piggies* (New York: W. W. Norton, 1993), 371–81.

In addition, many professionals among the eugenic leaders felt that "the mind is more important than the body" (*NYT*, 26 November 1915, 8). Sociology professor Franklin H. Giddings explained more bluntly: "The idiotic child should mercifully be allowed to die. The child with a good brain, however crippled otherwise, should be saved" (*Independent*, 3 January 1916, 23. For others with similar views, see *TNR*, 18 December 1915, 174; *NYT*, 18 November 1915, 4, and 25 November 1915; *CH*, 17 November 1915; *CT*, 18 November

1915; *New York American* (hereafter *NYAm*), 19 November 1915, 6; *New York Medical Journal* 100 (26 December 1914): 1247, 1249.

16 Fisher and Fisk, *How to Live*, 322; Wiggam, *Fruit of the Family Tree*, 275, emphasis added. See also Guyer, *Being Well-Born*, 438, passage retained from 1916 edition. For similar aesthetic efforts in German eugenics see Weindling, *Health, Race and German Politics*, 410–13.

The presumably unintended implication of communal living or polygamy in Wiggam's quote results from his diction, not my ellipsis.

17 Individual school districts continued to use *The Science of Life* for decades after 1937. For more on the film see Martin S. Pernick, "Sex Education Films, U.S. Government," *Isis* 84 (1993): 766–768. The last three reels focused on hygiene, human reproduction, VD, and eugenics.

I have identified over 40 films shown in the United States between 1900 and 1930 that dealt with aspects of eugenics and/or human heredity. Most were short one- and two-reelers not yet subject-indexed in any reference guide and so largely unknown to scholars. Almost all these films are now considered lost, though I have discussed and analyzed them from written records (see Pernick, *Black Stork*, chap. 7).

18 *Science of Life*, reel 12, *General Hygiene*, National Archives (hereafter NA), Motion Picture Division, College Park, MD, reel number 90.26. The following discussion is also based on two versions of reel 11, *Personal Hygiene for Young Men* and *Personal Hygiene for Young Women*, NA reels 90.24 and 90.25.

NYT, 15 November 1923, 10; *American Journal of Public Health* 12 (December 1922): 1033, and 13 (September 1923): 737; *Journal of Social Hygiene* 14 (January 1928): 14; New York State Archives, Motion Picture Division Scripts, Albany, NY (hereafter NYSA-MPD), Box 2565, Folders 12,471 and 12,493, including a clipping from the *New York Herald*, 15 April 1923; Records of the United States Public Health Service, NA, Record Group 90, File 1350. Thanks to Peter Laipson and Aloha South for locating the NA material.

19 Charles Musser, *The Emergence of Cinema* (New York: Scribner, 1990); Francois Drag-ognet, *Etienne-Jules Maret* (New York: Zone Books, 1992); Marta Braun, *Picturing Time: The Work of Etienne-Jules Maret* (Chicago, IL: University of Chicago Press, 1992). Thanks to Rebecca Zurier for prompting these ideas.

20 This distinctive aesthetic mix reached its peak in *Way to Strength and Beauty*, a 1925 German film shown in the United States, which combined dramatically modern steep-angle cinematography with scenes of both classical and primitive Teutonic athletes. The film was produced by the UFA and is available from the Bundesarchiv in Cologne and the LC-MBRS. See also *Fit: Episodes in the History of the Body* (Straight Ahead Films, 1993); Lois Banner, *American Beauty* (New York: Alfred Knopf, 1983); and Martha Banta, *Imaging American Women* (New York: Columbia University Press, 1987).

21 Mann used the phrase to describe "the really characteristic and dangerous aspect of Na-tional Socialism," quoted in *New York Review of Books*, 30 January 1986, 21.

22 *CA*, 29 November 1915, and 30 November 1915, 2.

23 On photographic iconography see Martin Elks, "Visual Rhetoric: Photographs of the Feeble-Minded during the Eugenics Era, 1900–1930" (Ph.D. diss., Syracuse University, 1992). On the history of disability in entertainment film see Martin F. Norden, *The Cin-ema of Isolation: A History of Physical Disability in the Movies* (New Brunswick, NJ: Rutgers University Press, 1994); and Gaylyn Studlar, *This Mad Masquerade: Stardom and*

Masculinity in the Jazz Age (New York: Columbia University Press, 1996), chap. 4. On disability in recent horror films see Paul K. Longmore, "Screening Stereotypes: Images of Disabled People," *Social Policy* 16 (summer 1985): 31–37.

24 *CA*, 2 December 1915, 2. In many ways Haiselden's approach to art mimicked that of Thomas Eakins. On art and disfiguration of the canvas, see Michael Fried, *Realism, Writing, Disfiguration* (Chicago, IL: University of Chicago Press, 1987). For other comparisons see Pernick, *Black Stork*, 60–71 passim.

25 Wiggam, *Fruit of the Family Tree*, 262, 273–74.

26 *CA*, 24 November 1915; 30 November 1915, 2.

27 *TNR*, 18 December 1915, 173–74.

28 Kevles, *In the Name of Eugenics*, 12. For Karl Pearson's insistence that his diagnosis of Jewish inferiority was based on "the cold light of statistical inquiry," not "prejudice," see his paper in the 1925 inaugural *Annals of Eugenics*, Karl Pearson and M. Moul, "The Problem of Alien Immigration into Great Britain, Illustrated by an Examination of Russian and Polish Jewish Children," *Annals of Eugenics* 1 [1925], 5–127, quoted by Stephen Jay Gould, *Hen's Teeth and Horse's Toes* (New York: W. W. Norton, 1983), 296–98. Wiggam, *Fruit of the Family Tree*, 272–79.

29 While the responses of ordinary viewers are hard to document, movie reviewers and film censors demonstrate that such "unauthorized" interpretations were common. *CT*, 2 April 1917, 18; *New York Dramatic Mirror* (hereafter *NYDM*), 17 February 1917, 32; *Wid's Film Daily*, 5 April 1917, 220; *Motion Picture News* (hereafter *MPN*), 24 February 1917, 1256.

30 *Exhibitor's Trade Review* (hereafter *ExTrR*), 24 February 1917, 836; *Motography*, 24 February 1917, 424. For similar mixed reviews see *NYDM*, 17 February 1917, 32; *MPN*, 24 February 1917, 1256.

31 *Wid's*, 5 April 1917, 220–21.

32 Parsons in *CH*, 2 April 1917, 11; Kelly in *Chicago Examiner* (hereafter *CE*), 4 April 1917, 8. The *Chicago Tribune* admitted the "ideas may be all right," but found the film "as pleasant to look at as a running sore." Pursuing such clinical metaphors to the limit, *Photoplay* called Lait's screenplay "so slimy that it reminds us of nothing save the residue of a capital operation" (*CT*, 2 April 1917, 18; *Photoplay*, June 1917, 155).

33 The National Board of Review of Motion Pictures' advisors repeatedly used such language to describe the film's audiences as sick. See Andrew Edson of New York City's Education Department, 17 November; U. G. Manning, 18 November; Jonathan Dean, 18 November; Ernest Batchelder, 22 November; Maude Levy, 20 November; W. L. Percy, 21 November; and Robbins Gilman, 23 November; all 1916 and all in National Board of Review of Motion Picture Records, Controversial Film Correspondence, Rare Books and Manuscripts Division, the New York Public Library (hereafter *MBRMP*), Box 103.

34 *Chicago Daily News* (hereafter *CN*), 6 April 1917, 21.

35 The year it first rejected *The Black Stork*, the influential early Pennsylvania state film censor board adopted a list of aesthetic offenses that included any films about eugenics and a range of other medical topics (Pennsylvania State Board of Censors, *Rules and Standards* [Harrisburg, PA: J. L. L. Kuhn, 1918], 15–17). The first Production Code of the Motion Picture Producers and Distributors of America (1930), which synthesized this and similar state lists of forbidden topics, labeled "surgical operations" a "repellent subject" and included a catch-all restriction on all other "disgusting, unpleasant, though not necessarily

evil, subjects" that was used to eliminate most other graphic or unpleasant depictions of medical issues.

Garth Jowett, *Film: The Democratic Art* (Boston, MA: Little, Brown, 1976), chaps. 5, 7, 10. Code of 1930 reprinted, 468–72. On precode films and the rise of censorship see also Francis Couvares, "Hollywood, Main Street, and the Church: Trying to Censor the Movies before the Production Code," *American Quarterly* 44 (December 1992): 584–615; Stephen Vaughn, "Morality and Entertainment: The Origins of the Motion Picture Production Code," *Journal of American History* 77 (June 1990): 39–65; Edward De Grazia and Roger K. Newman, *Banned Films: Movies, Censors and the First Amendment* (New York: R. R. Bowker, 1982).

For aesthetic censorship of Tod Browning's *Freaks*, see NYT, 9 July 1932, 7; Robert Bogdan, *Freak Show* (Chicago: University of Chicago Press, 1988); Leslie Fiedler, *Freaks* (New York: Simon & Schuster, 1978).

36 For censorship history of *The Black Stork*, see MBRMP, Box 103; NYSA-MPD, Box 2565, Folders 383 and 12,421. Quotations are from letter of disapproval, Commissioner to H. J. Brooks, 4 April 1923, NYSA-MPD, Box 2565, Folder 383.

In a private straw poll of community leaders from across the country conducted by a film industry voluntary rating agency, the National Board of Review of Motion Pictures, 9 of the 52 respondents explicitly cited aesthetic objections as a major reason for not approving *The Black Stork*, MBRMP, Box 103.

On *Tomorrow's Children* see "Memo on Behalf of the Motion Picture Division to the Commissioner of Education," 4; and "Court of Appeals Brief for the Respondent," 6, both in NYSA-MPD, Box 333, Folder 28,361. The censors initially also declared the film "immoral" for showing audiences "methods that . . . prevent conception," but this argument was soon dropped; see letter of Irving Egmond, 24 August 1934, in Box 296, Folder 27,387.

For the role of VD and sex education films in the growth of film censorship, see De Grazia and Newman, *Banned Films*; and Annette Kuhn, *Cinema, Censorship and Sexuality, 1909–1925* (London: Routledge, 1988).

37 For the importance of this change see Carl Degler, *In Search of Human Nature* (New York: Oxford, 1991), part 1.

The new definition meant individual heredity was unchangeable. For the first time, science viewed heredity and environment as distinct and exclusive categories, and selective reproduction now became the only mechanism for changing the future genetic composition of the population.

38 A scene script of *Birth* is in LC-MBRS copyright records MU-835; quotes are from *Wid's*, 19 April 1917, 244–45. See also *Moving Picture World* (hereafter *MPW*), 28 April 1917, 609; *MPN*, 28 April 1917, 2687; *NYAm*, 8 April 1917, 7M, and 15 April 1917, 4M; *Motography*, 28 April 1917, 915; DN, 29 April 1917, 6, and 6 May 1917, 5. See also *New York Evening Journal*, 9 April 1917, 8, and advertisements; 11–14 April 1917, movie page; American Film Institute (hereafter AFI), *Catalog of Feature Films, 1911–1920* (Berkeley: University of California Press, 1989), 69–70.

See also the Children's Bureau film *Well Born: Child Health Magazine*, December 1923, 571–72, and September 1924, 407; *Educational Screen*, February 1924, 80; *American Journal of Public Health* 14 (1924): 276; *Bulletin of the National Tuberculosis Association*, January 1924, 4. Other Children's Bureau films of the 1920s are available at the National Archives, but no surviving copies of this one are known.

39   Quote from *Wid's*, 14 June 1917, 369–371. For promotion see *MPN*, June through August 1917.

40   Haller, *Eugenics*, 141–43; Kevles, *In the Name of Eugenics*, 100.

41   What were called environmental "germ poisons" were widely believed to cause inheritable mutations. Conversely, genetic factors might determine who was most susceptible to environmental damage. And some reputable scientists remained "Lamarckians" into the 1930s.

   On germ poisons see *Popular Science Monthly* 88 (1916): 84–85; Allan Brandt, *No Magic Bullet* (New York: Oxford University Press, 1987), 14–15; *Eugenics in Race and State: Scientific Papers of the Second International Congress of Eugenics . . . New York 1921* (Baltimore, MD: Williams & Wilkins, 1923), 309, 346–47. Anti-Lamarckian prohibitionist John Harvey Kellogg gave extensive publicity to alcohol as a germ poison: *Good Health Magazine* 51 (1916): 75–76; 52 (1917): 502–3; 54 (1919): 164, 219–224, 273–78, 717. For a Lamarckian view of this research, see Aldred Scott Warthin, *Creed of a Biologist* (New York: P. B. Hoeber, 1930), 57–58; Jean-Charles Sournia, *A History of Alcoholism* (Oxford: Basil Blackwell, 1990), chap. 7; L. Crowe, "Alcohol and Heredity: Theories about the Effects of Alcohol Use on Offspring," *Social Biology* 32 (1985): 146–61; R. H. Warner and H. L. Rosett, "Effects of Drinking on Offspring: An Historical Survey of the American and British Literature," *Journal of Studies of Alcohol* 36 (November 1975): 1395–1420.

   On environmental susceptibility see René and Jean Dubos, *The White Plague: Tuberculosis, Man and Society* (London: Victor Gollancz, 1953), 28–43, 125–28; Robert N. Proctor, *Racial Hygiene: Medicine under the Nazis* (Cambridge, MA: Harvard University Press, 1988), 215–17; *Eugenics in Race and State*, 300–301.

   For persistent Lamarckian beliefs in the 1930s see Warthin, *Creed of a Biologist*.

   Thus eminent scientists like psychologist G. Stanley Hall considered germ fighting part of eugenics. His plan for a "Department of Eugenics" specifically included infectious diseases and milk inspection among its responsibilities (Dorothy Ross, *G. Stanley Hall* [Chicago, IL: University of Chicago Press, 1972], 362–63, 413. Thanks to Alice Smuts for this reference). Similar examples include Fisher and Fisk, *How to Live*, 293–94; *Good Health Magazine* 54 (1919): 658; *Social Hygiene Bulletin* 2 (January 1916): 3, and 3 (November 1916): 4.

42   Many motion pictures explicitly defined "eugenics" as meaning "fit to marry." *The Black Stork* itself was retitled *Are You Fit to Marry?* when it was rereleased in 1918–19 and in 1927. See also "heredity" in *Oxford English Dictionary*, compact edition (New York: Oxford University Press, 1971).

   On the link between causality and morality see Thomas Haskell, *The Emergence of Professional Social Science* (Urbana: University of Illinois Press, 1977), esp. chap. 11; and Sylvia Tesh, *Hidden Arguments: Political Ideology and Disease Prevention Policy* (New Brunswick, NJ: Rutgers University Press, 1988).

43   Environment wins out in *Are They Born or Made?* (Warner, 1917), *A Daughter's Strange Inheritance* (Broadway Star-Vitagraph, 1917), *A Victim of Heredity* (Kalem, 1913), *The Power of Mind* (Mutual, 1916), *A Disciple of Nietzsche* (Thanhouser, 1915), and *The Red Circle* (Pathe, 1915).

   Heredity wins in *Heredity* (Biograph, 1912), *Heredity* (Broadway Star, 1915), *Inherited Sin* (Universal, 1915), *The Power of Heredity* (Rex, 1913), and *The Second Generation* (Pathe, 1914).

One of the first commercial melodramas to be billed as an explicitly "eugenic" film was D. W. Griffith's *The Escape* (Reliance-Majestic, 1914). Following a prologue by Dr. Daniel Carson Goodman that called for breeding humans as carefully as livestock, it traces in gruesome detail the awful consequences of human "mismating." The fictional "Joyce" family compresses into two generations all the defects and deviance found among two centuries of Jukes and Kallikaks.

The film's conclusion may have been based on Lamarckian concepts of heredity (critics disagreed on this point—see *MPW*, 13 June 1914, 1515, versus *NYDM*, 10 June 1914, 42). The physician-hero cures a lunatic strangler surgically and redeems the lunatic's prostitute sister by marrying her. But whatever definition of heredity it was using, what made the film "eugenic" was its dramatization of the effects of bad parenting. AFI, *Catalog 1911–20*, 244; *Variety*, 5 June 1914, 19; *NYT*, 2 June 1914, 11; William K. Everson, *American Silent Film* (New York: Oxford University Press, 1978), 76; Robert Connelly, *The Motion Picture Guide: Silent Film* (Chicago, IL: Cinebooks,, 1986), 74.

44 Fisher in *Eugenics in Race and State*, 318, 464–65. Robie in *A Decade of Progress in Eugenics: Scientific Papers of the Third International Congress of Eugenics* (Baltimore, MD: Williams & Wilkins, 1934), 202; for similar views of the American Eugenics Society in 1935 see Ellsworth Huntington, *Tomorrow's Children* (New York: John Wiley, 1935), 41–42, quoted in Barry Mehler, "Eliminating the Inferior," *Science for the People*, November–December 1987, 16.

45 These concerns retain their influence today, even among those leading the return to supposedly biological explanations. Thus Richard Herrnstein and Charles Murray assert in *The Bell Curve* (New York: Free Press, 1994), "If women with low scores are reproducing more rapidly than women with high scores, the distribution of scores will, other things equal, decline, *no matter whether the women with the low scores came by them through nature or nurture*" (emphasis added). Quoted by Malcolm Browne, *New York Times Book Review*, 16 October 1994, 1.

46 Ernst Haeckel, *The Wonders of Life* (New York: Harper & Brothers, 1905), 21, 114–20; Haeckel, *The History of Creation*, vol. 1 (1868; reprint, New York; D. Appleton, 1876), 170–71; I. van der Sluis, "The Movement for Euthanasia, 1875–1975," *Janus* 66 (1979): 134–37; Daniel Gasman, *The Scientific Origins of National Socialism* (London: MacDonald, 1971), 91. On Haeckel's follower Ploetz, see Stephen Trombley, *The Right to Reproduce: A History of Coercive Sterilization* (London: Weidenfeld & Nicolson, 1988), 71.

Other eugenic professionals who advocated such views prior to 1910 included Hungarian welfare expert Sigmund Engel, British physicians Charles E. Goddard and Robert Rentoul, Chicago dentist Eugene Talbot, Yale law professor Simeon Baldwin, physicians William D. McKim and Edward Wallace Lee, Chicago surgeon G. Frank Lydston, psychologist G. Stanley Hall, and psychiatrist Walter Kempster. The first effort to legislate such proposals was introduced by Link Rodgers in Michigan in 1903, and similar bills were debated in Iowa and Ohio in 1906.

Sigmund Engel, *The Elements of Child-Protection*, trans. Eden Paul (New York: Macmillan, 1912). For Goddard, see O. Ruth Russell, *Freedom to Die: Moral and Legal Aspects of Euthanasia* (New York: Human Sciences Press, 1975), 59. For Rentoul, see Trombley, *Right to Reproduce*, 19. Simeon Baldwin, "The Natural Right to a Natural Death," *Journal of Social Science* 37 (1899): 1–17, quoted in Cynthia B. Cohen, "The Treatment of Impaired Newborns in American History: Implications for Public Policy" (Department of Philosophy, Villanova University, 1985), 87; Eugene S. Talbot, *Degeneracy* (London: Walter Scott, [1898]), 3–4. For other U.S. proposals to kill the mentally retarded, as early as 1883, see Russell Hollander, "Euthanasia and Mental Retardation," *Mental Retardation* 27 (April 1989): 53–61; William McKim, *Heredity and Human Progress* (New York: G. P. Putnam's Sons, 1900), 188–92; G. Stanley Hall, "What Is to Become of Your Baby?" *Cosmopolitan* 47 (April 1910): 661–668; Ross, *Hall*, 318–319; Philip Reilly, *The Surgical Solution* (Baltimore, MD: Johns Hopkins University Press, 1991), 37–38; for Lydston, see Stephen Louis Kuepper, "Euthanasia in America, 1890–1960" (PH.D. diss., Rutgers University, 1981), 65; for Lee, see *New York Medical Journal* 100 (26 December 1914): 1251. On the Michigan plan, see Curtis, "Eugenic Reformers," 69–70; *CE*, 22 May 1903; *DN*, 22 May 1903; on Rodgers see *Michigan State Gazeteer* (Detroit: R. L. Polk, 1903); *DN*, 21 May 1903, 3. For Kempster, *NYT*, 26 January 1906; for Dr. R. H. Gregory, van der Sluis, "Euthanasia," 135.

Infanticide for reasons including elimination of sickly infants had been practiced in the ancient world and in many non-Western cultures.

47 Davenport, *Heredity in Relation to Eugenics* (New York: Henry Holt, 1911), 4, quoted in Kuepper, "Euthanasia in America," 62. For Fisher, see National Conferences on Race Betterment, *Proceedings*, 1 (1914): 472, 475. For others with same point at the conference see *Proceedings* 1 (1914): 477, 500–501; (1915): 89–90 and addenda slip for 61.

48 *Independent*, 3 January 1916, 23. The same article also contained an endorsement from Raymond Pearl.

49 *Boston American*, 20 December 1915, 16; George Woodcock, *Anarchism* (Cleveland, OH: World Publishing, 1962), 328, 336, 462. For comparisons between Dr. Haiselden and Dr. Jack Kevorkian today see Pernick, *Black Stork*, 170–71.

50 *NYT*, 13 November 1917, 12.

51 Keller in *TNR*, 18 December 1915, 173–174. *CH*, 20 November 1915, 2, and 21 November 1915, 3. *Call*, 29 November 1915, 3. A Los Angeles proposal was reported as early as 20 November; see *CA*, 24 November 1915, 3. For Haiselden's use of consultants to confirm his nontreatment decisions, see *CA*, 22 December 1915 magazine page; *CE*, 24 July 1917, *NYT*, 16 November 1917, 4; *MRR* 23 (1917): 607; *CA*, 16 November 1917, 3. For modern parallels see Mary B. Mahowald, "Baby Doe Committees: A Critical Evaluation," *Clinics in Perinatology* 15 (December 1988): 789–800.

Occupational health pioneer Dr. Alice Hamilton noted the irony that mass culture demanded expanding the power of the profession. "Curiously enough it is not the medical profession which is seeking an extension of its rights; it is the laity which is trying to force upon physicians a power over life and death which they themselves shrink from." *Survey* 35 (4 December 1915): 266. But popular support for giving doctors this particular power itself depended on a broader Progressive-era faith in the methods of science, a faith that was actively promoted by medical and eugenic leaders.

52 *Independent*, 3 January 1916, 26; *NYT*, 16 July 1917, 10. Although the *Times* changed its position on nontreatment, the editors consistently maintained that the "wise" physician should make such decisions silently. *NYT*, 18 November 1915, 8; 22 November 1915, 14; 29 November 1915, part 2, 10.

Columbia University sociology chairman Franklin H. Giddings applauded the death of "molasses-minded" mental defectives but felt it was a "question that should be considered soberly, thoughtfully and by rigorous intellectual processes. To put it up to the general public in all the emotional and imaginative setting of a photo-play is, in my judgment, an utterly wrong thing to do." A series of legal investigations upheld Haiselden's refusal to treat impaired newborns, but he was expelled from the Chicago Medical Society for publicizing his actions. NYT, 18 November 1915, 4, and Giddings to W. D. McGuire, 20 November 1916, MBRMP, Box 103.

53 CT, 28 January 1918, 12. See chaps. 6 and 9 of Pernick, *The Black Stork.*

54 Fisher and Fisk, *How to Live,* 12th ed., 294. Even Dr. William J. Robinson, one of Haiselden's most vigorous supporters in 1915–16, wrote in 1917 that "no eugenic considerations will induce us to adopt Spartan-like methods and to neglect or kill off the weak and puny. . . . Every child that is born . . . is entitled to the very best of care." William J. Robinson, *Eugenics and Marriage* (New York: Critic & Guide, 1917), 138, see also 73–76. For similar disavowals see Wiggam, *Fruit,* 283; Eden Paul, "Eugenics, Birth Control, and Socialism," in *Population and Birth Control* (New York: Critic & Guide, 1917), 142.

Extra Chromosomes and Blue Tulips:
Medico-familial Interpretations
Rayna Rapp

OMG !

So they diagnosed Amelia right away, on the delivery table, she was barely out, I barely got a chance to catch my breath or marvel at my first baby when this doctor pours this bad news all over us. "She's got Down syndrome," he says to us, very coldly. And after he tells us about blood tests and confirmations and all this stuff, we say to him, "But what does that *mean*? What should we *expect*?" And just as coldly he says, "Don't expect much. Maybe she'll grow up to be an elevator operator. Don't expect much." So we clung to each other, and cried. (April Schwartz, white lawyer, mother of a four-year-old with Down syndrome)

My doctor was so angry with me, he couldn't believe I didn't take that test, "How could you let this happen?" he yelled at me. "You're 40!" But I think something else: Even though he's mentally retarded, he could be a good person. . . . It's just like finding out you have a new job. You just do it, and you accept it, that's all there is to it. (Anna Morante, Puerto Rican nurse's aide, mother of a seven-year-old with Down syndrome)

In humans, the twenty-first chromosome suffers nondisjunction at a remarkably high frequency, with unfortunately rather tragic effect. . . . These unfortunate children suffer mild to severe mental retardation and have a reduced life expectancy. . . . We have no clue as to why an extra twenty-first chromosome should yield the highly specific set of abnormalities associated with trisomy-21. But at least it can be identified in utero by counting the chromosomes in fetal cells, providing an option for early abortion. (Gould 1980)

The smiling face of the Mongolian Imbecile suggests the possession of some secret source of joy. (Sutherland 1900: 23)

With the discovery of the complement of normal human chromosomes in 1958, and the development and widespread use of amniocentesis and related prenatal diagnostic technologies over the last 25 years, epidemiological knowledge and public health screening of Down syndrome have become routinized. In North America, Down's is the iconic condition described by geneticists and genetic counselors when explaining their diagnostic technologies to potential patients. Yet despite widespread popular recognition of this condition, expanded access to prenatal diagnosis, and a high rate of elective abortion following upon diagnosis, the birth of individual babies with Down syndrome is always a shock. It provides an occasion for intense medical and familial discussions of what "causes" the condition, and how children born with it are to be treated. There is a gap between epidemiological description, clinical services, and individual understandings of affliction which is continuously open to speculation and practical intervention. Technologies of diagnosis, therapies of intervention, and systems of support are all enacted and interpreted within that gap.

This essay explores that gap, focusing on the traffic between biomedical and familial understandings of the presence of Down syndrome in newborns and children. It is based on two years' participant-observation in New York City in a support group for parents whose children have this condition, as well as interviews conducted through an early intervention program. The 38 families who were kind enough to share their thoughts and family time with me are part of a larger study of the social impact and cultural meaning of prenatal diagnosis.[1]

Here, my analysis begins with the observation that the realm of technoscientific knowledge and practice is rapidly expanding: we all find ourselves increasingly inside of science, heir to its immense benefits and ambiguous burdens, whether as researchers, service providers, patients, and caretakers of patients, or anthropologists who occasionally occupy any and all of these roles. The clinicians and parents whose ideas fill this essay are differently located in relation to new technologies like prenatal diagnosis, chromosome karyotyping, and neonatal surgery, all of which are likely to loom large when a newborn is diagnosed as having Down syndrome. What counts as a new biomedical technology to one constituency may be quite routinized for another. And new technologies are deployed and understood by parents and practitioners in relation to their funds of social as well as individual knowledge. Thus medico-familial interpretations of the extra chromosome which produces Down syndrome are shaped at intersections which are unstable and continuously subject to claims of expert, expansive knowledge.

The Unexpected Baby

When parents narrate the natural history of learning to live with a child's hereditary disabilities, they almost always spontaneously begin by describing the birth, and whether or not a diagnosis was quickly made. As the first two stories which open this chapter suggest, the birth and diagnosis of a newborn with Down syndrome is an event which is vividly remembered not only by the birthing woman and her partner, but by medical practitioners as well. Indeed, the third quotation points toward a lengthy medical commentary on the mysterious nature of births gone awry: doctors may have strong personal and professional responses to delivering and treating babies who cannot be seen as normal, and whose ills cannot be cured, investing them with symbolic meaning which sometimes supersedes their individual characteristics. Birthing mothers recalled their attendants' words and deeds in great detail, judging the quality of response:

> So I had a section and my doctor came in seven hours later and I was still pretty wiped out and he stood there with me and he says to me with tears in his eyes, he says, "Well, you have a Down syndrome child." And I didn't know what he meant, I says, "Is it a cold, does it go away, what the hell is it?" And he says, "Patsy, the baby is mongoloid." I mean, it hits home, it's like, "Are you for real?" And then he looks me square in the eye and he says, "We have some papers, you could award him to the state if you don't want him." And I looked at my doctor that just delivered my son, my doctor that I loved, we had such a friendship, and I says, "Get the hell out of this room." (Patsy DelVecchio, white bus driver, mother of a six-year-old with Down syndrome)

> So my husband didn't make it home for the delivery but he called from the airport and the doctor got on the phone right away and gave

him all this bad news. But you know it's like the doctor was more upset than we were, like he couldn't bring himself to say "here's this baby and we don't know for sure." It's very hard for professional people not to see the down side, you know, to see the worst possible, this could have been the Down's kid that was gonna have an IQ of 100 and make it to Harvard. We don't know the future when it's first born. But the doctor was seeing maybe his next door neighbor's kid who can't do anything, or something, so it was very hard that he painted this gloomy terrible picture. (Lydia Sellers, white homemaker and dressmaker, mother of a nine-year-old with Down syndrome)

She was tiny but she was great, like she was just the cutest thing and then my husband came in and he looked weird and immediately he said, "The baby, something's wrong. . . ." And all I could think of was that she's blind, I guess that was probably the worst thing I could ever have imagined. But the doctor had just called him and told him that Rose was mongoloid. It took a half hour to get it out of him, like he couldn't finish telling me the story, and then the doctor came and said, "What your husband just told you is right." He was, like very down on the whole thing, very negative, he said, "The only blessing is they don't tend to live very long." So he thought it would be a good thing if our new baby would die. What more can I say? (Flora Taglitone, white homemaker, mother of a six-year-old with Down syndrome)

As such stories indicate, Down syndrome babies are "wrong babies," marked almost from the moment of birth by medical scrutiny as incurably damaged. Many women across class lines and from diverse ethnic backgrounds told similar stories of medical dismay at their children's births. It is not hard to spot the despair at having delivered a child most people consider frighteningly marred, and for which technological surveillance and interventions are available prenatally. Nor is it hard to pick up (as Lydia Sellers's words suggest) the attitudes toward mental retardation expressed by many medical professionals. I should also note that while the majority of birth stories I collected pointed an accusatory finger at awkward, cold, or downright insensitive obstetricians, a few families felt very well served by both obstetricians and pediatricians, whose calm discretion they recalled with appreciation:

We're so lucky we had Robin at the Birthing Center, and not in the hospital. I mean, in a hospital, he would have been examined to death by a cast of thousands, they surely would have picked it up. But at the Center, they missed it. So I got to take him home, to nurse him, we stayed at home for four days quietly, all together, and then we took him to meet the pediatrician. And he made the diagnosis immediately. He was excellent, really excellent. It's such an important thing, how the professional handles it, the initial comment, I can't emphasize how important it is. . . . He was just very positive and sensitive, he just said, "I have to tell you this, there are some things I'm concerned about," and I said, "Well, what?," and he said, "Well, let's look at his eyes and, of course, there's this crease in his palm. It's a simian crease." I don't know how I knew that, but I just knew what he was talking about, so I turned to my husband and I said, "Do you know what he's talking about?" and Paul said, "No," and I said, "Well, he's talking about Down syndrome." So I guess he didn't really ever have to tell me, he just got me to the point where I knew for myself. And then he hooked us up with all sorts of people, genetic counselors, heart specialists, and we always felt he just wanted the best for our son. (Polly Denton, white actress, mother of a five-year-old with Down syndrome)

Laura and Dan Schulmann were also quite satisfied with the straightforward explanation their pediatrician offered when he made the diagnosis of Down syndrome one hour after Ashley's birth:

He caught Dan at the telephone, calling everyone, and stopped him. "Don't make any more calls till after we've had a moment to talk," he said. And once he was done explaining, he warned us, "Don't touch the literature. It's badly out of date, it will only scare you." And he got us some other parents to talk to.

We should note the presence of the simian crease, a term of differential diagnosis, to whose history I will return, and the auto-critique of the medical literature in these very positive doctor/patient stories. Several women went out of their way to also describe the sensitivity and compassion with which nurses, rather than doctors, embedded a diagnostic situation in a more optimistic message that their babies would receive help rather than judgment.

Medicalization

In the realm of biomedicine, newborns tentatively diagnosed with Down syndrome have their blood samples sent immediately for karyotyping. Once diagnosed, they are intensively and technologically scrutinized for specific conditions that range from mild to life-threatening. Regulation is considered key to normalizing the life chances of babies and young children with Down syndrome. Whether the individual story of diagnosis is coded as negative or positive, virtually all parents of a newborn with Down syndrome find themselves stitched into medical networks. Because babies with this condition are at high risk for heart problems, intestinal blockages, and a host of less life-threatening disabilities, a diagnosed baby is a medicalized baby, tied to appointments with specialists and scheduled for high-technology testing from the moment a diagnosis is tentatively made: geneticists, pediatric cardiologists, neurologists, and pediatric surgeons are all likely to see the baby shortly after birth; audiology, ophthalmology, podiatry, and behavioral psychology are among the services to which most parents of children with Down syndrome are routinely introduced. All are likely to be accompanied by a range of biomedical technologies. While some new parents find this attention reassuring, others find it invasive and disheartening:

> Then they send you to the Heredity Department, that's when they give you the low-down, when you're at your lowest. That's when they say, "Heart problems. Leukemia. The works." (Johnella Cornell, African American hairdresser, mother of an 18-month-old with Down syndrome)

Diagnosed babies and their parents are also likely to be "social-worked," connected to early intervention services not only in the realm of medicine, but in educational, physical, occupational, and speech therapies for infants and young children. These, too, include technologies which are likely to be new to families, whether as low-tech as the physio balls physical therapists use with floppy newborns, or as cutting-edge as computer learning programs for correcting toddler speech pathology. Funding for such interventions comes through the Family Court (in New York State, where my research was conducted), tying families into a bureaucratic web of services and paperwork from the moment of diagnosis. While we might want to note that all newborns are conscripts to modern bureaucratic record-keeping and discipline via birth records, immunization schedules, the establishment of contracts, wills, and the like, diagnosed babies are fused with public services at an intense and often bewildering rate. This, too, is a realm where technology enters the lives of families with disabled newborns and older children.

For some families, learning to speak the highly medicalized physical therapy language of hypotonia, proprioception, and subluxation provides a vocabulary around which early interventions may be affected. And exposure to the range of helping therapists available through early intervention programs also provides aid for families coming to terms with how to handle and what to expect from a "different" or "wrong" baby. As one physical therapist who works extensively with developmentally delayed newborns and young children put it, "With a handicapped baby, we now know how important it is to go all out, to shoot for the moon. That way, the kid will achieve whatever is best for them."

The optimistic energy and realistic sense of possibility expressed by such therapists are usually extremely beneficial to family members. Yet early intervention services also have shadow effects. When I praised the high-quality services available to parents of newborns and infants to the director of an early intervention program, herself the mother of a teenager with Down syndrome, she told me this story:

> When Debbie was born, the pediatrician said, "Well, she has mongoloid tendencies." I knew what he meant. He knew that I knew. But no one talked about mental retardation or heart defects all the time. I went for weeks without anyone mentioning it; it was a keen eye that picked up Downs in babies then. I had a couple of years to grow into my baby, to grow with her. Now, every parent that's referred here is waiting for the results of chromosome studies, hoping it's "only mosaicism," and thinking about facial surgery. What kind of information do you really need to handle a six-week-old? I didn't look at my daughter every day and say, "She has Downs." Today, they get more services, and more support. But they've got less ability to forget it, to just get on with knowing the child.

New technical knowledge both opens and closes doors, a point forcefully made by Barbara Katz Rothman more than a decade ago, in speaking of amniocentesis (1986). Here, I underline the increasing biomedical routinization of diagnostic technological capacities such as chromosome karyotyping and cardiac echosonography of newborns, which make both doctors and parents more quickly aware of the specificity of a newborn's membership in a taxonomy of pathology. In both positive and negative terms, I have been describing a system of continuous interventions marking difference in medical and kinship language. In the shadow of such difference, establishing the child's bone fide presence inside a system of connection, that is, as a family member, is a major cultural accomplishment. There are many barriers—both subtle and overt—to normalizing kin ties with disabled children. Medical and other professional language may constitute the first barrier, for it often separates Down syndrome and other hereditarily disabled newborns from the category of normalcy, imposing descriptions that create distance. One Haitian mother, for example, who gave birth to a child with a rare and anomalous chromosomal diagnosis, a partial trisomy, was asked to bring her newborn son to the genetics laboratory. There, geneticists discussed the oblique palpebral fissure and micrognathia of her six-week-old which led them to label his condition as trisomy 9, while she genealogized his features, assimilating them to various aunts and uncles. Likewise, one white mother of a newly diagnosed Down syndrome baby boy kept insisting that his father was black and had the same low-hung ears as the baby, linking the child to his familial heritage over the pathologizing discourse of the pediatricians. Another African American mother said of her newly diagnosed baby, "They wanna talk about trisomy something, I need to deal with a sick kid. My kid's got a heart problem. Let me deal with that first, then I'll figure out what all this Down's business means." An interpretive clash on the terrain of medico-familiar explication is always a strong possibility.

Alienated Kinship

When mothers of children with Down syndrome tell the story of their pregnancies, births and diagnoses, one common theme is explicit disconnection, or lack of familial resemblance, as orchestrated by medical attendants:

> So I had a home delivery and the midwife was very cool. Like she suspected something, but she didn't want to say anything, she just wanted me to enjoy the birth, to bond with Laney. But he was too sleepy, so she knew something was wrong, she called the doctor, and the pediatrician came and she said, "I hate to bring this up, I just have the vague suspicion he doesn't look like he's related to anyone in this family, I just don't think he resembles any of you." . . . At first, I just

blocked what she was saying, and then I looked, and well, I had this uneasy feeling 'cause he didn't look like us. He looked like he belonged to some other family. (Judy Kaufman, white nurse)

The first thing the doctor said was, he said, "If you had a lot of Irish moon faces in your family, I'd be happier about seeing this child. But she doesn't look like you, she doesn't look like she's from your gene pool at all." Then he explained why he thought it was Down's. (April Schwartz, white lawyer)

An activist couple who were parents of a child with Down syndrome interrupted our interview in midstream when the mother exclaimed, "Shit! I just told you that Leslie doesn't have all the stigmata associated with Down's! There I go, sounding just like them!" The father commented that it was almost impossible to avoid pathological language, despite their pride in their daughter's accomplishments. And many families noted that the language used to diagnose and describe Down syndrome includes references to a "simian crease," obviously grouping its bearers with apes rather than humans. We will return to this problem of animal identification and a "throwback" language of evolution below.

The claims of kinship must be articulated not only against the technicist diagnostic discourse of biomedicine, but sometimes against other kinsfolk and community members who blame mothers for giving birth to "wrong" babies: "My husband would have left me if I'd done that," said the mother-in-law of one mother of a newborn with Down's. Two African American fathers believed that their babies caught mental retardation from retarded neighbors from whom they had warned their wives to keep a distance during their pregnancies lest it "mark the baby." Gloria Hurwitz, an Orthodox Jew, told almost none of her relatives that her baby had been diagnosed with mosaic trisomy 18. Beyond initial medical evaluations, she mainly consulted a geneticist who belonged to the same temple. "Jewish people don't accept mental retardation," she told me. But she expected to send Hershel to Hebrew school, along with her other children. Susan Lee, estranged from her parents after a religious conversion and marriage to someone of another faith, didn't initially tell her parents that their first grandchild had Down syndrome. "What's the point? They were already set to reject her, this will only make it worse," she reasoned. Marilyn Trainer (1991), whose widely published essays on life with a Down syndrome son present a consistent message of acceptance, never told her elderly parents that her fourth child had this disability. She didn't want to burden them with what she expected to be sorrowful news. Some women without privileged educational backgrounds had to convince their partners and other family members that they'd done nothing to "deserve" or "cause" the "wrong baby."

Indeed, the existential problem of what causes hereditary disabilities haunted many in the early days of parenting anomalous babies, when biomedical explanation often cannot assuage experiential confusion and pain. Susan Lee, newly fundamentalist Christian and antiabortion, thought her prior abortion was being redressed by a Down syndrome birth; Patsy Del-Vecchio, a recovering alcoholic, believed that she was being punished for earlier drinking habits. Johnella Cornell told me she was refused amniocentesis at five city hospitals because she was too young; but in her recurrent dreams she gave birth to a damaged baby again and again, and she wanted the test to confirm the vision. When her son was born with Down syndrome, she considered it a sign, and was relieved to have discovered the root cause of the dream. Pat Carlson decided to keep a Down syndrome pregnancy after a positive prenatal diagnosis. She believed that her son Stevie was put on earth for a mysterious and only partly revealed reason; his mission will become clearer as he grows up. Many practicing Catholics and churchgoing Protestants told me, "God only gives burdens to the strong." Some parents used medical language against itself, to explain their children's special qualities:

> I think it's like something positive, they're always feeding you all this negative stuff about the extra chromosome, all these disabilities, but I think it's something positive. Maybe the extra genetic stuff carries some mutation that causes positive things, too. I think that all that heart, that generosity, the lovingness, the feeling one with the world, those qualities, that's the positive side they never talk about. And it's got to be genetically built into them. Those are traits, too. (Judy Kaufman, white nurse, mother of a seven-year-old with Down syndrome)

> My son just has a different brain, it's got different inhibitors built in to it. The point is not that he's stupid, that he can't learn. He learns really well, but really slowly. The brain connections are just different, he doesn't inhibit, he isn't limited, his brain just doesn't inhibit certain emotional expressions the way the rest of us do. His feelings are much more available to be expressed by this brain. What's so bad about that? (Bonnie D'Amato, mother of a five-year-old with Down syndrome)

Finding alternative meaning within biomedical discourses is a capacity exercised by many parents of youngsters with hereditary disabilities.

Acceptance of stigmatized difference is an achievement that surely belongs to parents, but it is also dependent on larger social groups and forces. Johnella Cornell's dream of a disabled baby and her strong criticisms of "being sent to Heredity" after her son's birth should also be contextualized by her long-standing residence in Harlem. There, her mother received a White House commendation for having fostered 12 community children, many with disabilities. There, too, Johnella described dense interactions with neighbors who had nonspecific mental retardation or cerebral palsy, both of which are diagnosed at high rates in poor communities. This working knowledge of disability gave Johnella pause to worry about how her son with Down syndrome might be teased as he grew up; but it also gave her confidence in his ability to survive as a member of his community. Likewise, three of the parents I interviewed through the Down Syndrome Parent Support Group were teachers of special education; they had considerable professional knowledge of mild mental retardation.

Professional knowledge doesn't necessarily imply acceptance; among the 50 stories I collected of women who chose to abort after receiving what is so antiseptically labeled a "positive" diagnosis, teachers of special education are well represented (Rapp 1999: chap. 9). But it does suggest that when babies are born with developmental delays, those with prior knowledge are likely to be quite resourceful about how to cope:

> I spent the first month on the telephone. By that time, I had Amy connected to every retarded service in the Bronx and lower Westchester. There was never any question: my kid was gonna get the best special services the whole world had to offer. (Linda Hornstein, white special education consultant, mother of a six-year-old with Down syndrome)

When viewed from a wider context beyond the clinic, access to early intervention and its many services is a (relatively) new technology, too.[2]

Imagined Communities

The communities within which parents form alliances and receive support or judgment are not only geographically, professionally, or religiously based: some are associational as well. Throughout this chapter, I have referred to some parents as activists; their particular activities, orientations, and aspirations for their disabled children are powerfully reorganized by participation in support groups. Parents are encouraged by a host of professionals—geneticists and genetic counselors, pediatricians and social workers—to join voluntary family support groups. Such groups are historically rooted in at least three intersecting traditions. One historic precursor to these groups lies in the tradition of immigrant self-help groups of the late 19th century. These shared with Alcoholics Anonymous, a WASP invention of the 1930s, certain practices of what might be labeled "early-identity politics." A strong belief that "it takes one to know one," or, in this case, "to help one," was present in the birth of both those social movements. Endemic to this tradition is the valorization of "experience" (cf. Scott 1992) and the (often appropriately justified) suspicion of the availability or good-will of public agencies to solve what are widely perceived to be intractable problems and recurrent crises.

National public interest in mental retardation was surely amplified by the well-publicized stories of the Kennedy family, beginning in the 1960s: an elder sister with mental retardation, and a child who died young with the same condition are part of the family legacy. So, too, are the scores of centers for research and clinical services to mentally retarded Americans which are found coast to coast. Many have been generously funded by the Kennedys, and some bear variants on their name. Legislative transformations in the Kennedy-Johnson years also affected the increase of Social Security coverage in the 1970s; and Section 504 of the National Rehabilitation Act of 1973 mandated that states cover an appropriate education for all handicapped children. The Americans with Disabilities Act of 1990, now winding its way into enforcement via federal and state regulations and court-based challenges, provides the most comprehensive protections to date.

Lay support groups clearly grew out of and responded to all these legal, medical, and social developments. Self-help organizations for those with specific physical and mental health concerns (rather than generic veterans' groups, or research service charities like the Easter Seal Society) are a relatively recent phenomenon, a product of the 1950s and 1960s, and becoming ever more specialized as more differentiating and disabling conditions take on specific medical nomenclature (Weiss and Mackta 1996). In this newer tradition of grouping and differentiating support groups and networks according to diagnostic categories, there are at least four important national organizations, and scores of state-based and local associations, which grow from a fusion of familial and professional concern with

Down syndrome. The two largest national organizations offer 800 telephone help-lines. The National Down Syndrome Congress was founded in 1971. It maintains a parent hotline, publishes a newsletter, holds conventions, and lobbies on national policy issues. The National Down Syndrome Society, founded in 1979, raises funds to support biomedical researchers whose work will enrich the understanding of Down's. Both groups offer pamphlets, videos, and other resources which are widely available to parents of newly diagnosed Down syndrome children. Local chapters of the ARC (formerly, the Association of Retarded Citizens) and Down Syndrome Parent Support Groups provide informal networks for parent-to-parent peer counseling.

Local support groups offer rich and reassuring resources for parents learning to normalize a child as a family member, not only as a medical diagnosis. Paradoxically, as I hope to show, medical worldview and resources figure large in the repertoire of such groups, even as they contest their exclusive dominion over definitions of disabled family members. New identities as well as new knowledge of services are modeled by parent-activists for their recently conscripted peers. During the two years in which I attended meetings of the Down Syndrome Parent Support Groups of Manhattan and the Bronx, and occasional meetings of other groups, I was particularly impressed by the many levels on which parent peer support was mobilized and extended,

Doubled Discourses

In attending public meetings, hearing uplifting success stories, and participating in peer counseling, parents who rely on support groups often come to speak a doubled discourse of both difference and normalization. On the one hand, they must individually come to terms with a baby who wasn't expected, a baby whose developmental trajectory is largely unknown, and known to be different from other family and community members. On the other hand, families in the support group are given a rich array of resources for the acceptance and incorporation of their Down syndrome children, and taught that they should have high aspirations for their success.

In describing this doubled trajectory of acceptance and normalization of difference, many parents told me a story which circulates widely among families with disabled children. I myself first heard it from activist Emily Kingsley at a parent support group. Some said an obstetrician or pediatrician first recounted the parable, while others attributed it to a caring nurse or social worker. It is Xeroxed and distributed in many hospital pediatric wards:

> Imagine you have planned a vacation to Italy, to see the rose gardens of Florence. You are totally excited, you have read all the guidebooks, your suitcases are packed, and off you go. As the plane lands, the pilot announces, "Sorry, ladies and gentlemen, but this flight has been rerouted to the Netherlands." At first you are very upset: the vacation you dreamed about has been canceled. But you get off the plane, determined to make the best of it. And you gradually discover that the blue tulips of Holland are every bit as pretty as the red roses you had hoped to see in Florence. They may not be as famous, but they are every bit as wonderful. You didn't get a red rose. But you got a blue tulip, and that's quite special, too.

The parable of the blue tulip opens up for me a discussion of "doubled discourses," in which recognition of difference is substituted for judgments of abnormality, and enlightenment occurs. Like all metaphorical journeys of enlightenment, the one which many parents describe is time-consuming, fraught with tests and challenges, and, of course, leads to great rewards. It entails a movement away from focusing on abnormality in their children to accepting differences variously described as physical, mental, emotional, and, sometimes, spiritual. Thus the eye and facial bone structure or low muscle tone so characteristic of Down syndrome becomes perceived as adorable and appealing rather than stigmatized in infants and toddlers; their eagerness and good humor are valued as signs of openness to experience rather than as simple-minded; their affectionate presence and ability to appeal to strangers are resignified as special "gifts" of a disabled child. In journeying narratives, doubled discourses provide maps, metaphors, and images of the normal and abnormal, sometimes described in terms of sameness and difference, human and animal, or even innocence and savagery. Doubled discourses inform not only parental perceptions, but professional attitudes and activist aspirations as well.

These ideas pertaining to doubled, hegemonic, and resistant discourses are highly abstract, but the processes they describe are quite concrete.[3] Nature/culture oppositions, for example, are commonly found in the ordinary language with which mentally retarded children are described by parents and professionals alike. Even those most committed to nurturing and serving developmentally delayed children spontaneously deploy nature/culture oppositions when they use the language of animal imagery to merge them with other species:

> Aleem was born with a lot of hair. I said, "Nurse, is this gonna fall off before I bring him home from the hospital?" Because I didn't want nobody to look at Aleem and think he was a little monkey, not a boy. (Johnella Cornell, African American hairdresser, mother of an infant with Down syndrome)

> Having him in the house, it's like having a gorilla. (Cynthia Foreman, white law professor, mother of a toddler with a chromosome anomaly)

Evolutionary Thought as Diagnostic Technology

Among the 10 common characteristics used for medical diagnosis of Down syndrome in newborns is the presence of a simian crease. The label refers to a single deep fold which runs across the palm, common among people with Down syndrome, in contrast to the multiple angular folds which most people without this condition carry. The medical use of the term "simian" carries with it a devolutionary implication: people with Down syndrome share some physical characteristics with monkeys. Like the racial label of "mongol" to which I turn below, "simian" indexes similarities in its bearers which group and segregate them from people without this characteristic, recategorizing them as closer to the nonhuman primates than to their immediate human kin. Several parents alluded to the problem of "monkey business" in labeling this "stigmata" (another word still widely used in medical texts and practice to describe the signs of Down syndrome). One mother, however, inverted the discourse, resignifying the simian crease:

> He's all heart, like he's such a lovely person, even now, he'll make me stop the car if his brother is crying, so he can get out of the car seat to hug him. He's pure love. He's right there in the moment, all 100% of him, which most normal people don't have that capacity. . . . The simian crease, well, according to palmistry, there are two lines, the head and the heart. The two lines should go across, one's the head, one's the heart. And they (kids with Down syndrome) only have one. So it's like they're merged, the head and the heart, all in one line. And I think that's true of all Down syndrome people, right across the

board. They're all heart. And it shows in the crease. (Judy Kaufman, white nurse, mother of a child with Down syndrome)

In her view, the purity of Down syndrome children's love, vested in their "heart," corresponds to the single, deep crease, when read through the counterdiscourse of palmistry. A covertly negative label is thus reprocessed through an alternative grid to yield a positive attribute.

The idea that children with this condition are less evolved, hence closer to animals and to the "savage races," has a long history. Most famously, John Langdon Haydon Down, for whom the condition was medically named, served as the medical supervisor of the Earlswood Asylum for Idiots in Surrey, England, for a decade beginning in 1858. Later, he ran a private home for retarded adults in Teddington until his death in 1897 (Brain 1967). In keeping with the humanist scientific fashions of his era, Down devoted considerable time to observing and categorizing his patients, whom he divided by what he perceived to be their similarities to various ethnic races. Some were classified as "Ethiopians," some as "Malay." But the largest group contained "Mongols," and it is worth considering Down's reasoning at some length:

> A very large number of congenital idiots are typical Mongols. So marked is this that, when placed side by side, it is difficult to believe that the specimens compared are not children of the same parents. . . . [Down then describes hair, facial, skin, and limb characteristics typical of the population under observation.] The ethnic classification of idiocy which I indicated is of extreme interest philosophically as well as of value practically. Philosophically because it throws light on the question which very much agitated public opinion about the time of the American Civil War. The work of Nott and Glidden labored to prove that the various ethnic families were distinct species, and a strong argument was based on this to justify a certain domestic institution [slavery]. If, however, it can be shown that from some deteriorating influence the children of Caucasian parents can be removed into another ethnic type, it is a strong corroborative argument that the difference is a variable and not a specific one. (Down 1887: 213)

Down's classification thus exhibits a doubled discourse which has perhaps "gone underground" but is by no means banished from popular understanding: on the one hand, "defectives" and "idiots" resemble races which are ranked (here, by the English) as inferior to "Caucasians." Retarded people and exotic races are thus condensed together as evolutionary throwbacks to a prior, intellectually inferior stage. This is the dominant message of the racial classification of retarded patients, and the one which continues to be projected whenever the label of "mongoloid" is used, as it was in the U.S.A. in medical books through the 1970s, and through the 1980s in analogous texts in England (Lippman and Brunger 1991; Gould 1980). Likewise, other medical writers from the third quarter of the 19th century onward commented on the affectionate personalities and amiable humor of people with Down syndrome. Such commentary suggests that scientific practitioners and authors were no less heir to deeply held cultural imagery than were their less-educated contemporaries. To labor an obvious point: we need to recognize that today's biomedical and social scientists, too, live through and in the sociocultural horizons of their own times, including its genetic and prenatal testing technologies.

While I am claiming that the problem of infantilization is linked to pervasive evolutionary paradigms in the history of Western intellectual thought, many authors and activists concerned with disability rights contest a more straightforward present-day version of this problem. They have objected to the infantilization of disabled people in general: criticisms have been leveled against a wide range of "disabling images," including "Jerry's Kids"–style telethons; poster children as fundraisers; and, more grimly, the rigid and punitive practices of enforced dependency encoded in more than a century's history of institutions designed to both protect and contain disabled citizens; as well as in policies and laws limiting the autonomy and choices—in education, jobs, housing, and even sexual, reproductive, and marital relations (Shapiro 1993; Finger 1990). This discourse of infantilization in all its complexity is particularly salient in representations of mentally retarded children, especially those with Down syndrome. Parents of disabled children fall heir to this complex discursive heritage for they spontaneously speak a doubled discourse of both accepting difference and actively working for normalization. Indeed, as many of the stories recounted in this essay suggest, activist parents are particularly articulate in deploying both sides of this worldview.

Bio-Techno-Sociality?

The connections between biomedical and technicist discourses and familial knowledge stand at the center of this chapter. I have implicitly argued that our understandings of new biomedical technologies are significantly enhanced when we examine them in a wide social framework and do not confine our investigation to the clinic. This broader perspective enables us to see technologies in play, as they are understood, appropriated, and occasionally resisted by the parties who deploy them. I am particularly interested in how a language of science (and social science) harking back to 19th-century evolutionary thought and forward to molecular biology is incorporated, and occasionally contested in the fund of social knowledge which families of children with Down syndrome develop. As I have tried to show throughout this essay, modern community-based public institutions like early intervention programs and parent support groups offer powerful resources for parents to become scientifically literate as they seek the best possible services and outcomes for their children. In the process, they also normalize biomedical definitions of the problems and solutions within which a disabling condition is assimilated into family and community life.

Parents (and children) who resculpt their identities using the resources of peer support groups are participating in a process which Paul Rabinow has labeled "biosociality," the forging of a collective identity under the emergent categories of biomedicine and allied sciences (1992). Throughout this essay I have also tried to describe older and deeper traditions of doubled discourses through which children labeled abnormal or anomalous can be reconfigured and integrated into social life. Biomedicine provides discourses with hegemonic claims over this social territory, encouraging enrollment in the categories of biosociality. Its influential technologies provide precise diagnoses, clinical interventions, and statistical pictures of risk and benefit for those who live under the sign of difference. In an emergent worldview of geneticization (Lippman 1991), new claims on identity are powerfully produced through biotechnical interventions. Yet these claims do not go uncontested. Religious orientations and practices, informal folk beliefs, class-based and ethnic traditions, as well as scientifically inflected counter discourses, also lay claim to the interpretation of extra chromosomes. Moreover, not all families of children with Down syndrome rely on support groups, nor are all families equally likely to traffic in scientific worldviews and categories. At stake in the analysis of the traffic between biomedical and familial discourses is an understanding of the inherently uneven seepage of technoscience and its multiple uses and transformations into contemporary social life.

Notes

Acknowledgments: Funding for this study was provided by: the National Endowment for the Humanities, the National Science Foundation, the Rockefeller Foundation's "Changing Gender Roles Program," the Institute for Advanced Studies, the Spencer Foundation, and a semester's sabbatical from the Graduate Faculty, New School for Social Research. I am deeply grateful for their support, and absolve them from any responsibility for the uses to which I have put it. I especially thank the scores of pregnant women, health care providers, and family members who took the time and energy to engage my research questions. Pseudonyms have been used when quoting directly from interviews and conversations.

1   Other aspects of this study are discussed in Rapp 1988, 1993, 1995, 1998, 1999; Marfatia et al. 1991.

2   The work of Alice Hayden and her colleagues, which pioneered infant stimulation for developmentally delayed young children, dates from the 1970s.

3   The influence of Raymond Williams's analysis (1977) of language-borne traditions of political and cultural agency deserves acknowledgment here.

References

Black, R. B., and J. O. Weiss. 1990. "Genetic Support Groups and Social Workers as Partners." *Health and Social Work* 15(2): 91–9.

Brain, L. 1967. "Chairman's Opening Remarks: Historical Introduction." In G. E. W. Wolstenholme and R. Porter (eds.), *Mongolism*. CIBA Foundation Study Group, 25. Boston: Little Brown and Company, pp. 1–5.

Down, J. Langdon. 1887. *Mental Afflictions of Childhood and Youth*. London: J&A Churchill.

Ferguson, T. 1996. *Health Online: How to Find Health Information, Support Groups, and More in Cyberspace*. Reading, MA: Addison-Wesley.

Finger, A. 1990. *Past Due: A Story of Disability, Pregnancy and Birth*. Seattle: Seal Press.

Gould, Stephen Jay. 1980. "Dr. Down's Syndrome." In *The Panda's Thumb: More Reflections in Natural History*. New York: W. W. Norton, pp. 160–8.

Lippman, Abby. 1991. "Prenatal Genetic Testing and Screening: Constructing Needs and Reinforcing Iniquities." *American Journal of Law and Medicine* 17 (1 and 2): 15–50.

Lippman, Abby, and F. Brunger. 1991. "Constructing Down Syndrome: Texts as Informants." *Santé Culture Health* 8 (1–2): 109–31.

Marfatia, L., D. Punales-Morejon, and R. Rapp. 1990. "When an Old Reproductive Technology Becomes a New Reproductive Technology: Serving Underserved Populations." *Birth Defects* 26:109–26.

Nadel, L., and D. Rosenthal (eds.). 1995. *Down Syndrome: Living and Learning in the Community*. New York: John Wiley.

Rabinow, Paul. 1992. "Artificiality and Enlightenment: From Sociobiology to Biosociality." In Jonathan Crary and Sanford Kwinter (eds.), *Incorporations*. New York: Zone (distrib: MIT Press), pp. 234–52.

Rapp, Rayna. 1988. "Chromosomes and Communication: The Discourse of Genetic Counseling." *Medical Anthropology Quarterly* 2 (1): 27–45.

Rapp, Rayna. 1993. "Accounting for Amniocentesis" In Shirley Lindenbaum and Margaret

Lock (eds.), *Knowledge, Power and Practice: The Anthropology of Medicine and Everyday Life. Comparative Studies of Health Systems and Medical Care.* Berkeley: University of California Press, pp. 55–76.

Rapp, Rayna. 1995. "Heredity, or: Revising the Facts of Life." In S. Yanagisako and C. Delaney (eds.), *Naturalizing Power: Essays in Feminist Cultural Analysis.* New York: Routledge, pp. 69–86.

Rapp, Rayna. 1998. "Refusing Prenatal Diagnosis: The Uneven Meanings of Bioscience in a Multicultural World." *Science, Technology, and Human Values* 23 (1): 45–70.

Rapp, Rayna. 1999. *Testing Women, Testing the Fetus: the Social Impact of Amniocentesis in America.* New York: Routledge.

Rothman, B. K. 1986. *The Tentative Pregnancy: Prenatal Diagnosis and the Future of Motherhood.* New York: W. W. Norton.

Scott, Joan W. 1992. "Experience." In Judith Butler and Joan W. Scott (eds.), *Feminists Theorize the Political.* New York: Routledge, pp. 22–40.

Shapiro, J. 1993. *No Pity: How the Disability Rights Movement Is Changing America.* New York: Times Books.

Sutherland, G. A. 1900. "The Differential Diagnosis of Mongolism and Cretinism in Infancy." *The Lancet* 6 January: 23–24.

Trainer, Marilyn. 1991. *Differences in Common: Straight Talk on Mental Retardation, Down Syndrome, and Life.* Rockville, MD: Woodbine House.

Weiss, J. O., and J. Mackta. 1996. *How to Start and Sustain Genetic Support Groups.* Baltimore: Johns Hopkins University Press.

Williams, Raymond. 1977. *Marxism and Literature.* Oxford: Oxford University Press.

Young, Allan. 1995. *The Harmony of Illusions: Inventing Post-Traumatic Stress Disorder.* Princeton, NJ: Princeton University Press.

On Being a Cripple
Nancy Mairs

To escape is nothing. Not to escape is nothing.—Louise Bogan

The other day I was thinking of writing an essay on being a cripple. I was thinking hard in one of the stalls of the women's room in my office building, as I was shoving my shirt into my jeans and tugging up my zipper. Preoccupied, I flushed, picked up my book bag, took my cane down from the hook, and unlatched the door. So many movements unbalanced me, and as I pulled the door open I fell over backward, landing fully clothed on the toilet seat with my legs splayed in front of me: the old beetle-on-its-back routine. Saturday afternoon, the building deserted, I was free to laugh aloud as I wriggled back to my feet, my voice bouncing off the yellowish tiles from all directions. Had anyone been there with me, I'd have been still and faint and hot with chagrin. I decided that it was high time to write the essay.

First, the matter of semantics. I am a cripple. I choose this word to name me. I choose from among several possibilities, the most common of which are "handicapped" and "disabled." I made the choice a number of years ago, without thinking, unaware of my motives for doing so. Even now, I'm not sure what those motives are, but I recognize that they are complex and not entirely flattering. People—crippled or not—wince at the word "cripple," as they do not at "handicapped" or "disabled." Perhaps I want them to wince. I want them to see me as a tough customer, one to whom the fates/gods/viruses have not been kind, but who can face the brutal truth of her existence squarely. As a cripple, I swagger.

But, to be fair to myself, a certain amount of honesty underlies my choice. "Cripple" seems to me a clean word, straightforward and precise. It has an honorable history, having made its first appearance in the Lindisfarne Gospel in the 10th century. As a lover of words, I like the accuracy with which it describes my condition: I have lost the full use of my limbs. "Disabled," by contrast, suggests any incapacity, physical or mental. And I certainly don't like "handicapped," which implies that I have deliberately been put at a disadvantage, by whom I can't imagine (my God is not a Handicapper General), in order to equalize chances in the great race of life. These words seem to me to be moving away from my condition, to be widening the gap between word and reality. Most remote is the recently coined euphemism "differently abled," which partakes of the same semantic hopefulness that transformed countries from "undeveloped" to "underdeveloped," then to "less developed," and finally to "developing" nations. People have continued to starve in those countries during the shift. Some realities do not obey the dictates of language.

Mine is one of them. Whatever you call me, I remain crippled. But I don't care what you call me, so long as it isn't "differently abled," which strikes me as pure verbal garbage designed, by its ability to describe anyone, to describe no one. I subscribe to George Orwell's thesis that "the slovenliness of our language makes it easier for us to have foolish thoughts." And I refuse to participate in the degeneration of the language to the extent that I deny that I have lost anything in the course of this calamitous disease; I refuse to pretend that the only differences between you and me are the various ordinary ones that distinguish any one person from another. But call me "disabled" or "handicapped" if you like. I have long since grown accustomed to them; and if they are vague, at least they hint at the truth. Moreover, I use them myself. Society is no readier to accept crippledness than to accept death, war, sex, sweat, or wrinkles. I would never refer to another person as a cripple. It is the word I use to name only myself.

I haven't always been crippled, a fact for which I am soundly grateful. To be whole of limb is, I know from experience, infinitely more pleasant and useful than to be crippled; and if that knowledge leaves me open to bitterness at my loss, the physical soundness I once enjoyed (though I did not enjoy it half enough) is well worth the occasional stab of regret. Though never any good at sports, I was a normally active child and young adult. I climbed trees, played hopscotch, jumped rope, skated, swam, rode my bicycle, sailed. I despised team sports, spending some of the wretchedest afternoons of my life, sweaty and humiliated, behind a field hockey stick and under a basketball hoop. I tramped alone for miles along the bridle paths that webbed the woods behind the house I grew up in. I swayed through countless dim hours in the arms of one man or another under the scattered shot of light from mirrored balls, and gyrated through countless more as Tab Hunter and Johnny Mathis gave way to the Rolling Stones, Creedence Clearwater Revival, Cream. I walked down the aisle. I pushed baby carriages, changed tires in the rain, marched for peace.

When I was 28 I started to trip and drop things. What at first seemed my natural clumsiness soon became too pronounced to shrug off. I consulted a neurologist, who told me that I had a brain tumor. A battery of tests, increasingly disagreeable, revealed no tumor. About a year and a half later I developed a blurred spot in one eye. I had, at last, the episodes "disseminated in space and time" requisite for a diagnosis: multiple sclerosis. I have never been sorry for the doctor's initial misdiagnosis, however. For almost a week, until the negative results of the tests were in, I thought that I was going to die right away. Every day for the past nearly 10 years, then, has been a kind of gift. I accept all gifts.

Multiple sclerosis is a chronic degenerative disease of the central nervous system, in which the myelin that sheathes the nerves is somehow eaten away and scar tissue forms in its place, interrupting the nerves' signals. During its course, which is unpredictable and uncontrollable, one may lose vision, hearing, speech, the ability to walk, control of bladder and/or bowels, strength in any or all extremities, sensitivity to touch, vibration, and/or pain, potency, coordination of movements—the list of possibilities is lengthy and, yes, horrifying. One may also lose one's sense of humor. That's the easiest to lose and the hardest to survive without.

In the past 10 years, I have sustained some of these losses. Characteristic of MS are sudden attacks, called exacerbations, followed by remissions, and these I have not had. Instead, my disease has been slowly progressive. My left leg is now so weak that I walk with the aid of a brace and a cane; and for distances I use an Amigo, a variation on the electric wheelchair that looks rather like an electrified kiddie car. I no longer have much use of my left hand. Now my right side is weakening as well. I still have the blurred spot in my right eye. Overall, though, I've been lucky so far. My world has, of necessity, been circumscribed by my losses, but the terrain left me has been ample enough for me to continue many of the activities that absorb me: writing, teaching, raising children and cats and plants and snakes, reading, speaking publicly about MS and depression, even playing bridge with people patient and honorable enough to let me scatter cards every which way without sneaking a peek.

Lest I begin to sound like Pollyanna, however, let me say that I don't like having MS. I hate it. My life holds realities—harsh ones, some of them—that no right-minded human being ought to accept without grumbling. One of them is fatigue. I knew of no one with MS who does not complain of bone-weariness; in a disease that presents an astonishing variety of symptoms, fatigue seems to be a common factor. I wake up in the morning feeling the way most people do at the end of a bad day, and I take it from there. As a result, I spend a lot of time *in extremis* and, impatient with limitation, I tend to ignore my fatigue until my body breaks down in some way and forces rest. Then I miss picnics, dinner parties, poetry readings, the brief visits of old friends from out of town. The offspring of a puritanical tradition of exceptional venerability, I cannot view these lapses without shame. My life often seems a series of small failures to do as I ought.

I lead, on the whole, an ordinary life, probably rather like the one I would have led had I not had MS. I am lucky that my predilections were already solitary, sedentary, and bookish—unlike the world-famous French cellist I have read about, or the young woman I talked with one long afternoon who wanted only to be a jockey. I had just begun graduate school when I found out something was wrong with me, and I have remained, interminably, a graduate student. Perhaps I would not have if I'd thought I had the stamina to return to a full-time job as a technical editor; but I've enjoyed my studies.

In addition to studying, I teach writing courses. I also teach medical students how to give neurological examinations. I pick up freelance editing jobs here and there. I have raised a foster son and sent him into the world, where he has made me two grandbabies, and I am still escorting my daughter and son through adolescence. I go to Mass every Saturday. I am a superb, if messy, cook. I am also an enthusiastic laundress, capable of sorting a hamper full of clothes into five subtly differentiated piles, but a terrible housekeeper. I can do italic writing and, in an emergency, bathe an oil-soaked cat. I play a fiendish game of Scrabble. When I have the time and the money, I like to sit on my front steps with my husband, drinking Amaretto and smoking a cigar, as we imagine our counterparts in Leningrad and make sure that the sun gets down once more behind the sharp childish scrawl of the Tucson Mountains.

This lively plenty has its bleak complement, of course, in all the things I can no longer do. I will never run again, except in dreams, and one day I may have to write that I will never walk again. I like to go camping, but

I can't follow George and the children along the trails that wander out of a campsite through the desert or into the mountains. In fact, even on the level I've learned never to check the weather or try to hold a coherent conversation: I need all my attention for my wayward feet. Of late, I have begun to catch myself wondering how people can propel themselves without canes. With only one usable hand, I have to select my clothing with care not so much for style as for ease of ingress and egress, and even so, dressing can be laborious. I can no longer do fine stitchery, pick up babies, play the piano, braid my hair. I am immobilized by acute attacks of depression, which may or may not be physiologically related to MS but are certainly its logical concomitant.

These two elements, the plenty and the privation, are never pure, nor are the delight and wretchedness that accompany them. Almost every pickle that I get into as a result of my weakness and clumsiness—and I get into plenty—is funny as well as maddening and sometimes painful. I recall one May afternoon when a friend and I were going out for a drink after finishing up at school. As we were climbing into opposite sides of my car, chatting, I tripped and fell, flat and hard, onto the asphalt parking lot, my abrupt departure interrupting him in mid-sentence. "Where'd you go?" he called as he came around the back of the car to find me hauling myself up by the door frame. "Are you all right?" Yes, I told him, I was fine, just a bit rattly, and we drove off to find a shady patio and some beer. When I got home an hour or so later, my daughter greeted me with "What have you done to yourself?" I looked down. One elbow of my white turtleneck with the green froggies, one knee of my white trousers, one white kneesock were blood-soaked. We peeled off the clothes and inspected the damage, which was nasty enough but not alarming. That part wasn't funny: The abrasions took a long time to heal, and one got a little infected. Even so, when I think of my friend talking earnestly, suddenly, to the hot thin air while I dropped from his view as though through a trap door, I find the image as silly as something from a Marx Brothers movie.

I may find it easier than other cripples to amuse myself because I live propped by the acceptance and the assistance and, sometimes, the amusement of those around me. Grocery clerks tear my checks out of my checkbook for me, and sales clerks find chairs to put into dressing rooms when I want to try on clothes. The people I work with make sure I teach at times when I am least likely to be fatigued, in places I can get to, with the materials I need. My students, with one anonymous exception (in an end-of-the-semester evaluation), have been unperturbed by my disability.

Some even like it. One was immensely cheered by the information that I paint my own fingernails; she decided, she told me, that if I could go to such trouble over fine details, she could keep on writing essays. I suppose I became some sort of bright-fingered muse. She wrote good essays, too.

The most important struts in the framework of my existence, of course, are my husband and children. Dismayingly few marriages survive the MS test, and why should they? Most 22- and 19-year-olds, like George and me, can vow in clear conscience, after a childhood of chicken pox and summer colds, to keep one another in sickness and in health so long as they both shall live. Not many are equipped for catastrophe: the dismay, the depression, the extra work, the boredom that a degenerative disease can insinuate into a relationship. And our society, with its emphasis on fun and its association of fun with physical performance, offers little encouragement for a whole spouse to stay with a crippled partner. Children experience similar stresses when faced with a crippled parent, and they are more helpless, since parents and children can't usually get divorced. They hate, of course, to be different from their peers, and the child whose mother is tacking down the aisle of a school auditorium packed with proud parents like a Cape Cod dinghy in a stiff breeze jolly well stands out in a crowd. Deprived of legal divorce, the child can at least deny the mother's disability, even her existence, forgetting to tell her about recitals and PTA meetings, refusing to accompany her to stores or church or the movies, never inviting friends to the house. Many do.

But I've been limping along for 10 years now, and so far George and the children are still at my left elbow, holding tight. Anne and Matthew vacuum floors and dust furniture and haul trash and rake up dog droppings and button my cuffs and bake lasagna and Toll House cookies with just enough grumbling so I know that they don't have brain fever. And far from hiding me, they're forever dragging me by racks of fancy clothes or through teeming school corridors, or welcoming gaggles of friends while I'm wandering through the house in Anne's filmy pink babydoll pajamas. George generally calls before he brings someone home, but he does just as many dumb thankless chores as the children. And they all yell at me, laugh at some of my jokes, write me funny letters when we're apart—in short, treat me as an ordinary human being for whom they have some use. I think they like me. Unless they're faking. . . .

Faking. There's the rub. Tugging at the fringes of my consciousness always is the terror that people are kind to me only because I'm a cripple. My mother almost shattered me once, with that instinct mothers have—

blind, I think, in this case, but unerring nonetheless—for striking blows along the fault lines of their children's hearts, by telling me, in an attack on my selfishness, "We all have to make allowances for you, of course, because of the way you are." From the distance of a couple of years, I have to admit that I haven't any idea just what she meant, and I'm not sure that she knew either. She was awfully angry. But at the time, as the words thudded home, I felt my worst fear, suddenly realized. I could bear being called selfish: I am. But I couldn't bear the corroboration that those around me were doing in fact what I'd always suspected them of doing, professing fondness while silently putting up with me because of the way I am. A cripple. I've been a little cracked ever since.

Along with this fear that people are secretly accepting shoddy goods comes a relentless pressure to please—to prove myself worth the burdens I impose, I guess, or to build a substantial account of goodwill against which I may write drafts in times of need. Part of the pressure arises from social expectations. In our society, anyone who deviates from the norm had better find some way to compensate. Like fat people, who are expected to be jolly, cripples must bear their lot meekly and cheerfully. A grumpy cripple isn't playing by the rules. And much of the pressure is self-generated. Early on I vowed that, if I had to have MS, by God I was going to do it well. This is a class act, ladies and gentlemen. No tears, no recriminations, no faint-heartedness.

One way and another, then, I wind up feeling like Tiny Tim, peering over the edge of the table at the Christmas goose, waving my crutch, piping down God's blessing on us all. Only sometimes I don't want to play Tiny Tim. I'd rather be Caliban, a most scurvy monster. Fortunately, at home no one much cares whether I'm a good cripple or a bad cripple as long as I make vichyssoise with fair regularity. One evening several years ago, Anne was reading at the dining-room table while I cooked dinner. As I opened a can of tomatoes, the can slipped in my left hand and juice spattered me and the counter with bloody spots. Fatigued and infuriated, I bellowed, "I'm so sick of being crippled!" Anne glanced at me over the top of her book. "There now," she said, "do you feel better?" "Yes," I said, "yes, I do." She went back to her reading. I felt better. That's about all the attention my scurviness ever gets.

Because I hate being crippled, I sometimes hate myself for being a cripple. Over the years I have come to expect—even accept—attacks of violent self-loathing. Luckily, in general our society no longer connects deformity and disease directly with evil (though a charismatic once told me that I have MS because a devil is in me), and so I'm allowed to move largely at will, even among small children. But I'm not sure that this revision of attitude has been particularly helpful. Physical imperfection, even freed of moral disapprobation, still defies and violates the ideal, especially for women, whose confinement in their bodies as objects of desire is far from over. Each age, of course, has its ideal, and I doubt that ours is any better or worse than any other. Today's ideal woman, who lives on the glossy pages of dozens of magazines, seems to be between the ages of 18 and 25; her hair has body, her teeth flash white, her breath smells minty, her underarms are dry; she has a career but is still a fabulous cook, especially of meals that take less than twenty minutes to prepare; she does not ordinarily appear to have a husband or children; she is trim and deeply tanned; she jogs, swims, plays tennis, rides a bicycle, sails, but does not bowl; she travels widely, even to out-of-the-way places like Finland and Samoa, always in the company of the ideal man, who possesses a nearly identical set of characteristics. There are a few exceptions. Though usually white and often blonde, she may be black, Hispanic, Asian, or Native American, so long as she is unusually sleek. She may be old, provided she is selling a laxative or is Lauren Bacall. If she is selling a detergent, she may be married and have a flock of strikingly messy children. But she is never a cripple.

Like many women I know, I have always had an uneasy relationship with my body. I was not a popular child, largely, I think now, because I was peculiar: intelligent, intense, moody, shy, given to unexpected actions and inexplicable notions and emotions. But as I entered adolescence, I believed myself unpopular because I was homely: my breasts too flat, my mouth too wide, my hips too narrow, my clothing never quite right in fit or style. I was not, in fact, particularly ugly, old photographs inform me, though I was well off the ideal; but I carried this sense of self-alienation with me into adulthood, where it regenerated in response to the depredations of MS. Even with my brace I walk with a limp so pronounced that, seeing myself on the videotape of a television program on the disabled, I couldn't believe that anything but an inch-worm could make progress humping along like that. My shoulders droop and my pelvis thrusts forward as I try to balance myself upright, throwing my frame into a bony S. As a result of contractures, one shoulder is higher than the other and I carry one arm bent in front of me, the fingers curled into a claw. My left arm and leg have wasted into pipe-stems, and I try always to keep them covered. When I think about how my body must look to others, especially to men, to whom I have been trained to display myself, I feel ludicrous, even loathsome.

At my age, however, I don't spend much time thinking about my appearance. The burning egocentricity of adolescence, which assures one that all the world is looking all the time, has passed, thank God, and I'm generally too caught up in what I'm doing to step back, as I used to, and watch myself as though upon a stage. I'm also too old to believe in the accuracy of self-image. I know that I'm not a hideous crone, that in fact, when I'm rested, well dressed, and well made up, I look fine. The self-loathing I feel is neither physically nor intellectually substantial. What I hate is not me but a disease.

I am not a disease.

And a disease is not—at least not singlehandedly—going to determine who I am, though at first it seemed to be going to. Adjusting to a chronic incurable illness, I have moved through a process similar to that outlined by Elizabeth Kübler-Ross in *On Death and Dying.* The major difference—and it is far more significant than most people recognize—is that I can't be sure of the outcome, as the terminally ill cancer patient can. Research studies indicate that, with proper medical care, I may achieve a "normal" life span. And in our society, with its vision of death as the ultimate evil, worse even than decrepitude, the response to such news is, "Oh well, at least you're not going to *die.*" Are there worse things than dying? I think that there may be.

I think of two women I know, both with MS, both enough older than I to have served me as models. One took to her bed several years ago and has been there ever since. Although she can sit in a high-backed wheelchair, because she is incontinent she refuses to go out at all, even though incontinence pants, which are readily available at any pharmacy, could protect her from embarrassment. Instead, she stays at home and insists that her husband, a small quiet man, a retired civil servant, stay there with her except for a quick weekly foray to the supermarket. The other woman, whose illness was diagnosed when she was 18, a nursing student engaged to a young doctor, finished her training, married her doctor, accompanied him to Germany when he was in the service, bore three sons and a daughter, now grown and gone. When she can, she travels with her husband; she plays bridge, embroiders, swims regularly; she works, like me, as a symptomatic-patient instructor of medical students in neurology. Guess which woman I hope to be.

At the beginning, I thought about having MS almost incessantly. And because of the unpredictable course of the disease, my thoughts were always terrified. Each night I'd get into bed wondering whether I'd get out again the next morning, whether I'd be able to see, to speak, to hold a pen between my fingers. Knowing that the day might come when I'd be physically incapable of killing myself, I thought perhaps I ought to do so right away, while I still had the strength. Gradually I came to understand that the Nancy who might one day lie inert under a bedsheet, arms and legs paralyzed, unable to feed or bathe herself, unable to reach out for a gun, a bottle of pills, was not the Nancy I was at present, and that I could not presume to make decisions for that future Nancy, who might well not want in the least to die. Now the only provision I've made for the future Nancy is that when the time comes—and it is likely to come in the form of pneumonia, friend to the weak and the old—I am not to be treated with machines and medications. If she is unable to communicate by then, I hope she will be satisfied with these terms.

Thinking all the time about having MS grew tiresome and intrusive, especially in the large and tragic mode in which I was accustomed to considering my plight. Months and even years went by without catastrophe (at least without one related to MS), and really I was awfully busy, what with George and children and snakes and students and poems, and I hadn't the time, let alone the inclination, to devote myself to being a disease. Too, the richer my life became, the funnier it seemed, as though there were some connection between largesse and laughter, and so my tragic stance began to waver until, even with the aid of a brace and a cane, I couldn't hold it for very long at a time.

After several years I was satisfied with my adjustment. I had suffered my grief and fury and terror, I thought, but now I was at ease with my lot. Then one summer day I set out with George and the children across the desert for a vacation in California. Part way to Yuma I became aware that my right leg felt funny. "I think I've had an exacerbation," I told George. "What shall we do?" he asked. "I think we'd better get the hell to California," I said, "because I don't know whether I'll ever make it again." So we went on to San Diego and then to Orange, up the Pacific Coast Highway to Santa Cruz, across to Yosemite, down to Sequoia and Joshua Tree, and so back over the desert to home. It was a fine two-week trip, filled with friends and fair weather, and I wouldn't have missed it for the world, though I did in fact make it back to California two years later. Nor would there have been any point in missing it, since in MS, once the symptoms have appeared, the neurological damage has been done, and there's no way to predict or prevent that damage.

The incident spoiled my self-satisfaction, however. It renewed my grief and fury and terror, and I learned that one never finishes adjusting to MS. I don't know now why I thought one would. One does not, after all, finish adjusting to life, and MS is simply a fact of my life—not my favorite fact, of course—but as ordinary as my nose and my tropical fish and my yellow Mazda station wagon. It may at any time get worse, but no amount of worry or anticipation can prepare me for a new loss. My life is a lesson in losses. I learn one at a time.

And I had best be patient in the learning, since I'll have to do it, like it or not. As any rock fan knows, you can't always get what you want. Particularly when you have MS. You can't, for example, get cured. In recent years researchers and the organizations that fund research have started to pay MS some attention even though it isn't fatal; perhaps they have begun to see that life is something other than a quantitative phenomenon, that one may be very much alive for a very long time in a life that isn't worth living. The researchers have made some progress toward understanding the mechanism of the disease: it may well be an autoimmune reaction triggered by a slow-acting virus. But they are nowhere near its prevention, control, or cure. And most of us want to be cured. Some, unable to accept incurability, grasp at one treatment after another, no matter how bizarre: megavitamin therapy, gluten-free diet, injections of cobra venom, hypo-thermal suits, lymphocytopharesis, hyperbaric chambers. Many treatments are probably harmless enough, but none are curative.

The absence of a cure often makes MS patients bitter toward their doctors. Doctors are, after all, the priests of modern society, the new sha-mans, whose business is to heal, and many an MS patient roves from one to another, searching for the "good" doctor who will make him well. Doctors too think of themselves as healers, and for this reason many have trouble dealing with MS patients, whose disease in its intransigence defeats their aims and mocks their skills. Too few doctors, it is true, treat their patients as whole human beings, but the reverse is also true. I have always tried to be gentle with my doctors, who often have more at stake in terms of ego than I do. I may be frustrated, maddened, depressed by the incurability of my disease, but I am not diminished by it, and they are. When I push myself up from my seat in the waiting room and stumble toward them, I incarnate the limitation of their powers. The least I can do is refuse to press on their tenderest spots.

This gentleness is part of the reason that I'm not sorry to be a cripple. I didn't have it before. Perhaps I'd have developed it anyway—how could I know such a thing?—and I wish I had more of it, but I'm glad of what I have. It has opened and enriched my life enormously, this sense that my frailty and need must be mirrored in others, that in searching for and shaping a stable core in a life wrenched by change and loss, change and loss, I must recognize the same process, under individual conditions, in the lives around me. I do not deprecate such knowledge, however I've come by it.

All the same, if a cure were found, would I take it? In a minute. I may be a cripple, but I'm only occasionally a loony and never a saint. Anyway, in my brand of theology God doesn't give bonus points for a limp. I'd take a cure; I just don't need one. A friend who also has MS startled me once by asking, "Do you ever say to yourself, 'Why me, Lord?' " "No, Michael, I don't," I told him, "because whenever I try, the only response I can think of is 'Why not?' " If I could make a cosmic deal, who would I put in my place? What in my life would I give up in exchange for sound limbs and a thrilling rush of energy? No one. Nothing. I might as well do the job myself. Now that I'm getting the hang of it.

Tell Me, Tell Me
Irving Kenneth Zola

Now I was the one who was nervous. Here we were alone in her room thousands of miles from my home.

"Well, my personal care attendant is gone, so it will all be up to you," she said sort of puckishly, "Don't look so worried! I'll tell you what to do."

This was a real turn-about. It was usually me who reassured my partner. Me who, after putting aside my cane, and removing all the clothes that masked my brace, my corset, my scars, my thinness, my body. Me who'd say, "Well, now you see 'the real me.'" How often I'd said that, I thought to myself. Saying it in a way that hid my basic fear—that this real me might not be so nice to look at . . . might not be up to "the task" before me.

She must have seen something on my face, for she continued to reassure me, "Don't be afraid." And as she turned her wheelchair toward me she smiled at me that smile that first hooked me a few hours before. "Well," she continued, "first we have to empty my bag." And with that brief introduction we approached the bathroom.

Anger quickly replaced fear as I realized she could get her wheelchair into the doorway but not through it.

"Okay, take one of those cans," she said pointing to an empty Sprite, "and empty my bag into it."

Though I'd done that many times before it wasn't so easy this time. I quite simply couldn't reach her leg from a sitting position on the toilet and she couldn't raise her foot toward me. So down to the floor I lowered myself and sat at her feet. Rolling up her trouser leg I fumbled awkwardly with the clip sealing the tube. I looked up at her and she laughed, "It won't break and neither will I."

Irving Kenneth Zola, "Tell Me, Tell Me," from *Ordinary Lives.* © 1982 by Irving Zola. Reprinted by permission of the author.

I got it open and her urine poured into the can. Suddenly I felt a quiver in my stomach. The smell was more overpowering than I'd expected. But I was too embarrassed to say anything. Emptying the contents into the toilet I turned to her again as she backed out. "What should I do with the can?" I asked.

"Wash it out," she answered as if it were a silly question. "We try to recycle everything around here."

Proud of our first accomplishment we headed back into the room. "Now comes the fun part . . . getting me into the bed." For a few minutes we looked for the essential piece of equipment—the transfer board. I laughed silently to myself. I seemed to always be misplacing my cane—that constant reminder of my own physical dependency. Maybe for her it was the transfer board.

When we found it leaning against the radiator I reached down to pick it up and almost toppled over from its weight. Hell of a way to start, I thought to myself. If I can't lift this, how am I going to deal with her? More carefully this time, I reached down and swung it onto the bed.

She parallel parked her wheelchair next to the bed, grinned, and pointed to the side arm. I'd been this route before, so I leaned over and dismantled it. Then with her patient instructions I began to shift her. The board had to be placed with the wider part on the bed and the narrower section slipped under her. This would eventually allow me to slip her across. But I could do little without losing my own balance. So I laid down on the mattress and shoved the transfer board under her. First one foot and then the other I lifted toward me till she was at about a 45 degree angle in her wheelchair. I was huffing but she sat in a sort of bemused silence. Then came the scary part. Planting myself as firmly as I could behind her, I leaned forward, slipped my arms under hers and around her chest and then with one heave hefted her onto the bed. She landed safely with her head on the pillow, and I joined her wearily for a moment's rest. For this I should have gone into training, I smiled silently. And again, she must have understood as she opened her eyes even wider to look at me. What beautiful eyes she has, I thought, a brightness heightened by her very dark thick eyebrows.

"You're blushing again," she said.

"How can you tell that it's not from exhaustion?" I countered.

"By your eyes . . . because they're twinkling."

I leaned over and kissed her again. But more mutual appreciation would have to wait, there was still work to be done.

The immediate task was to plug her wheelchair into the portable recharger. This would have been an easy task for anyone except the technical idiot that I am.

"Be careful," she said. "If you attach the wrong cables you might shock yourself."

I laughed. A shock from this battery would be small compared to what I've already been through.

But even this attaching was not so easy. I couldn't read the instructions clearly, so down to the floor I sank once more.

After several tentative explorations, I could see the gauge registering a positive charge. I let out a little cheer.

She turned her head toward me and looked down as I lay stretched out momentarily on the floor, "Now the real fun part," she teased. "You have to undress me."

"Ah, but for this," I said in my most rakish tones, "we'll have to get closer together." My graceful quip was, however, not matched by any graceful motion. For I had to crawl on the floor until I could find a chair onto which I could hold and push myself to a standing position.

As I finally climbed onto the bed, I said, "Is this trip really necessary?" I don't know what I intended by that remark but we both laughed. And as we did and came closer, we kissed, first gently and then with increasing force until we said almost simultaneously, "We'd better get undressed."

"Where should I start?" I asked.

My own question struck me as funny. It was still another reversal. It was something I'd never asked a woman. But on those rare occasions on which I'd let someone undress me, it was often their first question.

"Wherever you like," she said in what seemed like a coquettish tone.

I thought it would be best to do the toughest first, so I began with her shoes and socks. These were easy enough but not so her slacks. Since she could not raise herself, I alternated between pulling, tugging, and occasionally lifting. Slowly over her hips, I was able to slip her slacks down from her waist. By now I was sweating as much from anxiety as exertion. I was concerned I'd be too rough and maybe hurt her but most of all I was afraid that I might inadvertently pull out her catheter. At least in this anxiety I was not alone. But with her encouragement we again persevered. Slacks, underpants, corset all came off in not so rapid succession.

At this point a different kind of awkwardness struck me. There was something about my being fully clothed and her not that bothered me. I was her lover, not her personal care attendant. And so I asked if she minded if I took off my clothes before continuing.

I explained in a half-truth that it would make it easier for me to get around now 'without all my equipment.' "Fine with me," she answered and again we touched, kissed and lay for a moment in each other's arms.

Pushing myself to a sitting position I removed my own shirt, trousers, shoes, brace, corset, bandages, undershorts until I was comfortably nude. The comfort lasted but a moment. Now I was embarrassed. I realized that she was in a position to look upon my not so beautiful body. My usual defensive sarcasm about 'the real me' began somewhere back in my brain but this time it never reached my lips. "Now what?" was the best I could come up with.

"Now my top . . . and quickly. I'm roasting in all these clothes."

I didn't know if she was serious or just kidding but quickness was not in the cards. With little room at the head of the bed, I simply could not pull them off as I had the rest of her clothes.

"Can you sit up?" I asked.

"Not without help."

"What about once you're up?"

"Not then either . . . not unless I lean on you."

This time I felt ingenious. I locked my legs around the corner of the bed and then grabbing both her arms I yanked her to a sitting position. She made it but I didn't. And I found her sort of on top of me, such a tangle of bodies we could only laugh. Finally, I managed to push her and myself upright. I placed her arms around my neck. And then, after the usual tangles of hair, earrings and protestations that I was trying to smother her, I managed to pull both her sweater and blouse over her head. By now I was no longer being neat, and with an apology threw her garments toward the nearest chair. Naturally I missed . . . but neither of us seemed to care. The bra was the final piece to go and with the last unhooking we both plopped once more to the mattress.

For a moment we just lay there but as I reached across to touch her, she pulled her head back mockingly, "We're not through yet."

"You must be kidding!" I said, hoping that my tone was not as harsh as it sounded.

"I still need my booties and my night bag."

"What are they for?" I asked out of genuine curiosity.

"Well my booties—those big rubber things on the table—keep my heels from rubbing and getting irritated and the night bag . . . well that's so we won't have to worry about my urinating during the night."

The booties I easily affixed, the night bag was another matter. Again it was more my awkwardness than the complexity of the task. First, I removed the day bag, now emptied, but still strapped around her leg and replaced it with the bigger night one. Careful not to dislodge the catheter I had to find a place lower than the bed to attach it so gravity would do the rest. Finally, the formal work was done. The words of my own thoughts bothered me for I realized that there was part of me that feared what "work" might still be ahead.

She was not the first disabled woman I'd ever slept with but she was, as she had said earlier, "more physically dependent than I look." And she was. As I prepared to settle down beside her, I recalled watching her earlier in the evening over dinner. Except for the fact that she needed her steak cut and her cigarette lit, I wasn't particularly conscious of any dependence. In fact quite the contrary, for I'd been attracted in the first place to her liveliness, her movements, her way of tilting her head and raising her eyebrows. But now it was different. This long process of undressing reinforced her physical dependency.

But before I lay down again, she interrupted my associations. "You'll have to move me. I don't feel centered." And as I reached over to move her legs, I let myself fully absorb her nakedness. Lying there she somehow seemed bigger. Maybe it was the lack of muscle-tone if that's the word—but her body seemed somehow flattened out. Her thighs and legs and her breasts, the latter no longer firmly held by her bra, flapped to her side. I felt guilty a moment for even letting myself feel anything. I was as anxious as hell but with no wish to flee. I'm sure my face told it all. For with her eyes she reached out to me and with her words gently reassured me once again, "Don't be afraid."

And so as I lay beside her we began our loving. I was awkward at first, I didn't know what to do with my hands. And so I asked. In a way it was no different than with any other woman. In recent years, I often find myself asking where and how they like to be touched. To my questions she replied, "My neck . . . my face . . . especially my ears. . . ." And as I drew close she swung her arms around my neck and clasped me in a surprisingly strong grip.

"Tighter, tighter, hold me tighter," she laughed again. "I'm not fragile. . . . I won't break."

And so I did. And as we moved I found myself naturally touching other parts of her body. When I realized this I pulled back quickly, "I don't know what you can feel."

"Nothing really in the rest of my body."

"What about your breasts," I asked rather uncomfortably.

"Not much . . . though I can feel your hands there when you press."

And so I did. And all went well until she told me to bite and squeeze harder, then I began to shake. Feeling the quiver in my arm, she again reassured me. So slowly and haltingly where she led, I followed.

I don't know how long we continued kissing and fondling, but as I lay buried in her neck, I felt the heels of her hands digging into my back and her voice whispering, "tell me . . . tell me."

Suddenly I got scared again. Tell her what? Do I have to say that I love her . . .? Oh my God. And I pretended for a moment not to hear.

"Tell me . . . tell me," she said again as she pulled me tighter. With a deep breath, I meekly answered, "Tell you what?"

"Tell me what you're doing," she said softly, "so I can visualize it." With her reply I breathed a sign of relief. And a narrative voyage over her body began; I kissed, fondled, caressed every part I could reach. Once I looked up and I saw her with her head relaxed, eyes closed, smiling.

It was only when we stopped that I realized I was unerect. In a way my penis was echoing my own thoughts. I had no need to thrust, to fuck, to quite simply go where I couldn't be felt.

She again intercepted my own thoughts—"Move up, please put my hands on you," and as I did I felt a rush through my body. She drew me toward her again until her lips were on my chest and gently she began to suckle me as I had her a few minutes before. And so the hours passed, ears, mouths, eyes, tongues inside one another.

And every once in a while she would quiver in a way which seemed orgasmic. As I thrust my tongue as deep as I could in her ear, her head would begin to shake, her neck would stretch out and then her whole upper body would release with a sigh.

Finally, at some time well past one we looked exhaustedly at one another. "Time for sleep," she yawned, "but there is one more task—an easy one. I'm cold and dry so I need some hot water."

"Hot water!" I said rather incredulously.

"Yup, I drink it straight. It's my one vice."

And as she sipped the drink through a long straw, I closed my eyes and curled myself around the pillow. My drifting off was quickly stopped as she asked rather archly, "You mean you're going to wrap yourself around that rather than me?"

I was about to explain that I rarely slept curled around anyone and certainly not vice-versa but I thought better of it, saying only, "Well, I might not be able to last this way all night."

"Neither might I," she countered. "My arm might also get tired."

We pretended to look at each other angrily but it didn't work. So we came closer again, hugged and curled up as closely as we could, with my head cradled in her arm and my leg draped across her.

And much to my surprise I fell quickly asleep—unafraid, unsmothered, and more importantly rested, cared for, and loved.

Finch the Spastic Speaks
Gordon Weaver

The doctor's achievements with problems like mine are famous; his connection with the university—research and occasional lectures—accounts for my choice of this state, city, school. I had, of course, my pick of institutions. He is, I think, basically kind, but too great a scientist to obscure his ministrations with mercy or pity, and for this I am grateful. Though we have met each month for the past five years, we have no . . . what you would call *rapport.*

Answer a leading question: what is Finch? Is he the body, the badly made bundle of nerve ends and motor responses? Or is he the mind, the intelligence, the scholarships and fellowships, the heap of plaques, medallions, scrolls, given in testimony to his brilliance? Or is he something even more than these, a total greater than the sum of his parts? I ask you, does not Finch . . . feel?

Ah, you mock! Finch, you say, Finch of all people! Finch? Poor, pathetic Finch, with his tested and recorded intelligence quotient of 233, locked forever in his prison of chaotic muscles. Poor Finch, who falls as easily over a curbstone as an infant toddler over a toy. Unfortunate Finch, whose large, staring eyes often roll wildly behind his thick glasses. Tragic Finch, who must choke and strain like some strangling madman if he is to ask for so much as a drink of water.

You underestimate me.

Stripped to shorts and undershirt, I sit on the edge of the doctor's examination table, legs dangling. With an ordinary tape measure, he checks my calves, thighs, forearms, biceps, to see if any disparity has developed. Kneeling, he exerts pressure on each foot as I pull up against him, testing

Gordon Weaver, "Finch the Spastic Speaks," from *The Entombed Men of Thule.* © 1972 by Gordon Weaver. Reprinted by permission of Louisiana State University Press.

for any distinction in muscular strength. "Okey doke," he says, pausing to jot conclusions in the thick folder bearing my name that will doubtless one day yield monographs, to his ever-spreading renown. "Ready?" he says, handing pen and folder to the attentive nurse. I do not speak needlessly.

He stands near me, raises his hands, spreads his fingers like a wrestler coming to close with an opponent in the center of the ring. And I see it just that way, a contest, for my amusement. I am very strong.

Relaxation is the secret. I half-close my eyes to concentrate, bombarding my shoulders, arms, hands, fingers, with commands: relax! Gradually, the fingers twitch, release the edge of the table, and slowly my arms rise, fingers open to meet his. He meets me halfway, interlocks his fingers with mine, and we push, face to face. I watch his skin flush, eyes protrude ever so slightly, teeth clench. We push, as earnest as two fraternity boys arm wrestling for a pitcher of beer. I am very strong.

He grunts without meaning to, catches himself, pushes again, then gives up, exhales loudly. "Okay," he says. I smell the aroma of some candied lozenge on his breath. Is there a trace of sweat on his tanned brow? "Okay," he says, "okay now." To save time, the nurse helps him unlace our fingers.

There was an impressive formal reception when I came to the university, five years ago. Not for me alone, of course. Invited were perhaps a hundred new students with some claim to distinction: merit scholars, recipients of industrial science fellowships, national prize-winning essayists, valedictorians in great number. But, except for a small covey of timid and meticulous Negro boys and girls, to whom all the dignitaries paid solemn if perfunctory court, I was easily the center of attention.

Imagine Finch, the spastic, dressed for the occasion. (The habitual fraternity jacket was not to come until my sophomore year, when Delta Sigma Kappa, campus jocks, coming to know me from my work at the gymnasium, adopted me as something of a mascot, perhaps their social service project for the year—the jacket was free, as are the passes to football and basketball games. I could, if I cared to, sit on the players' bench.) I wear a dark suit with vest, and the dormitory housemother has tied a neat, hard little knot in my tie for me. I stand near the refreshment table, as erect as my balance will permit. My left arm is locked into place, palm up, whereon I place a napkin, a saucer, and a clear glass cup of red punch which I have no interest in tasting. With utmost care, I have tenderly grasped the cup's handle between thumb and forefinger, and there I stand, listening, questioning, answering, discussing (I speak extraordinarily well this day!) with a crowd of deans, departmental chairmen, senior professors, polite faculty wives, the president of the student body, and a handful of upper-class and graduate honor students. From time to time a few wander away to make a ritual obeisance to the Negroes, but they return.

Finch, Finch is the main attraction! Finch, with his certified intelligence quotient of 233, Finch who probes and reveals yawning gaps in the reading of graduate students 10 years his senior, Finch who speaks with authority of science, literature, and contemporary politics, Finch who dares to contradict the holder of the endowed chair in history! Oh, there is glory in this! Finch, who cannot tie a shoelace, cannot safely strike a match, has trouble inserting dimes in vending machine slots—Finch is master here!

The other new students stand on the fringe of my audience, bewildered, or stroll off to stare dumbly at the obligatory portraits of past university presidents and trustees that dot the walls. I grow weary, but the tremor of my head can pass for judicious nodding, the tick in my cheek for chewing gum. The punch in my cup rocks a little. Who is the free man here?

Is it the scholar-professor who must think hard to recall specific points in his dissertation if he is to answer me? Is it the hatchet-faced, balding Dean of Letters and Science who carefully defends the university against its out-of-state rival, which also sought Finch? Is it the beautiful girl who won a regional science fair, but stands here, open-mouthed and silent as Finch explicates the relationship between set theory and symbolic logic? Is it the faculty wife with bleached hair, calculating her sitter's wages, who dares not depart for fear of offending Finch? Or is it Finch, whose brain roars with commands of discipline to his muscles, achieved only with the excruciating tenuous force of his will?

What you might think a disaster was actually the climax of my triumph. I had almost no warning. I felt the spasm that plunged my chin down against my chest, felt a stiffening come over my arms and hands, but no more. As nicely as if I wished it, I tossed my cup of punch up and back over my shoulder, while the saucer snapped in two in my left hand, giving me a rather nasty cut across the palm. There was a fine spray of punch in the air, the cup shattering harmlessly against the wainscoted wall behind me. Only the beautiful winner of the regional science fair forgot herself so far as to shriek as if she had been goosed.

I allowed no time for tension or embarrassment. I spoke quickly, clear as a bell, "Please excuse me," and reached up with the napkin to wipe punch from my forehead and hair. I asked for a chair, was seated, and the conversation continued as before while my hand was bandaged.

Which of you, I ask, would dare such a thing outside your dreams? When I smiled they laughed. And the winner of the science fair blushed, mortified by her outburst, as I related other such experiences in my past for their entertainment.

Above all, do not underestimate me.

The doctor breathes heavily. At my sides, my hands still hold their clawlike, grappling shape. A small victory, I am stronger than he; something to savor for a short time each month. He writes again, says, "I trust you're keeping up with the schedule." I nod, or what passes for a nod. The nurse helps me into my shirt and trousers.

"I can't emphasize that enough, James," the doctor said. He has called me by my first name since I met him; I was, after all, only 17 when my parents arranged the first consultation.

"I don't want to alarm you," he said, "but there is evidence of unilateral deterioration—" I know the jargon as well as he—"your right side's progressing fairly rapidly. I want you to stay with the schedule, and don't miss the medication. I'm going to write your folks. . . ."

I have always kept the schedule. Ever since I can remember, there has been a schedule, exercises, work with weights, isometrics, special breathing and relaxation drills. At home, in my dormitory room, in classes, on regular visits to the gymnasium, I have faithfully kept the schedule. And medication. Pills, occasional injections as new serums and theories prevail. My wristwatch is equipped with a small but persistent buzzer to keep me precisely on the schedule.

"You know the literature on progression yourself . . . ," he is saying. The nurse is fastening the buckles on my shoes; I once counted it a great breakthrough to go from snaps to buckles. I looked forward to laces, but no longer care about such matters. The nurse brings my fraternity jacket.

"You do understand the import of what I'm saying, James?" the doctor said. I realized he wanted more than a nod or flutter of eyelids. I must speak.

I did not forget the beautiful winner of the regional science fair. I saw her now and again during my first quarter at the university. We passed in corridors, joined the same lines in the cafeteria and bookstore, and once, sat in the same aisle in the auditorium to watch a foreign film. Whether she seemed to notice me or not (how, I ask, does one *not notice* Finch?), I never forgot her face as I saw it when my hand was being bandaged at the reception, flushed with distress for her unmannerly and callous shriek at my misfortune with the punch cup. I understood she was emotionally in my debt until I should release her.

As these weeks passed, I began to pay attention, to sometimes go out of my way to meet her as she left a class or walked one of the narrow paths crossing the wide, green campus on her way to or from her dormitory. I found stations, fixed and concealed points, from which to observe her at length. It was not until the first long vacation, however, that I recognized how affected I was by her beauty. Her name was Ellen.

Picture Finch: his father or mother drives him to the public library for a day's work, and he burrows into his books and three-by-five notecards with a determination the envy of any serious scholar. A librarian helps him carry books to a far, quiet corner near a window, where the sun's warm rays belie the frozen, cold stillness of the snow-covered streets and buildings outside. He begins, reads, writes, outlines, and time passes without his knowing it, or caring. But a dingy cloud throws him into shade, or the day has already faded to that dark, chill cast that is a deep winter afternoon. He lifts his trembling head, closes his eyes, sore with strain, and suddenly sees nothing, thinks of nothing, but the beautiful Ellen. History or political science or biology evaporate, and his reality consists only of her pale blond hair, the hazel tint of her bright, large eyes, the unbelievably fresh smoothness of her skin, the light downy hair on her arm, the sparkle of her white, even teeth; to the exclusion of even his life-long awareness of his insane, spastic body, Finch knows only this beautiful Ellen!

I see, I *feel* the beauty of her movement: her hand glides to gesture, her fingers curl around a pencil, artless as the flow of water, no more self-conscious than the law of gravity; her head tilts, or she throws it to cast her hair back out of her eyes; she sits, crosses one long, sleek leg over the other, and it bobs in time to the animation of her conversation; she arches her back, thrusts out her breasts, and lets her coat slide down her stiffened arms as if they were greased rails; she climbs the steps to her dormitory, her knees churning like pistons, and pauses before the door to stomp snow from her high, black boots; alone on a path (but Finch, hidden, watches!) she holds her books against her stomach, runs, slides like a tightwire walker on a streak of silvery ice.

Ah, thinks Finch, oblivious to his books and the dry, clean smell of the library, *beauty!* She walks and runs, this beautiful Ellen, sits, jumps, with the floating, liquid perfection of some gaudy reptile.

It was Christmas, and I was home with my family, and I had reading and research papers to do, but I—why should I not say it—was in love. Finch was eighteen, and in love for the first time in his life. Yes, *Finch loves!* Or, thought he did. Loved, once.

"Jim?" says a voice outside this absorbing, warming reality—it is his father, or his mother, come at the agreed hour. "Jim, it's time to go, we'll be late for supper." Finch opens his eyes, and it is winter again, cars make slushy noises outside the window, and he must reorder his mind, recall where he left off his research, stack his cards and papers, answer questions, think of real things, when and where and what he is.

It is Christmas Eve night, and my family gathers at the huge tree that dominates our living room. There are special things to eat, and I am allowed a little whiskey for the occasion. My mother is happy in her Christmas way, tears in her eyes as she hands me many expensive gifts, elaborately wrapped—a new fountain pen, made in Germany, with a thick barrel, so much easier for the fingers to circle; a cowhide briefcase with a manacle fitted to the handle so I can lock it to my wrist (this will require new feats of balance, but, to please her, I say nothing of it); an astrakhan hat, in vogue among students this year—she will not have me lack what others have!

I appear to enjoy this annual ceremony as much as they. I give, and get, an enthusiastic hug and kiss as I open each gift, being careful not to too badly smash or tear the fluffy bows and ribbons and bright paper as I unwrap each package, labeled, as always, *To Jim from Santa*. I faithfully follow my father's direction as he films all this, stooped behind his camera and tripod, his words just a bit thick with too much whiskey. I pose, seated on the floor between my younger brother and sister (they are both perfectly ordinary), put my arms around their necks, do my best to smile so that I will not look drunk or half-witted in the movie.

But I go to bed early, pleading fatigue, the ritual splash of whiskey, the research to be done even on Christmas day. I leave them, to seek Ellen, to be alone in my bed and nourish this thrilling, weakening sensation of love that for the first time in my life lets me, makes me, forget myself. My taut body relaxes in stages, by degrees, while my brain whirls gently with real and imaginary visions of this exquisite Ellen. I still hear music, the rattle of happy, sentimental talk as my parents sit up late, drinking and watching old Christmas films—and for the first time in my life, I am not ashamed of the erection that keeps me from sleep.

The good doctor has just informed me that my future is limited. The paralysis, unknown to me as I labor faithfully at my schedules, as I dose myself to the point of nausea, has been progressing. Subtle as a tiny worm, my malady has eaten away at this comic body, devouring days of my life. The figures noted in my folder already record the shrinkage from atrophy. The ultimate and sure end, if progression is not arrested, will be a spasm of sufficient duration, somewhere vital, the throat, the diaphragm, and I will suffocate in a final paroxysm, no different than if I had swallowed a fish-bone. Yet he asks me to speak now, reassure him that I understand and face his diagnosis calmly.

He waits, brows lifted, expectant, needing; the nurse returns my file to the cabinet drawer. I speak, for us both, a lie.

"I'm . . . not . . . alarmed," I say, almost effortlessly. True, my mouth twists in shapes wholly unrelated to the words. My tongue emerges as I finish, and I am in danger of drooling idiotically, but the words, slow-paced, are only a little distorted, like the stridency in the voices of the deaf when they sing.

True, no one could take me for normal, but that I speak at all is a minor wonder.

"Good," the doctor said, "good," washing his hands. The nurse has left the room.

I have said, does not Finch feel? But feeling brings on paralysis, in-terrupts the constant stream of impulses from brain to muscle—feeling means stasis, immobility. I must be alone if I am to allow myself grief or wonder. Solitude waits only on my tortured passage through the waiting room, a perilous descent of the stairs, a short ride on my bicycle to the dormitory.

Back at the university, I determined to call her. Though I might have known she would not refuse me, I shook as if I suffered Saint Vitus' dance, telephone receiver in hand, until she said yes, she would accompany me to a movie. "Will we be walking, Jimmy?" she asked. I faltered, choked, not having thought to the point of specific arrangements. Finch, pride of the history department, flustered like any juvenile! *No*, I managed to stammer: even the closest theater was a trek across the campus, far enough to be humiliating. I cringed, imagining us, arm in arm perhaps, floundering and swaying on the icy paths. "Oh," Ellen said, and waited for me to speak. I rocked fitfully on the small seat in the booth in the empty dormitory corridor. It might have sounded, in her ear, like the wild and frantic banging of someone prematurely buried.

I nearly mentioned my bicycle, but this was unsafe in winter for me alone—with her, perched on the handlebars, it would have been macabre. "I have a car, Jimmy," she said sweetly. And so we went in her car.

I do not remember what film we saw, for through most of the feature I sat rigid, inching my hand closer and closer to hers. Something happened in the film, something loud, action with bombastic musical accompaniment, and damning myself eternally a coward if I failed to act, at last, with a short, convulsive, clutching thrust, I slipped my hand over hers. She was kind enough to turn her head to me, and smile. We sat that way until the house lights came up, my sweaty palm covering the back of her smooth, cool hand. Surreptitiously, I breathed her delicious perfume, and from the corner of my eye, exulted in the delicate turn of her ear, her nostril, the way her blond hair swept upward on the back of her neck, the soft line of her throat, the faint heaving of her bosom.

We parked at the dormitory complex. It was very cold, and the other cars raised thick, steady clouds of exhaust. Their occupants, clasped in long, intense embraces, moved as shadows behind the frosted windows, all about us. Every few minutes, an engine died, a door opened, and a couple emerged to walk to one or another of the buildings. In the doorway lights we saw clearly their final kissing and fondling.

Ellen left the motor running, and we sat, silent. She wore a heavy coat, open, with a hood, a ring of snowy rabbit fur framing her face. We sat, quiet, while my brain raced, wondering what I should, or would, or could do. I did not want, at first, to touch her, but felt I must. I could feel the tick in my cheek grow worse, knew my limbs were frozen, hands balled in fists in my lap.

"Do you want me to walk with you to your dorm, Jimmy?" she said, and quickly, she leaned toward me, perhaps to open the door for me, I do not know. Somehow it terrified me, and I lurched, as if I had been given an electrical shock, and I spoke.

"No!" I said. I did not mean to touch her, not at first.

My left arm came up, swiftly enough to have given her a jarring slap, but stopped short, and I caressed her cheek and chin. She seemed to lean further toward me. I willed my right hand to take her shoulder and turn her fully toward me. I think she wanted me to kiss her, or thought I wanted to—I looked into her face, and she was, again, smiling, as she had in the theater. Her mouth was open slightly, her eyelids fluttering.

It was then I decided to kiss her, and let myself feel fully the love I had not permitted myself before, ever. I think I may have begun to cry.

I was not in love, I understand now, not in love with this beautiful Ellen, this precocious student of science, with her skin like milk, her grace of movement so inherent and unconscious as to put a dancer or an animal to shame. I did not love her, I say. I felt, then, as I moved my head closer to hers, the welling up of my response to all the love showered on me before, by my family, doctors, nurses, therapists, teachers.

Should not Finch, like you, feel?

I was, surely, crying, making a grotesque sound like the growling of a beast. I was moved by the collective force of all that love—my weepy mother, standing at the end of the parallel handrails, holding back her tears, whispering, *step Jimmy, step, one more step to mother, Jimmy*; my father, carrying me high on his shoulders in the teeth of a biting wind at a football game, cheering, *look at him go, Jimmy!*, suddenly letting me drop into his arms, hugging me to his chest, saying, *it's okay, Jim, it's okay*, because he thought I felt hurt, unable ever to run like that anonymous halfback; my teachers, *see, James knows, you're all so smart aleck, but James always has the right answer*; my sister, *Jimmy, are you the smartest person in the world?*; an auditorium filled with parents, the state superintendent of education saying, *I cannot say enough in praise of James Finch*, rolls of applause as I move, like some crippled insect, to the podium, everyone's eyes wet . . . I draw Ellen's face close to mine, my hand tightening on her shoulder. Stupidly, I try to speak.

Kiss me, I want to say, with all the force muted by all the tenderness of my need. And I am betrayed once more by my odious body. Ellen's mouth is closed to meet mine, and I gargle some ugly distortion of my intention: *Kwaryoup*, I say, and her eyes pop open in horror. I hold her tightly, feel her resistance, try again—*Keeeebryumbeel* erupts from my throat. She tries to release herself. *Sochavadeebow*, I am saying, trying to reassure her.

"Jimmy!" she says, and pulls at my wrists. "Let go, Jimmy!" I want to comply, but my left hand, nerves along my arm seeming to explode like a string of firecrackers, raises, comes down on her breast. "Jimmy!" she shrieks, and is crying now. "Get away from me, Jimmy, let go of me! Get your hands off me, you're hurting me, Jimmy!"

And it is over, mercifully. The door is open, I crawl or fall out, scramble through the snow on my hands and knees, slobbering, falling, thrashing. Behind me, I hear Ellen's nearly hysterical sobbing.

Ah, Finch, to think you might love! I no longer need to remember this, but when I do, am amused, recalling fairy tales of frogs and princesses, recited, sometimes hour after hour, in an effort to relax me for sleep, by my patient mother. A student of history, I remind myself, should have known better.

No matter. Before the following year was out, I had ceased avoiding her. When we meet now, we can even smile, though we do not speak.

As I leave, other patients in the waiting room pretend not to see me. An old woman with a cane and a platform shoe covers her eyes with a magazine. A palsied man, no more than forty, looks down at his shuddering hands. Another woman, younger, with a perfectly healthy-looking child on her lap, suddenly becomes interested in her son's hair, like a grooming, lice- and salt-seeking primate. Yet another woman, her face set in a lopsided grimace, one shoulder permanently higher than the other, merely yawns, closes her eyes, pinches the bridge of her nose between two fingers until I am beyond her, as if she cannot bear her affliction so long as I am before her to remind her of it.

I walk to the door. I stagger like an old wino, head whipping from side to side with the thrust of each leg, as if I keep time to some raucous, private music. My arms are cocked, ready to catch me if I slip. My feet point inward, and my torso tips forward to provide the continuity of momentum, my broad shoulders thrown back to maintain a risky balance.

It is a gait to embarrass, to make children laugh, a clumsy cantering locomotion that results from only the most exacting and determined attention to control. Inside my rolling head, behind my shocked, magnified eyeballs, my brain orders, with utmost precision, each awkward jerk of thigh, leg, foot. Just as I reach the door to the stairs, a voice greets me cheerfully.

"Hello, Jimmy," sings out in a lilting feminine rush of genuine delight. I bang loudly against the door as I stop, gripping the knob with both hands for support. My head nearly hits the panel of thick, opaque glass. I turn with difficulty. "Hello, Jimmy," she says again.

I know her, but not well. She is a disgusting thing to see, a fellow-student. Fat of face and body, her legs are little more than pale pink, waxy skin stretched over bone, her feet strapped to the steel platform of her wheelchair. One arm is horribly withered, the thin, useless fingers held curled in her broad lap. The other is braced for strength to allow her to work the levers that steer her chair. Beneath her seat squats a large, black battery, her source of power. Her neck angles slightly to one side. Someone has recently given her jet black hair a hideous pixie cut.

I know her. She is one of the small, cohesive platoon of handicapped, crippled, maimed university students. They have an association of sorts, advised by a conscientious faculty member who lost an eye in Korea. The university provides a specially equipped Volkswagen van to take them about campus. They have keys to operate freight elevators, and the buildings have ramps to accommodate them. When I came to the university I was invited, by the one-eyed professor, to join their ranks. I even attended one meeting—mostly polio victims and amputees. The agenda was devoted to a discussion of whether or not to extend membership to an albino girl whose eyesight was so bad she could not read mimeographed class handouts. I declined to join, of course, but still receive their randomly published newsletter. We have nothing in common.

She smiles now, lipstick and powder, rouge and eyebrow pencil making a theater mask of her face. "I've never seen you up here before, Jimmy, have you just started coming?" I am struck, suddenly with the awareness that she has an . . . an *interest* in me! I grope frantically to open the door.

I must, and do, speak, but badly, without thinking, so shaken am I with my understanding. *Haroyoup* comes groaning from my lips, like the creaking of a heavy casket lid. Startled and embarrassed, she smiles all the harder, and I push open the door to begin the slow descent of the steep stairs leading to the street where my bicycle waits. Mad Finch, who dared to think he might feel!

At the top of the stairs I turn around, for I must descend backwards. I take the rail with both hands, regulate my breathing, concentrate, then step back, into the air, with one foot . . . I have a special sense of freedom, for I can never know if the foot will find the stair just below, or if I will step backward into space, find nothing, and fall. I am, for an instant, like a blindfolded highdiver who steps off the springboard, uncertain if there is water below.

I am able, momentarily at least, to forget my self-pity in this kind of freedom only I know.

I must not despair! Though Finch wields the chalk no better than a child does a crayon, he cuts surely as a surgeon to the heart of the problem on the blackboard. Though his pronunciation is atrocious, his syntax is exact, his structure flawless, vocabulary well beyond his years. Though his eyes, enlarged behind thick lenses, stare, sometimes roll up in his head, no one reads more or faster, and for amusement he will commit a paragraph or a page to memory in record time.

It is Finch who is free to traverse the lines of caste and class in our community. Finch is the locker room pet of brainless athletes. They challenge him to feats of strength, and lose goodnaturedly. From the heights of their chicken wire and toilet paper float thrones, Junoesque sorority queens wave to Finch in the crowd, call him by name. Filthy and morose, the bearded politicals and bohemians, who lurk in the basement of the student union, will take time to read Finch their latest throwaway or poem. Serious students, praying for futures in government or academia, consult Finch before submitting seminar reports.

Oh, I am not lonely!

So, with an effort of will, informed by the discipline of my regimen in physical therapy, weightlifting, my schedules, I heave, lifting my center of balance upward with an exaggerated shrug of my broad, strong shoulders; then, at the exact moment, a second divided into several parts for precision, I lean to the right, forcing all my weight onto my right leg, onto the raised pedal of my bicycle. There is no continuity, no fluid evolving process of motion, but my timing is correct—my mind has once more concentrated this fool's body into a preconceived pattern—the pedal depresses, the bike rolls forward.

There is an instant when disaster is possible—I am thrown forward with the bike, but my locked left hand grips the handlebar, stops me short of an ignominious and bruising tumble to the pavement. I remember to pull with my right arm, to isolate the individual muscles that will steer out, away from the curb, past the hulk of a parked florist's truck.

I move. Out now, near the center line, I assert the series of stiff, dramatic thrusts of hip and leg that pump me along, past the campus shops, the bus stop.

Students throng the sidewalk, and they call to me. The frat boys, the unmercifully attractive girls, golden and creamy in their expensive clothes, jocks in their letter sweaters and windbreakers, malcontents in old military jackets. They call: "Ho Finch!" "Jimbo!" "Hi Jimmy!" They grin, wave. "Baby Jim boy!" "Hi Jim," they call.

With careful, paced breathing, I multiply the complexity of my ordeal. Almost one by one, I unlock my fingers from the handlebar. With the strained deliberation of a weight-lifter, I raise it above my head, steering and balance both entrusted to my left arm. Aloft, the tingling spasms are sufficient to produce a casual wave. Like a swimmer shaking water from his inner ear, I rock my head, once, twice, three times, until I face them. Opening my jaw is enough to pull my lips back over my teeth: a smile.

In this instant I am helpless. Were a car to swerve into my path, a pedestrian dart in front of me, all would end in an absurd, theatrical collision—perhaps serious injury. But I prevail.

Now, the breeze in my ears, my glasses vibrating on the bridge of my nose, threatening to fall across my mouth, I speak. My tongue bucks and floats, the stiff planes of my throat shiver, and I respond.

"Jimmy!" they cry. "How you doing, Jimbo!"

Hyaroul explodes my voice, and I can almost see their delight, the fullness of quick and easy tears of sentimental pity form in their eyes. *Hyarouffa!* I say, already plotting how I will lower my right hand, face the road again. *Haluff!* I make an unexpelled breath, not knowing if it is my cry of joy at being alive, known, loved, or a curse far more terrible than any profane cliché they will ever know—because . . . I suspect . . . simply because I cannot answer my own questions, cannot know what is, or is not, Finch.

PART II

Social Factors and Inequality

Introduction to *Infections and Inequalities: The Modern Plagues*
Paul Farmer

Medical statistics will be our standard of measurement: we will weigh life for life and see where the dead lie thicker, among the workers or among the privileged.
—Rudolf Virchow, 1848

What Killed Annette Jean?

Early on the morning of her death, Annette Jean was feeling well enough to fetch a heavy bucket of water from a spring not far from her family's hut. In the weeks prior to that day, she had been complaining of a "cold." It was not serious, she thought, although night sweats and a loss of appetite were beginning to trouble her. Annette's brothers later recalled that she was cheerful, "normal," that morning. She made everyone coffee and helped her mother load up the donkey for market. It was an overcast day in October of 1994, and Haiti's rainy season was drawing to a close.

Shortly after Annette's brothers left for their garden, the young woman abruptly began coughing up blood. A young cousin, watching from across the yard, saw her throw off a bright red arc and then collapse on the dirt floor of the tiny house. The child ran for Annette's three brothers, who tried in vain to rouse her; the young woman could do no more than gurgle in response to their panicked cries. The brothers then hastily confected a stretcher from sheets and saplings. It would take them more than an hour, carrying their inert sister, to reach the nearest clinic, situated in the village of Do Kay far below their mountaintop garden.

Half there, it began to rain. The steep path became slippery, further impeding progress. Two-thirds of the way there, Annette coughed up clots of darker blood and then stopped gurgling. By the time they reached the clinic, it was raining heavily. The larger clots refused to melt, hardening on her soaked shirt, and Annette was motionless in a puddle of diluted blood. She was not yet 20 years old.

I was in the clinic on that rainy day, conversing with a patient near the building's main entrance when the Jean brothers and a fourth man passed into the clinic's courtyard with their terrible cargo. A single rivulet of blood was falling from somewhere under the stretcher onto the paved courtyard. They approached me wordlessly, and I, also silent, reached for the young woman's wrist. It was an easy, joyless diagnosis—death from massive hemoptysis due, almost certainly in a woman her age, to tuberculosis—and Annette was already cold. Her brothers, who had been numbed into silence by the hope that something might still be done, began wailing, each taking up in turn a shrill cry of grief as I pronounced her dead.

One of the women from Do Kay had been mopping the floor of the clinic, but she had stopped to stare. When the men began to weep, she lifted her apron to her eyes and turned away. She had never met Annette Jean or her brothers, but she had seen plenty of tuberculosis. Her own sister, the mother of five children, had died of the same disease in October of 1988. One of those children also died years later from complications of tuberculosis, but not before going stone deaf from one of the medications used to treat it.

I had seen a lot of tuberculosis, too, even though the little clinic in Do Kay was built to serve only a tiny region of the Central Plateau. In 1993 alone, we had diagnosed over 400 cases of tuberculosis, more than were registered in the entire state of Massachusetts that same year. Diagnosing tuberculosis is something I expect to do on a daily basis. But I too was shaken by the blood, the rain, and by the brothers' sharp grief.

The story does not end with Annette's dramatic agony. Another sister, I learned, had also succumbed to tuberculosis. And a few months after Annette's death, one of her brothers, Marcelin, returned to the clinic with a case of shingles (herpes zoster). From our interview I soon learned that he—like Annette, the child of a peasant family—had been working as a servant in Port-au-Prince, Haiti's capital city. This employment history in a person with herpes zoster has come to suggest, for many of us, early HIV disease, a suspicion confirmed in Marcelin's case by a laboratory test. Although, unlike his sisters, Marcelin was fortunate enough to receive treatment for the active tuberculosis that he later developed, he has told his family that he will die.

I could tell that Annette's family did not—*could* not—comprehend why they should be so unfortunate. To lose two young, previously healthy members of a close-knit family seemed both insufferable and unfair; so did Marcelin's illness. But their incomprehension eventually gave way first to hypotheses and then to conclusions. They were the victims of sorcery, they surmised. Someone had it in for them, and that someone was likely to be another villager.

After a decade of medical practice in the same village, I was accustomed to ferreting out accusations of sorcery and had previously spent some years trying to make sense of them.[1] And that, paradoxically, is the primary function of such accusations: to make sense of suffering. The anthropologist within me is perfectly satisfied to analyze such explanations, but to a physician it is nothing less than punishing to see preventable or treatable pathologies chalked up to village-level squabbles.

The doctor in me insists that no one should die of tuberculosis today; it's completely curable. Yet it is, at the same time, the world's leading infectious cause of death among young adults. An estimated 3 million people are dying each year from tuberculosis.[2] This figure comes as a surprise to many, who read more frequently in their newspapers about Ebola or "flesh-eating bacteria" than about tuberculosis. Exacting its toll among the world's poor, tuberculosis has ceased to occasion much interest, either in scientific circles or in the popular press. Barry Bloom puts it even more strongly: tuberculosis, he writes, "has been virtually ignored for 20 years and more."[3]

Many are also surprised to learn that infectious diseases remain the world's single most common cause of death. In 1995, for example, a year in which an estimated 52 million people died worldwide, about 17.3 million of these deaths were due to bacterial, viral, or parasitic infections.[4] And although the majority of deaths occurred in the developing world, infectious diseases also remain a major killer of the U.S. poor. One study of New York City welfare recipients revealed staggeringly high rates of tuberculosis and AIDS: of 858 clients enrolled in 1984, 47 developed tuberculosis and 84 were diagnosed with AIDS. The study thus revealed tuberculosis and AIDS incidence rates well in excess of those found in many poor countries and 70 times higher than the U.S. national rate. In fact, simply being on welfare and having a history of drug or alcohol abuse were strongly associated with death: fully 183 clients—21.3% of the cohort—died within 8 years. The mean age at death was less than 50 years.[5]

Infections and Inequalities

Amartya Sen has observed that the first question in any critical examination of equality is "equality of *what*?"[6] This book examines inequalities in the distribution and outcome of infectious diseases. It asks why people like Annette Jean and her siblings are likely to die of infections such as tuberculosis and AIDS and malaria, while others are spared this risk. It explores the creation and maintenance of such disparities, which are biological in their expression but are largely socially determined. This book also explores social responses to infectious diseases, responses ranging from quarantine to accusations of sorcery.

This exploration leads me to examine various, often discrepant explanations for these disparities of risk and outcome, including those proffered by officialdom and by academics. I argue that scholars often weaken their contributions to an understanding of infectious diseases by making "immodest claims of causality" regarding the distribution and course of these disorders. These claims are immodest because they are wrong or misleading. They are immodest because they distract attention from the modest interventions that could treat and, often enough, cure people like Annette Jean. And they are immodest because they distract attention from the preventable social disorder that exacerbates biological disorders.

Using data from Haiti, the United States, Peru, and elsewhere, this volume calls into question many such claims. *Infections and Inequalities* is intended as a corrective and a complement to the growing literature on "emerging infectious diseases." Although many who study the dynamics of infectious disease will concede that, in some sense, disease emergence is a socially produced phenomenon, few have examined the contribution of specific social inequalities. Yet such inequalities have powerfully sculpted not only the distribution of infectious diseases but also the course of health outcomes among the afflicted.

Strikingly patterned outbreaks of HIV, tuberculosis, and even Ebola—and the social responses to these outbreaks—all suggest that models of disease emergence need to be dynamic, systemic, and critical. They need to be critical of facile claims of causality, particularly those that scant the pathogenic roles of social inequalities. Critical perspectives on emerging infections must ask how large-scale social forces come to have their effects on unequally positioned individuals in increasingly interconnected populations; a critical epistemology needs to ask what features of disease emergence are obscured by dominant analytic frameworks. Such models must strive to incorporate change and complexity and must be global in scope, yet alive to local variation.

This critique leads inevitably to questions about my own disciplinary perspectives. Although this book is the work of a full-time clinician who is also an anthropologist, these essays are neither clinical nor ethnographic. They are instead lodged between medicine and anthropology, drawing freely on both disciplines and on several others, including the sociology of knowledge. This willed "interdisciplinarity" is not meant to free the author from the responsibilities of discipline. Rather, it is clear to me that the disparities of risk and outcome described here are embedded in complex *biosocial* realities. To understand these realities, nothing less than a biosocial analysis will do—an analysis that draws freely on clinical medicine and on social theory, linking molecular epidemiology to history, ethnography, and political economy. Of course, such a synthesis is easy to demand but harder to produce: Fineberg and Wilson have termed it the "Holy Grail" of epidemiology.[7]

Finally, this book is lodged as a protest. The inequalities of outcome I describe are, by and large, biological reflections of social fault lines. Annette Jean's death could and should have been averted; effective interventions might have ranged from the clinical to the political. To conclude otherwise is to engage, wittingly or unwittingly, in delusion or obfuscation.

Visual-Field Defects in Anthropology and Medicine

In reexamining anthropology and medicine from the vantage point of Haiti, there often seems to be no shortage of delusion and obfuscation. At the very least, a good deal of selective blindness exists. The exact nature of the visual-field defect seems to depend on what sort of anthropologist or physician one is. The histories of both anthropology and medicine show these disciplines to be notable for their lack of attention, respectively, to oppression (and, perhaps, to human suffering in general) and to the sicknesses of the poor.[8]

Take anthropology, for starters. Not too long ago, in her study of hunger in Brazil, Scheper-Hughes wrote that "everyday violence, political and domestic horror, and madness . . . are strong words and themes for an anthropologist."[9] Why is this so, if anthropologists work in the same regions from which television exports its images of famine and strife? The killing fields described by journalists were the training fields for generations of anthropologists. What exactly *were* we talking about when we were not talking about "everyday violence, political and domestic horror, and madness"? We were talking a lot about "culture," and part of the problem lies in the ways this term was used. "The idea of culture," explained one authority approvingly in a 1975 book on the subject, "places the researcher in a position of equality with his subjects: each 'belongs to a culture.'"[10]

The tragedy, of course, is that this equality, however comforting to the anthropologist, is entirely illusory. Anthropologist and informant are not separate and equal; both are caught up in a global web of unequal relations. But such illusions reveal an important means by which key misreadings are sustained. A blindness to inequality and structural violence, often the local manifestation of transnational (or at least extraregional) forces, has long marred anthropology.

In a much-quoted essay, "Missing the Revolution," Orin Starn examines the ethnographies coming from highland Peru on the eve of the country's guerrilla war. Working in the very same villages that would later prove sympathetic to the Shining Path (Sendero Luminoso), how was it that anthropologists failed to see what was happening? Following Said, Starn writes of an "Andeanism" that appreciatively stressed the highland peasants' continuity with Incan ancestors. Concerned with ecology and ritual, with depicting remoteness rather than discerning links, a generation of anthropologists seemed to have missed the revolution:

> Ethnographers usually did little more than mention the terrible infant mortality, minuscule incomes, low life expectancy, inadequate diets, and abysmal health care that remained so routine. To be sure, peasant life was full of joys, expertise, and pleasures. But the figures that led other observers to label Ayacucho a region of "Fourth World" poverty would come as a surprise to someone who knew the area only through the ethnography of Isbell, Skar, or Zuidema. They gave us detailed pictures of ceremonial exchanges, Saint's Day rituals, weddings, baptisms, and work parties. Another kind of scene, just as common in the Andes, almost never appeared: a girl with an abscess and no doctor, the woman bleeding to death in childbirth, a couple in their dark adobe house crying over an infant's sudden death.[11]

A more systemic view of highland Peru, and its many economic and administrative links to Lima and beyond, might have corrected this myopia. But, as Starn points out, "this economic nexus was one that most anthropologists—largely depending on the categories of 'culture' and 'community'—were unprepared to explore"[12]

A decade earlier, many of the classic ethnographies of anthropology—including those by Evans-Pritchard, Malinowski, and Lévi-Strauss—were critiqued as similarly shortsighted. But more recent studies have also shown a disturbing tendency to offer misreadings of oppression and suffering. Common indeed are the ethnographies in which poverty and inequality, the end result of a long process of impoverishment, are reduced to a form of cultural difference. We were sent to the field to look for different cultures. We saw oppression; it looked, well, *different* from our comfortable lives in the university; and so we called it "culture." We came, we saw, we misdiagnosed.

These omissions were the result, it's been argued, of theoretical fashions, of the ways in which anthropology "makes its object," and of the ways in which ethnography was written.[13] Most now agree that the omissions were also the result, in part, of anthropologists' relations with colonial or neocolonial power. On the level of the individual researcher, however, the visual-field defects of anthropology are rarely a question of motives but rather, as Asad suggests, a question of our "mode of perceiving and objectifying alien societies."[14] Three decades ago, today's truisms triggered acrimonious debate within anthropology. But debates that focused on the image of the anthropologist as the willing stooge of power often failed to address the more subtle effects of hegemony. This book suggests that the myths and mystifications surrounding these issues often serve powerful interests, in spite of the best intentions of researchers.

The extent to which these critiques of anthropology are still valid is a matter of some debate. Perhaps Marcus and Fischer were correct when, more than a decade ago, they argued that "our consciousness has become more global and historical: to invoke another culture is to locate it in a time and space contemporaneous with our own, and thus to see it as a part of our world, rather than a mirror or alternative to ourselves, arising from a totally alien origin."[15] Perhaps scores of students are this minute studying, say, the plight of women like Annette Jean. Perhaps several Fulbrights have been awarded to study the effects of recent political and economic policies on health outcomes among the poor of Latin America and Africa. But I don't think we're battering down wide-open doors here, if working in Haiti and dealing with AIDS and tuberculosis are at all instructive.

In my first years of reading anthropology, I certainly "missed the revolution." But what better remedial training than that to be found in Haiti? Although I went there in the spring of 1983 with a host of pre-fab research questions, each tightly linked to a sanctioned desire to "contribute to the theory," I gradually developed a quite different set of questions, the ones addressed in this book. And in the course of a decade of research, reading, and writing, much of it in collaboration with very ecumenical colleagues, I came to discern disturbing patterns in much social-science writing on AIDS and tuberculosis.[16] For example, when we were face to face with sexual practices or AIDS outcomes that were manifestly linked to poverty and inequality, we wrote instead about the exotic reflections of cultural difference. Animal sacrifice, zoophilia, ritualized homosexuality, scarification, and ritual beliefs all figure prominently in the early anthropology of AIDS. The only problem was that none of this had any demonstrable relevance to HIV transmission or AIDS outcomes, and claims to the contrary were eventually revealed to be mistaken—not, however, before a certain amount of damage was done, as several of the chapters that follow suggest.

This conflation of structural violence and cultural difference has marred much commentary on AIDS, especially when that commentary focuses on the chief victims of the disease: the poor. A related trend is the exaggeration of the agency of those most likely to become infected. Often such exaggeration is tantamount to blaming the victim.[17] Explorations of AIDS have involved intense scrutiny of local factors and local actors, including the natives' conceptions and stated motives. But is it possible to explain the distribution of HIV by discussing only attitude or cognition? After more than 15 years in Haiti, I would not hazard to comment on the psychological makeup specific to Haitians with AIDS, and I suspect that quests for psychological "predispositions" are fundamentally misguided. On the makeup of Haiti's changing social conditions and their relation to AIDS, however, much can be said. On the nature of inequality and on the structure of poverty—increasingly a global process—much can be said. On the mechanisms by which these forces come to alter sexuality and sexual practices, much can be said. On Haitians' lack of access to both AIDS prevention and treatment, again, much *must* be said. It is thus unfortunate that these topics have been neglected in the social science and clinical literature on AIDS.

What about medicine's blind spots? If the anthropologist working in Haiti is faced with a host of theoretical and methodological dilemmas, it would seem, at first blush, that the physician's task would be somewhat easier. To a certain extent, it is. There is, first, the wonderful simplicity of the patient-healer dyad. The doctor's allegiance, goes the saw, is always to his or her patient. There is thus little need for angst over social theory: this allegiance holds whether that patient is an elderly, overweight U.S. businessman with coronary artery disease or a thin, coughing Haitian woman, still in her 20s and dying of tuberculosis and malnutrition.[18] Having had the privilege of caring for both of these patients, I can say only that a warm and caring rapport is possible, indeed necessary, in both cases. Furthermore, the warmth of clinical exchanges—the vitality of practice— can serve as a powerful corrective to the "experience-distant" models of economics, political science, and sociology.

That said, it is important to add, though perhaps not to one's patients, that North American men with coronary artery disease are apt to live much longer than Haitian women with tuberculosis. North American men with coronary artery disease are apt to live longer than Haitian women, period. And the former, even those who are uninsured, clearly have much greater access to top-quality care than do the latter: indeed, it may be true that few Haitian peasants have received state-of-the-art care for pulmonary tuberculosis or any other serious illness—ever.[19]

A warm patient-doctor relationship is surely indispensable to quality care. So too is a familiarity with the biomedical literature. The vast, if still largely potential, power of modern medicine stems in great measure from its focus on the biological sciences. No one who has access to the vast array of drugs and diagnostic tools of a modern hospital could fail to appreciate the century's remarkable return on investments in bench science. No one who confidently prescribes a new medication could fail to appreciate the double-blinded controlled trial. But the narrow or uncritical use of these tools is one reason for physicians' blindness to the large-scale forces that generate sickness. Such pathogenic forces were once the focus of social medicine, as the work of Rudolf Virchow and others can remind us:

> Virchow understood, as we his successors have not, that medicine, if it is to improve the health of the public, must attend at one and the same time to its biologic *and* to its social underpinnings. It is para-doxic that, at the very moment when the scientific progress of medi-cine has reached unprecedented heights, our neglect of the social roots Virchow so clearly identified cripples our effectiveness.[20]

Physicians again need to think hard about poverty and inequality, which influence *any* population's morbidity and mortality patterns and deter-mine, especially in a fee-for-service system, who will have access to care.

In short, all of the forces that bring a patient to a doctor (or keep a patient from a doctor), all of the processes leading to sickness and then to diagnosis and treatment, are related to a series of large-scale social factors. The diagnostic dilemma, in thinking about the health of populations, is not so very different from that faced by the anthropologist.

So how might humane and compassionate physicians work such perspectives into their practice? Many of the finest clinicians I know have neither the time nor the inclination to consider such large-scale questions. Obligated to keep up with the explosion of medical knowledge and increased administrative demands, they are (or feel) consumed by the task at hand—to see a patient through an acute illness or to diminish the suffering of the chronically ill. Their patients might prefer such an approach, I suspect, to the one advanced in this book; no one who is ill wants the doctor visibly distracted by the problems of others.

In a utopia, perhaps this would be enough. Others would make sure that everyone had access to high-quality medical services. Someone else would enforce standards of care and monitor the forces that generate sickness in a society. Others would make sure that medical care, broadly conceived, was designed to promote the full development of each member of society.

Alas, we live in a society that encompasses both Haiti and the United States. It is a society that includes both Harlem and the Lower East Side of Manhattan, Paris and Kinshasa, London and Bombay. Further, we live in a society that is poorly defined by national boundaries. Nowhere is this clearer than in the case of HIV, as I've tried to show in previous work:

> The ties that bind Haiti to urban North America have a historical basis, and they continue to change. These connections are economic and affective; they are political and personal. One reason this study of AIDS in rural Haiti returns again and again to urban Haiti and the United States is that the boundaries separating them are, at best, blurred. The AIDS pandemic is a striking reminder that even a village as "remote" as Do Kay is linked to a network that includes Port-au-Prince and Brooklyn, voodoo and chemotherapy, divination and serology, poverty and plenty. Indeed, the sexual transmission of HIV is as eloquent a testimony as any to the salience—and complicated intimacy—of these links.[21]

Such arguments are not inappropriate to the analysis of other diseases, including tuberculosis. Is it mere polemic to argue that in terms of social causation the coronary artery disease of millions of overfed northerners is linked to the tuberculosis of malnourished Haitian women?

Our society ensures that large numbers of people, in the United States and out of it, will be simultaneously put at risk for disease and denied access to care. In fact, the spectacular successes of biomedicine have in many instances further entrenched medical inequalities. This necessarily happens whenever new and effective therapies—from antituberculous drugs to protease inhibitors—are not made readily available to those in need. Perhaps it was in anticipation of late-20th-century technology that Virchow argued that physicians must be the "natural attorneys of the poor."

In any setting where medical injustice is a given, it is incumbent upon physicians and other healers to respond to the troubling questions posed by the destitute sick. These issues cannot be left to the leaders of the insurance and pharmaceutical industries, whose bottom line is not relief of suffering. Until doctors ask other types of questions—Who becomes sick and why? Who becomes a patient? Who has access to adequate services? How might inequalities of risk and outcome be addressed?—they will remain at least as blind as the anthropologists who "missed the revolution."

On Claims of Causality

Responses to these questions demand much more than careful phenomenology, a cornerstone of both good ethnography and clinical medicine. Studies compiled from the 12th century onward show that the poor, quite simply, are sicker than the nonpoor and that this is true in both rich and poor countries.[22] In a 1969 volume of papers addressing the issues of poverty and health, we read: "Clearly the poverty population is considerably less healthy than the rest of the population of [the United States]. It still experiences substantially higher rates of overall mortality (all ages and by age, and especially from the communicable diseases), infant mortality, and severe illness."[23] A more recent review argues that studies continue to point to the same conclusion:

> One of the most striking features of the relationship between [socioeconomic status] and health is its pervasiveness and persistence over time. This relationship is found in virtually every measure of health status: age-adjusted mortality for all causes of death as well as specific causes, the severity of acute disease and the incidence of severe infectious conditions, the prevalence and severity of nearly every chronic disease, and measures of disability and restricted activity.[24]

But how, precisely, are these inequalities of outcome explained? Also writing of the U.S. poor, Ryan puts it trenchantly: "The facts are plain: their health is bad. The cause is plain: health costs money, and they don't have money."[25] In the years since Ryan made this claim, we have learned that the relationship between poverty and health is more complicated.[26] But the complexities are often found in the diverse ways in which the health of the disenfranchised may be made to suffer. That is, poverty and other social inequalities come to alter disease distribution and sickness trajectories through innumerable and complicated mechanisms.

Take tuberculosis, with its persistence in poor countries and its resurgence among the poor of many industrialized nations. We cannot understand its markedly patterned occurrence—in the United States, for example, afflicting those in homeless shelters and in prison—without understanding how social forces, ranging from political violence to racism, come to be embodied as individual pathology.

Initially, poverty and racism increase the likelihood that one will become infected by *Mycobacterium tuberculosis*. The mechanisms by which this occurs include the prevalence of the disease among the poor and the fact that the poor are more likely to live together, often in the cramped, airless quarters that once characterized the "lung blocks" of industrializing cities and now describe the urban ghettoes in which tuberculosis is endemic. Various institutions designed to serve or contain the poor have in many instances been the settings for amplified outbreaks of tuberculosis. Nardell and Brickner argue, for example, that homeless shelters have become the lung blocks of the late 20th century.[27] Poverty and racism surely increase the likelihood that one will end up in a shelter, just as these forces arrange the chances that one will wake up in a crack house or a prison.

Once infected, the poor are more likely to progress to active disease. Again, the mechanisms are myriad. Cell-mediated immunity, which keeps tuberculosis quiescent in most persons, may be compromised by malnutrition, HIV infection (or other concurrent disease), or addiction to drugs or alcohol. Addiction, in turn, is usually not comprehensible without an understanding of subjugation and racism, at least not if historical and population-based studies are to be believed. Even reinfection with *M. tuberculosis* might play a role in ensuring that tuberculosis infection will progress to disease; the risk of reinfection is strongly influenced by the social factors just described.

These same factors determine outcomes among those with active tuberculosis disease. Poverty and racism increase the likelihood of dire outcomes among the sick by restricting access to effective therapy or rendering it less effective if patients are malnourished or addicted. Poverty clearly decreases the ability of patients to "comply" with demanding, lengthy regimens. Indeed, the advent of truly effective therapies only brings into starker relief the centrality of social inequalities, when unequal access to these therapies heightens the inequalities of infection and reactivation already described.

Thus do *fundamentally social forces and processes come to be embodied as biological events.* Throughout this book, I will make similar arguments in considering HIV and other infectious pathogens.

While underlining the essentially social nature of unequal health outcomes, I also want to avoid what might be termed the "Luddite trap." Addressing the social roots of disease is sometimes held to be incompatible with advocating the delivery of high-quality, high-tech care—an opinion often voiced by critics of private-sector medicine. But the facts are otherwise, as Paul Wise observes in a subtle discussion of racial disparities in infant mortality: "Too often, those who elevate the role of social determinants indict clinical technologies as failed strategies. But devaluing clinical intervention diverts attention from the essential goal that it be provided equitably to all those in need. Belittling the role of clinical care tends to unburden policy of the requirement to provide equitable access to such care."[28]

Nothing is wrong with high-tech medicine, except that there isn't enough of it to go around. It is, in fact, concentrated in precisely those areas where it will have the most limited effects. We need more and better clinical services for those marginalized by poverty and by discrimination. Annette Jean would no doubt be alive today had she been diagnosed and treated in a timely fashion. Combination antiretroviral therapy would—and, I hope, will—no doubt prolong her brother's life. The poor need access to the best clinical interventions available, and we are living in a time when double standards of care must be questioned. Indeed, this is one of the messages to be distilled from the voices cited in this book.

Another message is that, with effective clinical interventions, we can often hope to efface the embodied manifestations of social inequalities. This has certainly been the goal of many health care providers working in settings of great privation.[29] We can show that tuberculosis outcomes can be as good among the rural Haitian poor as they are anywhere else.[30] Others working in the U.S. inner cities have shown that inequalities of survival among those living with HIV can also be erased if high-quality AIDS care is afforded to all, regardless of ability to pay.[31]

Nevertheless, we must remember that effacing the inequality of outcomes is not the same as eliminating the underlying forces of inequality itself. And studying inequality is perhaps even further removed from this goal. But a desire for equality, whether avowed or hidden, often underpins such studies, as Sen points out: "When we assess inequalities across the world in being able to avoid preventable morbidity, or escapable hunger, or premature mortality, we are not merely examining differences in well-being, but also in the basic freedoms that we value and cherish."[32]

In a very real way, inequality itself constitutes our modern plague. The burdens of inequality are primarily borne by the poor and marginalized, for not everyone can claim victimhood, despite the self-serving identity politics and "soft relativism" of our times. But it is worth noting that even wealthy societies riven by great inequalities are bereft of social cohesion. This lack of cohesion is tightly linked to increased rates of morbidity and mortality: "It is now clear," writes Wilkinson in an important study of inequality in industrial societies, "that the scale of income differences in a society is one of the most powerful determinants of health standards in different countries, and that it influences health through its impact on social cohesion."[33]

In the United States, where this correlation is pronounced, one notes with alarm the widening income gap between worker and management: at this writing, the average CEO of a major company makes more than two hundred times what the average factory worker earns. This disparity, five times greater than it was 30 years ago, is growing. "You can almost hear the proletariat sharpening the guillotine," warned *Newsweek* in an article on the subject; but in truth there seems to be a monopoly of violence from above, not below.[34]

Notes

1 For a review of my conclusions, see Farmer 1992, chap. 18.
2 World Health Organization 1996.
3 Bloom 1992, p. 538.
4 These estimates are from the World Health Organization, which further reports that acute lower respiratory infections, diarrhea (including cholera, typhoid, and dysentery), tuberculosis, malaria, hepatitis B, HIV/AIDS, measles, neonatal tetanus, pertussis, and intestinal helminthiases top the list of infectious killers; see "Infectious Diseases" 1996.
5 Friedman, Williams, Singh, and Frieden 1996.

6   Sen 1992, p. ix.

7   Fineberg and Wilson 1996, p. 859.

8   There are, of course, many exceptions to this general rule. There are also signs that an anthropology of suffering and a greater attention to the sicknesses of the poor are of increasing importance in anthropology and medicine, respectively; see, for example, Kleinman, Das, and Lock 1997. That growing numbers of U.S. physicians are impatient with a health care system that fails to address the needs of the poor is suggested by statements such as that recently made by the Ad Hoc Committee to defend Health Care (1997).

9   Scheper-Hughes 1992, p. 21.

10 Wagner 1975, p. 2.

11 Starn 1992, p. 168.

12 Ibid., p. 163.

13 See Fabian's 1983 essay on "how anthropology makes its object." On ethnographic writing and its canon, see Geertz 1988, which offers a fairly complete, if somewhat dismissive, listing of other studies of the subject.

14 Asad 1975, p. 17.

15 Marcus and Fischer 1986, p. 134.

16 For a review of this literature, see Farmer, Connors, and Simmons 1996, chap. 5.

17 I have used the term "exaggeration of personal agency" throughout to indicate the failure, widespread in the social sciences and in popular commentary, to incorporate an understanding of how individual agency is constrained by poverty and inequality. In anthropology, such exaggeration was linked to the use of the notion of a "culture of poverty" (see Lewis 1969 and Valentine 1968). For a helpful overview of the ideological legacy of the "culture of poverty" debate, see Morris's trenchant 1996 essay.

18 It is important to note that risk for coronary artery disease, at least in the United States, is borne disproportionately by men in lower income brackets, not by prosperous businessmen with so-called Type-A personalities. For a review of the association between heart disease, race, and social class, see Ayanian, Udvarhelyi, Gatsonis, Pashos, and Epstein 1993; Escobedo, Giles, and Anda 1997; Giles, Anda, Caspar, Escobedo, and Taylor 1995; and Ferguson, Tierney, Westmoreland, Mamlin, Segar, Eckert, Zhao, Martin, and Weinberger 1997. See also two editorials on this topic by John Ayanian (1993, 1994). Some of the mechanisms underlying these associations are explored in Kawachi, Kennedy, Lochner, and Prothrow-Stith 1997.

19 Again, note that in the United States local inequalities—along lines of race, for example— are clearly associated with poor access to interventional cardiology. See, for example, the studies by Ayanian, Udvarhelyi, Gatsonis, Pashos, and Epstein (1993) and Giles, Anda, Caspar, Escobedo, and Taylor (1995).

20 Eisenberg 1984, p. 526.

21 Farmer 1992, p. 8.

22 I will draw upon this vast and heterogeneous literature throughout. For overviews, see Antonovsky 1967; Bunker, Gomby, and Kehrer 1989; Dutton and Levine 1989; Evans, Barer, and Marmor 1994; Haan, Kaplan, and Camacho 1987; Hahn, Eaker, Barker, Teutsch, Sosniak, and Krieger 1995; Kitagawa and Hauser 1973; Kosa, Antonovsky, and Zola 1969; Krieger, Rowley, Herman, Avery, and Phillips 1993; Pappas, Queen, Hadden, and Fisher 1993; Syme and Berkman 1976; Thiede and Traub 1997; Wilkinson 1992. A special issue of Dædalus (Fall 1994, vol. 123, no. 4) also reviews the subject of "health and wealth."

23   Lerner 1969, p. 111. See also Adler, Boyce, Chesney, et al. 1994, p. 15.

24   Dutton and Levine 1989, p. 31.

25   Ryan 1971, p. 163.

26   The often linear relationship between poverty and sickness changes as basic nutritional and sanitary needs are met. Wilkinson (1996) offers a critical overview of the association between income distribution—a key marker of social inequality—and health outcomes in wealthy and middle-income nations. In many of these settings, he argues, "health is almost unrelated to measures of economic growth and yet closely related to income distribution" (p. 221). For more on the association between high grades of inequality and increased morbidity and mortality, see Kawachi, Kennedy, Lochner, and Prothrow-Stith 1997; and Kennedy, Kawachi, and Prothrow-Stith 1996. In *Infections and Inequalities*, I have attempted to explore this topic from a transnational perspective, shedding light on some often obscured links between Latin America and the industrialized countries.

27   Nardell and Brickner 1996, p. 1259.

28   Wise 1993, p. 9.

29   Compare Paul Wise on infant mortality: "In a setting of profound poverty, the intention of clinical interventions is not to alleviate poverty but reduce its power to alter health outcomes; thus, clinical interventions' attack on the tragedy of infant mortality will be successful only when social influences are no longer expressed in differential outcomes" (ibid., p. 12).

30   See, for example, Farmer, Robin, Ramilus, and Kim 1991.

31   Chaisson, Keruly, and Moore 1995.

32   Sen 1992, p. 69.

33   Wilkinson 1996, p. ix.

34   Kadlec 1997, pp. 59–60.

References

Adler, N. E., T. Boyce, M. A. Chesney, et al. 1994. "Socioeconomic Status and Health: The Challenge of the Gradient." *American Psychologist* 49 (1): 15–24.

Antonovsky, A. 1967. "Social Class, Life Expectancy, and Overall Mortality." *Milbank Memorial Fund Quarterly* 45:31–73.

Asad, T., ed. 1975. *Anthropology and the Colonial Encounter*. London: Ithaca Press.

Ayanian, J. Z. 1993. "Editorial: Heart Disease in Black and White." *New England Journal of Medicine* 329 (9): 656–58.

Ayanian, J. Z. 1994. "Editorial: Race, Class, and the Quality of Medical Care." *Journal of the American Medical Association* 271 (15): 1207–8.

Ayanian, J. Z., S. Udvarhelyi, C. A. Gatsonis, C. L. Pashos, and A. M. Epstein. 1993. "Racial Differences in the Use of Revascularization Procedures After Coronary Angiography." *Journal of the American Medical Association* 269 (20): 2642–46.

Bloom, B. R. 1992. "Tuberculosis: Back to a Frightening Future." *Nature* 358: 538–39.

Bunker, J. P., D. S. Gomby, and B. H. Kehrer, eds. 1989. *Pathways to Health: The Role of Social Factors*. Menlo Park, Calif.: The Henry J. Kaiser Family Foundation.

Chaisson, R. E., J. C. Keruly, and R. D. Moore. 1995. "Race, Sex, Drug Use, and Progression of Human Immunodeficiency Virus Disease." *New England Journal of Medicine* 333 (12): 751–56.

Dutton, D. B., and S. Levin. 1989. "Socioeconomic Status and Health: Overview, Methodological Critique, and Reformulation." In *Pathways to Health: The Role of Social Factors*, edited
by J. P. Bunker, D. S. Gomby, and B. H. Kehrer, pp. 29–69. Menlo Park, Calif.: The Henry J.
Kaiser Family Foundation.

Eisenberg, L. 1984. "Rudolf Ludwig Karl Virchow, Where Are You Now That We Need You?"
American Journal of Medicine 77 (3): 524–32.

Escobedo, L. G., W. H. Giles, and R. F. Anda. 1997. "Socioeconomic Status, Race, and Death
from Coronary Heart Disease." *American Journal of Preventive Medicine* 13 (2):123–30.

Evans, R. G., M. L. Barer, and T. R. Marmor. 1994. *Why Are Some People Healthy and Others
Not? The Determinants of Health of Populations*. Hawthorne, N.Y.: Aldine de Gruyter.

Fabian, J. 1983. *Time and the Other: How Anthropology Makes Its Object*. New York: Columbia University Press.

Farmer, P. E. 1992. *AIDS and Accusations: Haiti and the Geography of Blame*. Berkeley: University of California Press.

Farmer, P. E., M. Connors, and J. Simmons, eds. 1996. *Women, Poverty, and AIDS: Sex, Drugs,
and Structural Violence*. Monroe, Maine: Common Courage Press.

Farmer, P. E., S. Robin, S. L. Ramilus, and J. Y. Kim. 1991."Tuberculosis, Poverty, and 'Compliance': Lessons from Rural Haiti." *Seminars in Respiratory Infections* 6: 373–79.

Ferguson, J. A., W. M. Tierney, G. R. Westmoreland, L. A. Mamlin, D. S. Segar, G. J. Eckert, X. H.
Zhao, D. K. Martin, and M. Weinberger. 1997. "Examination of Racial Differences in Management of Cardiovascular Disease." *Journal of the American College of Cardiology* 30 (7):
1707–13.

Fineberg, H. V., and M. E. Wilson. 1996. "Social Vulnerability and Death by Infection." *New
England Journal of Medicine* 334 (13): 859–60.

Friedman, L. N., M. T. Williams, T. P. Singh, and T. R. Frieden. 1996. "Tuberculosis, AIDS, and
Death Among Substance Abusers on Welfare in New York City." *New England Journal of
Medicine* 334 (13): 828–33.

Geertz, C. 1988. *Works and Lives: The Anthropologist as Author*. Stanford, Calif.: Stanford
University Press (1988).

Giles, W. H., R. F. Anda, M. L. Casper, L. G. Escobedo, and H. A. Taylor. 1995. "Race and Sex
Differences in Rates of Invasive Cardiac Procedures in U.S. Hospitals: Data from the National Hospital Discharge Survey." *Archives of Internal Medicine* 155:318–24.

Haan, M., G. A. Kaplan, and T. Camacho. 1987. "Poverty and Health: Prospective Evidence
from the Alameda County Study." *American Journal of Epidemiology* 125 (6): 989–98.

Hahn, R. A., E. Eaker, N. D. Barker, S. M. Teutsch, W. Sosniak, and N. Krieger. 1995. "Poverty
and Death in the United States—1973–1991." *Epidemiology* 6 (5): 490–97.

Kadlec, D. 1997. "How CEO Pay Got Away." *Newsweek*, 28 April, pp. 59–60.

Kawachi, I., B. P. Kennedy, K. Lochner, and D. Prothrow-Stith. 1997. "Social Capital, Income
Inequality, and Mortality." *American Journal of Public Health* 87 (9): 1491–98.

Kennedy, B. P., I. Kawachi, and D. Prothrow-Stith. 1996. "Income Distribution and Mortality: Test of the Robin Hood Index in the United States." *British Medical Journal* 312:
1004–8.

Kitagawa, E. M., and P. M. Hauser. 1973. *Differential Mortality in the United States: A Study in
Socioeconomic Epidemiology*. Cambridge, Mass.: Harvard University Press.

Kleinman, A., V. Das, and M. Lock, eds. 1997. *Social Suffering*. Berkeley: University of California Press.

Kosa, J., A. Antonovsky, and I. Zola, eds. 1969. *Poverty and Health: A Sociological Analysis*. Cambridge, Mass.: Harvard University Press.

Krieger, N., D. Rowley, A. Herman, B. Avery, and M. Phillips. 1993. "Racism, Sexism, and Social Class: Implications for Studies of Health, Disease, and Well-Being." *American Journal of Preventive Medicine* 9 (Suppl.): 82–122.

Lerner, M. 1969. "Social Differences in Physical Health." In *Poverty and Health: A Sociological Analysis*, edited by J. Kosa, A. Antonovsky, and I. Zola, pp. 69–112. Cambridge, Mass.: Harvard University Press.

Lewis, O. 1969. "The Culture of Poverty." In *On Understanding Poverty: Perspectives from the Social Sciences*, edited by D. P. Moynihan, pp. 187–200. New York: Basic Books.

Marcus, G., and M. Fischer. 1986. *Anthropology as Cultural Critique: An Experimental Moment in the Human Sciences*. Chicago: University of Chicago Press.

Morris, M. 1996. "Culture, Structure, and the Underclass." In *Myths About the Powerless: Contesting Social Inequalities*, edited by M. B. Lykes, A. Banuazizi, R. Liem, and M. Morris, pp. 34–49. Philadelphia: Temple University Press.

Nardell, E. A., and P. W. Brickner. 1996. "Tuberculosis in New York City—Focal Transmission of an Often Fatal Disease." *Journal of the American Medical Association* 276 (15): 1259–60.

Pappas, G., S. Queen, W. Hadden, and G. Fisher. 1993. "The Increasing Disparity in Mortality Between Socioeconomic Groups in the United States, 1960 and 1986." *New England Journal of Medicine* 329 (2): 103–9.

Ryan, W. 1971. *Blaming the Victim*. New York: Vintage.

Scheper-Hughes, N. 1992. *Death Without Weeping: The Violence of Everyday Life in Brazil*. Berkeley: University of California Press.

Sen, A. 1992. *Inequality Reexamined*. Cambridge, Mass.: Harvard University Press.

Starn, O. 1992. "Missing the Revolution: Anthropologists and the War in Peru." In *Rereading Cultural Anthropology*, edited by G. Marcus, pp. 99–112. Durham, N.C.: Duke University Press.

Syme, S. L., and L. F. Berkman. 1976. "Social Class, Susceptibility, and Sickness." *American Journal of Epidemiology* 104 (1): 1–8.

Thiede, M., and S. Traub. 1997. "Mutual Influences of Health and Poverty: Evidence from German Panel Data." *Social Science and Medicine* 45 (6): 867–77.

Valentine, C. A. 1968. *Culture and Poverty: Critique and Counter-Proposals*. Chicago: University of Chicago Press.

Wagner, R. 1975. *The Invention of Culture*. Englewood Cliffs, N.J.: Prentice-Hall.

Wilkinson, R. G. 1992. "National Mortality Rates: the Impact of Inequality?" *American Journal of Public Health* 82 (8): 1082–84.

Wilkinson, R. G. 1996. *Unhealthy Societies: The Afflictions of Inequality*. London: Routledge.

Wise, P. H. 1993. "Confronting Racial Disparities in Infant Mortality: Reconciling Science and Politics." *American Journal of Preventive Medicine* 9 (6): 7–16.

World Health Organization. 1996. "Infectious Diseases." *Groups at Risk: WHO Report on the Tuberculosis Epidemic*. Geneva: World Health Organization.

World Health Organization. 1996. *Groups at Risk: WHO Report on the Tuberculosis Epidemic*. Geneva: World Health Organization.

Unequal Treatment: What Healthcare Providers Need to Know about Racial and Ethnic Disparities in Healthcare
Brian D. Smedley, Adrienne Y. Stith, and Alan R. Nelson

News accounts of the state of healthcare delivery seem to be full of bad news, including concerns about rising healthcare costs, patient safety, and medical errors, and the growing numbers of uninsured Americans. To add to these problems, many recent news reports indicate that racial and ethnic minorities receive lower quality healthcare than whites, even when they are insured to the same degree and when other healthcare access-related factors, such as the ability to pay for care, are the same.

The Institute of Medicine (IOM) report *Unequal Treatment: Confronting Racial and Ethnic Disparities in Healthcare* added to the media fray when the IOM concluded that "(al)though myriad sources contribute to these disparities, some evidence suggests that bias, prejudice, and stereotyping on the part of healthcare providers may contribute to differences in care."

This finding was alarming to many healthcare professionals, the vast majority of whom work hard under very challenging conditions to ensure that patients receive the best possible healthcare to meet their needs. How could bias, prejudice, and stereotyping contribute to unequal treatment, particularly given that healthcare providers are sworn to beneficence and cannot, by law, discriminate against any patient on the basis of race, ethnicity, color, or national origin? This brief summary of the IOM *Unequal Treatment* report addresses this question, and summarizes other

Brian D. Smedley, Adrienne Y. Stith, and Alan R. Nelson, editors; Committee on Understanding and Eliminating Racial and Ethnic Disparities in Health Care, Board on Health Sciences Policy, Institute of Medicine. "Unequal Treatment: What Healthcare Providers Need to Know about Racial and Ethnic Disparities in Healthcare." © 2002 by the National Academy of Sciences. Permission is granted to reproduce this document in its entirety, with no additions or alterations.

relevant findings to help healthcare professionals meet the objective of providing high-quality care for all patients.

Do Racial and Ethnic Minorities Receive a Lower Quality of Healthcare?

In 1999, Congress requested that the IOM assess the extent of racial and ethnic disparities in healthcare, assuming that access-related factors—such as insurance status and the ability to pay for care are the same; identify potential sources of these disparities, including the possibility that overt or subtle biases or prejudice on the part of healthcare providers might affect the quality of care for minorities; and suggest intervention strategies.

To fulfill this request, an IOM study committee reviewed well over 100 studies that assessed the quality of healthcare for various racial and ethnic minority groups, while holding constant variations in insurance status, patient income, and other access-related factors. Many of these studies also controlled for other potential confounding factors, such as racial differences in the severity or stage of disease progression, the presence of co-morbid illnesses, where care is received (e.g., public or private hospitals and health systems) and other patient demographic variables, such as age and gender. Some studies that employed more rigorous research designs followed patients prospectively, using clinical data abstracted from patients' charts, rather than administrative data used for insurance claims. The study committee was struck by the consistency of research findings: even among the better-controlled studies, the vast majority indicated that minorities are less likely than whites to receive needed services, including clinically necessary procedures. These disparities exist in a number of disease areas, including cancer, cardiovascular disease, HIV/AIDS, diabetes, and mental illness, and are found across a range of procedures, including routine treatments for common health problems.

What Are the Sources of Healthcare Disparities?

Many factors may contribute to the healthcare disparities observed in these studies. Some researchers suggest that there may be subtle differences in the way that members of different racial and ethnic groups respond to treatment, particularly with regard to some pharmaceutical interventions, suggesting that variations in some forms of treatment may be justified on the basis of patient race or ethnicity. In addition, patients vary in help-seeking behavior, and some racial and ethnic minorities may be more likely than whites to avoid or delay seeking care. However, the majority of studies find disparities in clinical services that are equally effective for all racial and ethnic groups. Further, the studies that the IOM reviewed suggest that racial differences in patients' attitudes, such as their preferences for treatment, do not vary greatly and cannot fully explain racial and ethnic disparities in healthcare. A small number of studies, for example, find that African Americans are slightly more likely to reject medical recommendations for some treatments, but these differences in refusal rates are generally small (African Americans are only 3–6% more likely to reject recommended treatments, according to these studies). It remains unclear why African American patients are more likely to reject treatment recommendations. Are they refusing treatment because of a general mistrust of health care providers? Or do some decline treatment because of negative experiences in the clinical encounter or a perception that their doctor is not invested in their care? More research is needed to fully understand treatment refusal because the reasons for refusal may lead to different strategies to help patients make informed treatment decisions.

If minority patients' attitudes toward healthcare and preferences for treatment are not likely to be a major source of health care disparities, what other factors may contribute to these disparities? As shown in figure 1, the IOM study committee considered two other sets of factors that may be associated with disparities in healthcare, assuming that all populations have equal access to care. The first set of factors are those related to the operation of healthcare systems and the legal and regulatory climate in which they operate. These include factors such as cultural or linguistic barriers (e.g., the lack of interpretation services for patients with limited English proficiency), fragmentation of healthcare systems (as noted earlier, these include the possibility that minorities are disproportionately enrolled in lower-cost health plans that place greater per-patient limits on healthcare expenditures and available services), the types of incentives in place to contain costs (e.g., incentives to physicians to limit services), and where minorities tend to receive care (e.g., minorities are less likely to access care in a private physician's office, even when insured at the same level as whites).

The second set of factors emerges from the clinical encounter. Three mechanisms might be operative in healthcare disparities from the pro-

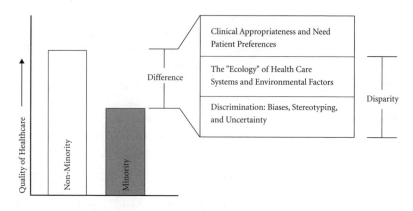

Figure 1. Differences, Disparities, and Discrimination:
Populations with Equal Access to Healthcare. Source: Gomes and McGuire, 2001.

vider's side of the exchange: bias (or prejudice) against minorities; greater clinical uncertainty when interacting with minority patients; and beliefs (or stereotypes) held by the provider about the behavior or health of minorities. Patients might also react to providers' behavior associated with these practices in a way that also contributes to disparities. Research on how patient race or ethnicity may influence physician decision-making and the quality of care for minorities is still developing, and as yet there is no direct evidence to illustrate how prejudice, stereotypes, or bias may influence care. In the absence of such research, the study committee drew upon a mix of theory and relevant research to understand how these processes might operate in the clinical encounter.

Clinical Uncertainty

Any degree of uncertainty a physician may have relative to the condition of a patient can contribute to disparities in treatment. Doctors must depend on inferences about severity based on what they can see about the illness and on what else they observe about the patient (e.g., race). The doctor can therefore be viewed as operating with prior beliefs about the likelihood of patients' conditions, "priors" that will be different according to age, gender, socioeconomic status, and race or ethnicity. When these priors are considered alongside information gathered in a clinical encounter, both influence medical decisions.

Doctors must balance new information gained from the patient (sometimes with varying levels of accuracy) and their prior expectations about the patient to make a diagnosis and determine a course of treatment. If the physician has difficulty accurately understanding the symptoms or is less sure of the "signal"—the set of clues and indications that physicians rely upon to make diagnostic decisions—then he or she is likely to place greater weight on "priors." The consequence is that treatment decisions and patients' needs are potentially less well matched.

The Implicit Nature of Stereotypes

A large body of research in psychology has explored how stereotypes evolve, persist, shape expectations, and affect interpersonal interactions. Stereotyping can be defined as the process by which people use social categories (e.g., race, sex) in acquiring, processing, and recalling information about others. The beliefs (stereotypes) and general orientations (attitudes) that people bring to their interactions help organize and simplify complex or uncertain situations and give perceivers greater confidence in their ability to understand a situation and respond in efficient and effective ways.

Although functional, social stereotypes and attitudes also tend to be systematically biased. These biases may exist in overt, explicit forms, as represented by traditional bigotry. However, because their origins arise from virtually universal social categorization processes, they may also exist, often unconsciously, among people who strongly endorse egalitarian principles and truly believe that they are not prejudiced. In the United States, because of shared socialization influences, there is considerable empirical evidence that even well-intentioned whites who are not overtly biased and who do not believe that they are prejudiced typically demonstrate unconscious implicit negative racial attitudes and stereotypes. Both implicit and explicit stereotypes significantly shape interpersonal interactions, influencing how information is recalled and guiding expectations and inferences in systematic ways. They can also produce self-fulfilling prophecies in social interaction, in that the stereotypes of the perceiver influence the interaction with others in ways that conform to stereotypical expectations.

Healthcare Provider Prejudice or Bias

Prejudice is defined in psychology as an unjustified negative attitude based on a person's group membership. Survey research suggests that among white Americans, prejudicial attitudes toward minorities remain more common than not, as over half to three-quarters believe that relative to whites, minorities—particularly African Americans—are less intelligent, more prone to violence, and prefer to live off of welfare. It is reasonable to assume, however, that the vast majority of healthcare providers find prejudice morally abhorrent and at odds with their professional values. But healthcare providers, like other members of society, may not recognize manifestations of prejudice in their own behavior.

While there is no direct evidence that provider biases affect the quality of care for minority patients, research suggests that healthcare providers' diagnostic and treatment decisions, as well as their feelings about patients, are influenced by patients' race or ethnicity. Schulman et al. (1999), for example, found that physicians referred white male, black male, and white female hypothetical "patients" (actually videotaped actors who displayed the same symptoms of cardiac disease) for cardiac catheterization at the same rates (approximately 90% for each group), but were significantly less likely to recommend catheterization procedures for black female patients exhibiting the same symptoms. In another experimental design, Abreu (1999) found that mental health professionals subliminally "primed" with African American stereotype-laden words were more likely to evaluate the same hypothetical patient (whose race was not identified) more negatively than when primed with neutral words. Further, in a study based on actual clinical encounters, van Ryn and Burke (2000) found that doctors rated black patients as less intelligent, less educated, more likely to abuse drugs and alcohol, more likely to fail to comply with medical advice, more likely to lack social support, and less likely to participate in cardiac rehabilitation than white patients, even after patients' income, education, and personality characteristics were taken into account. These findings suggest that while the relationship between race or ethnicity and treatment decisions is complex and may also be influenced by gender, providers' perceptions and attitudes toward patients are influenced by patient race or ethnicity, often in subtle ways.

Medical Decisions under Time Pressure
with Limited Information

Indeed, studies suggest that several characteristics of the clinical encounter increase the likelihood that stereotypes, prejudice, or uncertainty may influence the quality of care for minorities. In the process of care, health professionals must come to judgments about patients' conditions and make decisions about treatment, often without complete and accurate information. In most cases, they must do so under severe time pressure and resource constraints. The assembly and use of these data are affected by many influences, including various "gestalts" or cognitive shortcuts. In fact, physicians are commonly trained to rely on clusters of information that functionally resemble the application of "prototypic" or stereotypic constellations. These conditions of time pressure, resource constraints, and the need to rely on gestalts map closely onto those factors identified by social psychologists as likely to produce negative outcomes due to lack of information, to stereotypes, and to biases (van Ryn, 2002).

Patient Response: Mistrust and Refusal

As noted above, the responses of racial and ethnic minority patients to healthcare providers are also a potential source of disparities. Little research has been conducted as to how patients may influence the clinical encounter. It is reasonable to speculate, however, that if patients convey mistrust, refuse treatment, or comply poorly with treatment, providers may become less engaged in the treatment process, and patients are less likely to be provided with more vigorous treatments and services. But these kinds of reactions from minority patients may be understandable as a response to negative racial experiences in other contexts, or to real or perceived mistreatment by providers. Survey research, for example, indicates that minority patients perceive higher levels of racial discrimination in healthcare than non-minorities. Patients' and providers' behavior and attitudes may therefore influence each other reciprocally, but reflect the attitudes, expectations, and perceptions that each has developed in a context where race and ethnicity are often more salient than these participants are even aware of.

What Can Healthcare Providers Do to Help Eliminate Disparities in Care?

Given that stereotypes, bias, and clinical uncertainty may influence clinicians' diagnostic and treatment decisions, education may be one of the most important tools as part of an overall strategy to eliminate healthcare disparities. Healthcare providers should be made aware of racial and ethnic disparities in healthcare, and the fact that these disparities exist, often despite providers' best intentions. In addition, all current and future healthcare providers can benefit from cross-cultural education. Cross-cultural education programs have been developed to enhance health professionals' awareness of how cultural and social factors influence healthcare, while providing methods to obtain, negotiate and manage this information clinically once it is obtained. Cross-cultural education can be divided into three conceptual approaches focusing on *attitudes* (cultural sensitivity/awareness approach), *knowledge* (multicultural/categorical approach), and *skills* (cross-cultural approach), and has been taught using a variety of interactive and experiential methodologies. Research to date demonstrates that training is effective in improving provider knowledge of cultural and behavioral aspects of healthcare and building effective communication strategies.

Standardized data collection is also critically important in efforts to understand and eliminate racial and ethnic disparities in healthcare. Data on patient and provider race and ethnicity would allow researchers to better disentangle factors that are associated with healthcare disparities, help health plans to monitor performance, ensure accountability to enrolled members and payors, improve patient choice, allow for evaluation of intervention programs, and help identify discriminatory practices. Unfortunately, standardized data on racial and ethnic differences in care are generally unavailable, and a number of ethical, logistical, and fiscal concerns present challenges to data collection and monitoring, including the need to protect patient privacy, the costs of data collection, and resistance from healthcare providers, institutions, plans, and patients. In addition, health plans have raised significant concerns about how such data will be analyzed and reported. The challenges to data collection should be addressed, as the costs of failing to assess racial and ethnic disparities in care may outweigh new burdens imposed by data collection and analysis efforts.

Many other strategies must be undertaken, in conjunction with the training and educational strategies described here, to eliminate racial and ethnic disparities in healthcare. As noted in the report, these include, for example, policy and regulatory strategies that address fragmentation of health plans along socioeconomic lines, and health systems interventions to promote the use of clinical practice guidelines and promote the use of interpretation services where community need exists. In short, a comprehensive, multi-level strategy is needed to eliminate these disparities. Broad sectors—including healthcare providers, their patients, payors, health plan purchasers, and society at large—must work together to ensure all patients receive a high quality of healthcare.

Guide to Information Sources

An increasing number of resources are available to healthcare providers and their patients to increase awareness of racial and ethnic healthcare disparities and means to improve the quality of care for racial and ethnic minorities. The following is only a partial list of some of these resources, and is not intended as an endorsement of the products or individuals and groups that produced them:

American Board of Internal Medicine. (1998). *Cultural Competence: Addressing a Multicultural Society: The ABIM Report 1997–1998.* Philadelphia: American Board of Internal Medicine.

American Medical Association. (1999). *Cultural Competence Compendium.* Chicago, IL: American Medical Association. Product Number OP209199 / Phone 1-800-621-8335.

Betancourt, J. R., Like, R. C., and Gottlieb, B. R., eds. (2000). Caring for diverse populations: Breaking down barriers. *Patient Care,* Special Issue, May 15.

Lavizzo-Mourey, R., and Mackenzie, E. R. (1996). Cultural Competence: Essential Measurements of Quality for Managed Care Organizations. *Annals of Internal Medicine* 124, pp. 919–21.

National Alliance for Hispanic Health. (2002) *Quality Services for Hispanics: the Cultural Competency Component.* Rockville, MD: U.S. Department of Health and Human Services.

In addition to these sources, the Henry J. Kaiser Family Foundation and the Robert Wood Johnson Foundation have recently joined forces to sponsor an initiative to increase dialogue among physicians regarding healthcare disparities. To learn more about this initiative, please visit the "Why the Difference?" website at www.kff.org/whythedifference.

References

Abreu, J. M. (1999). Conscious and nonconscious African American stereotypes: Impact on first impression and diagnostic ratings by therapists. *Journal of Consulting and Clinical Psychology* 67(3):387–93.

Gomes, C., and McGuire, T. G. (2001). Identifying the sources of racial and ethnic disparities in health care use. Unpublished manuscript.

Schulman, K. A., Berlin, J. A., Harless, W., Kerner, J. F., Sistrunk, S., Gersh, B. J., Dube, R., Taleghani, C. K., Burke, J. E., Williams, S., Eisenberg, J., Escarce, J. J., Ayers, W. (1999). The effect of race and sex on physicians' recommendations for cardiac catherization. *New England Journal of Medicine* 340:618–26.

van Ryn, M., and Burke, J. (2000). The effect of patient race and socio-economic status on physician's perceptions of patients. *Social Science and Medicine* 50:813–28.

Beyond Cultural Competence:
Applying Humility to Clinical Settings
Linda M. Hunt

In recent years, the concept of "culture" has captured the imagination of a broad cross section of health care providers and policy makers. An increasingly diverse and multicultural society is inspiring health care providers to strive to develop cultural sensitivity and cultural competence. Virtually every health profession has made cultural competency a part of its curriculum, and many health care institutions are requiring cultural sensitivity training for personnel (American Medical Association, 1999). Such programs are generally designed to sensitize health providers to the special needs and vulnerabilities of different populations, with the goal of providing accessible and appropriate care to all.

The emphasis in this movement has clearly been focused on members of "underserved" and "underrepresented" racial and ethnic minority groups. Developing the cultural competence of health professionals is intended to minimize cultural barriers to health care and make health services more "user friendly" to culturally diverse subgroups, and thereby help to reduce their disproportionate burden of poor health. Health providers are encouraged to explore the traditional cultural concepts and practices of such patients, and to develop culturally appropriate models for clinical interactions, treatment protocols, and health education efforts (Carrillo, Green, and Betancourt, 1999).

Despite widespread popularity, cultural competency remains a vaguely defined goal, with no explicit criteria established for its accomplishment or assessment. This lack may in part be due to the elusive nature of its central construct: culture.

Linda M. Hunt, "Beyond Cultural Competence: Applying Humility to Clinical Settings," from *The Park Ridge Center Bulletin*, issue 24, 3–4. © 2001 by the Park Ridge Center for the Study of Health, Faith, and Ethics. Reprinted by permission of the publisher.

Defining Culture

Definitions of "culture" are multiple, broad, and notably ambiguous. While there is no agreed-upon definition of culture, the classic definition by E. B. Tylor in 1871 is widely cited in anthropology textbooks: "Culture . . . is that complex whole which includes knowledge, belief, art, morals, law, custom and any other capabilities and habits acquired by man as a member of society" (Tylor, 1871:1). Most definitions of culture emphasize that it is complex and dynamic, comprised of the shared solutions to problems faced by the group. These solutions include technologies, beliefs, and behaviors.

Culture does not determine behavior, but affords group members a repertoire of ideas and possible actions, providing the framework through which they understand themselves, their environment, and their experiences. Culture is a complex set of relationships, responses, and interpretations that must be understood, not as a body of discrete traits, but as an integrated system of orientations and practices generated within a specific socioeconomic context. Culture is ever changing and always being revised within the dynamic context of its enactment.

Culture is neither a blueprint nor an identity; individuals choose between various cultural options, and in our multicultural society, many times choose widely between the options offered by a variety of cultural traditions. It is not possible to predict the beliefs and behaviors of individuals based on their race, ethnicity, or national origin (O'Connor, 1996). Individuals' group membership cannot be assumed to indicate their culture because those who share a group label may variously enact culture.

In its zeal to encourage respect for cultural difference, the cultural competency movement has sometimes lost sight of these important features of the concept of culture. Instead it has too often represented culture as a decontextualized set of traits providing a template for the perceptions and behaviors of group members. A burgeoning literature on cultural diversity presents the reader with veritable laundry lists of traditional beliefs and practices ostensibly characteristic of particular ethnic groups. This approach encourages the questionable notion that immigrants and certain ethnic and racial minorities are particularly driven by traditionalism (Hunt, Schneider, and Comer, 2004). The emphasis in this genre is on difference, pitting the exotic and esoteric against mainstream or conventional beliefs that remain unnamed and unexplored.

The misconception, common in clinical settings, that culture can be understood as a set of discrete traits, has led some mistakenly to treat culture as an explanatory variable, subject to prediction and control. In such applications, specific ethnic cultures are represented as a codified body of characteristics that can be identified and then either modified or manipulated to facilitate clinical goals (Santiago-Irizarry, 1996).

Paradoxically, in such approaches, what originated in a desire to promote respect for individual differences may instead promote stereotyping and essentializing (Carillo, Green, and Betancourt, 1999). This process of reifying presumed difference may have the unintended consequence of bolstering a sense of group boundaries (Santiago-Irizarry, 1996). It may also reinforce the belief that culture can be diagnosed and treated, that exotic or unfamiliar beliefs and behaviors of members of already disempowered subgroups should be controlled and adjusted to resemble norms of the dominant group.

Cultural Humility

Such pitfalls may be avoided by more subtly integrating the concept of culture with the clinical agenda. The starting point for such an approach would not be an examination of the patient's belief system, but careful consideration by health care providers of the assumptions and beliefs that are embedded in their own understandings and goals in the clinical encounter (O'Connor, 1996). Training for cultural competency, with its emphasis on promoting understanding of the "cultural" client, has often neglected consideration of the providers' worldview. In the alternative approach, rather than learning to identify and respond to sets of culturally specific traits, the culturally competent provider would be taught to develop what might be called cultural humility.

Cultural humility has been described by Melanie Tervalon and Jann Murray-Garcia as a lifelong process of self-reflection and self-critique. Cultural humility does not require mastery of lists of "different" or peculiar beliefs and behaviors supposedly pertaining to certain groups of patients. Rather, the provider is encouraged to develop a respectful partnership with each patient through patient-focused interviewing, exploring similarities and differences between his own and each patient's priorities, goals, and capacities. In this model, the most serious barrier to culturally appropriate care is not a lack of knowledge of the details of any given cultural orientation, but the provider's failure to develop self-awareness and a respectful attitude toward diverse points of view.

Effectively exploring cultural issues in the clinic should begin with recognition that "cultural difference" refers to a relationship between two perspectives. Identifying difference requires contrasting two orientations: the provider's and the patient's. Culturally competent providers develop skills for exploring the existence and importance of differences in the basic assumptions, expectations, and goals they and their patients bring to any clinical interaction. This kind of reflexive attentiveness should not be limited only to those people who are perceived to be culturally "other," but can be useful in any clinical encounter.

The ideal conclusion of this kind of cross-cultural exploration would be to develop an approach to managing clinical problems based on negotiation between the two perspectives. Due to institutional, time, and other pragmatic limitations of the clinical setting, as well as social, economic, and other practical restrictions faced by patients, the ideal of reaching a negotiated plan of action may not be feasible. Still, following the principle of cultural humility, a culturally competent provider should be open and flexible enough to be able to identify the presence and importance of differences between her orientation and that of each patient, and to explore compromises that would be acceptable to both. This strategy does not call for the health care provider to become an expert in cultural minutiae, nor to act as a minister or an herbalist. Ideally, being appropriately cognizant of and responsive to cultural issues should not be thought of as reaching a "competency," so much as engaging in an ongoing process of honing and applying skills for self-awareness and for respectful recognition of the unique perspective each patient brings to the clinical encounter.

References

American Medical Association. 1999. *Cultural Competency Compendium*. Chicago: American Medical Association.

Carrillo, J. E., A. R. Green, and J. R. Betancourt. 1999. Cross-cultural primary care: A patient-based approach. [see comment]. *Annals of Internal Medicine* 130(10):829–834.

Hunt, L. M., S. Schneider, and B. Comer. 2004. Should "acculturation" be a variable in health research? A critical review of research on US Hispanics. *Soc.Sci.Med.* 59(5):973–986.

O'Connor, B. B. 1996. Promoting cultural competence in HIV/AIDS care. *Journal of the Association of Nurses in AIDS Care* 7 (Suppl 1):41–53.

Santiago-Irizarry, Vilma. 1996. Culture as cure. *Cultural Anthropology* 11(1):3–24.

Tervalon, M., and J. Murray-Garcia. 1998. Cultural humility versus cultural competence: A critical distinction in defining physician training outcomes in multicultural education. [Review] [32 refs]. *Journal of Health Care for the Poor & Underserved* 9(2):117–125.

Tylor, Edward B. 1871. *Primitive Culture: Researches into the Development of Mythology, Philosophy, Religion, Art and Custom*. London: John Murray.

Coming to Terms with Advanced Breast Cancer: Black Women's Narratives from Eastern North Carolina

Holly F. Mathews, Donald R. Lannin, and James P. Mitchell

I went to see the doctor because my arm was aching. He gave me a shot [of cortisone], but it kept on hurting. One day, I was chopping in the garden—I love to chop. It all began that night. It [breast] began to hurt. I thought I had jarred it with the hoe. All of a sudden it kept on hurting. That Saturday night I put a hot cloth on it. It began to run. Sunday, I kept putting cloths on it. It had a risen in it. It was running. That Monday I went to the doctor. He sent me to a surgeon doctor. He checked it over, and I went to the hospital . . . They took it off. I did not get scared. I took God with me . . . I don't have any thoughts about what could have caused it. First, it was a risen. It worked out that it was a risen and a cancer. You have to pray and give it to God. He will take care of it. If anybody's cancer is like mine, I would remove it. In three days it had lumps dripping out of it. I would tell others how I went through it. A lump and a tumor is not the same thing as a cancer. That's why I don't know for sure that mine was a cancer (Lydia, age 72 [1]).

"Coming to terms" is an interesting American expression. Technically, it means to 'compromise, arrive at an agreement, arbitrate' [2]; colloquially, it means to arrive at some understanding and acceptance of a problematic event or experience. Frequently, people come to terms with problematic experiences by putting their thoughts and feelings into words. This act of verbalization implies an attempt not only to conceptualize the experience, but also to define it so that the real work of understanding can begin.

In the narratives to be discussed in this paper, black women from eastern North Carolina draw on multiple sources of knowledge in order to come to terms with a diagnosis of advanced breast cancer—a biomedically

Holly Mathews, Donald R. Lannin, and James P. Mitchell, "Coming to Terms with Advanced Breast Cancer: Black Women's Narratives from North Carolina," from *Social Science and Medicine*, vol. 38, 512–515. © 1994. Reprinted by permission of Elsevier Science, Ltd.

defined disease entity that they often refuse to acknowledge or accept. Their narratives represent a debate over whose terms will be used to label and describe a disease which is new to many of them. This struggle for understanding is made more difficult by the lack of natural contexts for discussion about the nature of the disease since cancer, for a majority of these women, is a taboo topic to be concealed from others, even family and friends (see Balshem [3]). By asking these women to tell us their stories about breast cancer, we created a context in which many of them were able, for the first time, to talk openly about a frightening and often bewildering experience.

The narratives these women produced are the subject of this essay. They are very personal accounts of individual experiences of illness. Yet they also include explanatory commentaries which attempt to relate the meanings of these episodes to an indigenous model of health and disease found in many black communities in the South as well as to popular American notions about cancer and particular biomedical conceptions of breast disease and its treatment. As such, they provide us with an important window into the processes involved in adapting personal experience to pre-existent cultural models, in modifying such models in the light of new information, and in coming to terms with shifts in conceptual reality as perceived by the individual actor in a cultural system.

The narratives are part of a larger study investigating the reasons why some women delay seeking treatment for breast cancer. The study is described first to provide background and context for the narratives. A profile of the women interviewed is then presented along with a discussion of methodology. Finally, the results of the narrative analysis are interpreted in light of recent research on the use of narratives by individuals to conceptualize and understand the experience of illness.

Background for the Study

The narratives come from a study begun in 1988 by the Department of Surgery at the East Carolina University School of Medicine to investigate the reasons why women, and particularly black women in the region, tend in greater numbers than reported nationally, to present with advanced stages of disease when first seeking treatment for breast cancer [4]. Presentation with advanced stage disease is a major issue in breast cancer research because early detection and treatment are known to reduce mortality and suffering [5–7]. Moreover, the survival rates after treatment for breast cancer have been significantly lower for black than for white women primarily because black women present more often with advanced disease, a fact that has been well documented in a number of recent studies [8–10] and by the American College of Surgeons (ASC) Breast Cancer Surveys [11–13] and the Cancer Surveillance, Epidemiology, and End Results (SEER) Program [14].

Between 1 July, 1988, and 30 July, 1991, 400 women who sought treatment for breast cancer in eastern North Carolina received an hour-long, structured interview designed to explore a range of demographic, psychosocial, and cultural variables hypothesized to be associated with presentation for treatment with advanced stage disease [15]. In addition, all of these women were asked to complete open-ended, in-depth interviews about their own, personal experiences with breast disease, and their medical records were abstracted to record physician assessments of tumor size and stage at time of presentation as well as physician ratings of subsequent compliance with prescribed treatments.

The East Carolina University Medical School was established 10 years ago with a mandate to train family physicians for rural practice and to provide, in conjunction with the Pitt County Memorial Hospital, medical services and preventive care to the people living in the 33-county region of eastern North Carolina. Their jointly sponsored breast clinic is the major treatment site in the region for women with breast abnormalities and has a referral base of 1.5 million people, most of whom live in federally designated rural areas. Approximately one-third of the region's population is black, although the proportional resident concentration of blacks and whites varies by county. About 25% of this population lives below the poverty line, compared to 14.4% nationally [16].

Women patients entered the breast clinic in one of two ways: referral by a private physician or health department or self-referral directly to the breast clinic. The majority of private physicians and health departments in the rural eastern counties do not have the facilities available to provide advanced screening and treatment of breast disease and so rely on referrals to the ECU breast clinic. In the larger towns (all with populations under 50,000) located in close proximity to the medical center, some private physicians are able to provide advanced screening and treatment for their breast cancer patients. Consequently, the study was designed to draw a consecutive sample of all the women who were either physician- or self-referred to the ECU breast clinic over a three-year period while also interviewing a consecutive sample of women who sought treatment from a random sample of private physicians practicing in the three larger towns in eastern NC, including Greenville, site of the ECU breast clinic [17].

The 400 women interviewed came from 30 eastern NC counties. Of these 400, 133 or 30.4% were black. There were no significant demographic differences found between the patient population interviewed and the entire breast cancer patient population recorded in the Pitt County Hospital Tumor Registry for eastern North Carolina with regard to age, race, stage of disease, tumor size, patient residence, or insurance status [18, p. 25]. Preliminary analyses of the structured interview data focused upon categorizing patients by tumor stage at time of presentation and comparing this classification with the different variables measured in the structured interview. All tumors were staged according to the standardized TNM staging system as described in the 1988 version of the Staging Manual of the American Joint Committee on Cancer [19] using data from both physical examinations, mammography and other diagnostic techniques. For this study, *in situ* carcinomas representing stage 1 tumors are labeled as "Early Stage" presentation; *local* or invasive cancers localized to the breast representing stage 2 tumors are labeled as "Middle Stage" presentation; while *regional* cancers in the breast with spread to the regional lymph nodes or pectoral muscles representing stage 3 tumors and *remote* cancers with distant metastases representing stage 4 tumors are grouped and labeled as "Late Stage" presentation [19, p. 27].

Black women in the study were significantly more likely than white women to present with advanced or *Late Stage* disease (26% of black as opposed to 11% of white patients); or with *Middle Stage* disease (53% of black as opposed to 39% of white patients); while white women were significantly more likely to present with *Early Stage* disease (50% of white as opposed to 21% of black patients) [19, p. 26]. This strong association between race and late stage presentation persisted even when the group was stratified by income level, educational level, and method of cancer detection (i.e., breast self exam, physician exam, or mammography) and is consistent with results reported in other studies [8, 20].

In an effort to account for the specific effects of race on variation in tumor stage at time of presentation, interaction effects between race and the variables measured in the structured interview were assessed. The categories examined included demographic variables (age, education, residence, and occupation); access variables (income, physician utilization, insurance status, available transportation, and breast cancer knowledge); social support variables (overall size of social networks and perceived attitudes of male supports toward breast cancer); and psychosocial and cultural variables (fatalism, religiosity, and indigenous or "folk" medical beliefs). Those found to be most significantly correlated, in conjunction with race, to late stage presentation included, in order of significance, a high degree of fatalism, a strong sense that men were not supportive of women's suffering, a lack of knowledge of risk factors for breast cancer, lower educational levels overall, and a strong belief in the effectiveness of indigenous or folk treatments for breast disease [19, p. 32]. Access variables did not turn out to influence significantly stage at time of presentation, which dovetailed with our independent finding that no differences existed among the patients interviewed with regard to race, income, and educational levels in terms of rate of physician utilization with the only significant difference to emerge being one of age. Older women, of both races and all income levels, did utilize physicians significantly more often than younger women [19, p. 30].

In an effort to further understand the meaning of the findings reported from the quantitative data analysis, the in-depth narratives produced by those black women classified as presenting with late-stage disease were examined in the subsequent phase of the larger study.

Profile of the Patient Population and
Description of Methodology

Preliminary analysis of the in-depth interviews focused on 26 narratives produced by black women who presented with late-stage, advanced breast tumors (defined as TNM stage 3 or greater) and who were, therefore, assumed to have delayed a significant amount of time before seeking treatment for breast cancer. During the three-year period from 1988 to 1991, 34 or 26% of 133 black women patients presented for treatment at the breast clinic with advanced stage disease. After each woman completed the structured interview guide, she was asked to spend another 30 min to 1 hr, at a time convenient with her, telling the interviewer about her personal experiences with breast cancer. Of the 34 women contacted, 5 were very ill from breast cancer, having been immediately hospitalized after arrival at the breast clinic. Although most of them did the structured interview, none was able to finish in the in-depth portion. Four of the remaining 29 women contacted were unable to complete the in-depth interview because one became too ill, one died, one refused, and another dropped out of treatment and could not be located again. Consequently, the final data set consists of 26 completed in-depth interviews with black women with advanced disease.

Of these 26, 14 were completed prior to diagnosis around the time of biopsy, and the remaining 12 were done retrospectively with patients who had either completed treatment for breast cancer, were in the process of undergoing treatment, or who had refused treatment altogether. When possible, patients interviewed prior to diagnosis were contacted again on subsequent visits to the clinic as treatment progressed. In addition, those pre-biopsy patients who refused treatment were contacted in their homes for follow-up sessions.

The women interviewed ranged in age from 39 to 83 years with the majority being over the age of 50. There was no significant difference in the age distribution of advanced stage black patients and the rest of the cancer patient population. Although black women in the cancer study population tended overall to have significantly lower incomes than the white women, those grouped in the late stage category exhibited the same range of variation in income levels as the black women presenting with early and medium stage disease. There were also no significant differences in place of residence between the late and early/medium stage groups of black patients with similar proportions in each category coming from rural, small town, and large town locations. The one significant difference between the groups was educational level, with the late stage group having a significantly higher proportion of women with a low educational level (defining as having completed grade school or less) than the women in the early and medium stage categories, who were more likely to have completed high school.

A team of trained interviewers, matched to patients by race and sex, asked the women patients to talk about a standard set of topics related to their personal experience of breast cancer. These topics questioned them about when they had first noticed a breast problem and how; what actions they chose to follow and why; what perceptions they had about causes of the problem; how they felt about their experiences in the medical system; and ended by asking them for their suggestions about how patient care and cancer education efforts could be improved. The interviews employed a conversational style, with the standard topics introduced at points appropriate to the conversation, in order to allow women as much latitude as possible for generating their own narrative structures.

Once the interviews began, most women proceeded with little prompting to talk extensively about their thoughts and feelings. The average interview lasted an hour, but many went longer and were frequently very emotional experiences for both participants and interviewers. When possible, the interviews were tape-recorded; when this was not possible or the patients refused, detailed notes were taken and interview summaries written. The recorded interviews were transcribed onto the computer for software-aided analysis.

All of the coding and analysis was done by the anthropologist on the team using a twofold strategy. An examination of the overall structure of the narratives yielded insights into both the types of topics introduced and the sequencing of them produced by the respondents. This enabled a better sense of understanding about the issues these women found important, as well as about the goals they wanted to accomplish in the discussion. The subsequent stage of analysis focused on delineating from the discourse the important metaphors and propositions utilized by patients in conceptualizing and understanding breast cancer in order to try and ascertain the broader cultural models of health and disease that gave meaning to their discussions of individual episodes of illness. To assess the validity of these metaphors and propositions, an iterative procedure was employed. During the ongoing analysis, assumptions derived from the study of initial cases were tested on later interviewees. Second, an attempt was made whenever possible to reinterview patients in order to assess the validity of the analysis of the person's initial interview and to glean additional information to answer questions raised in the iterative process. Eventually, 20 of the 26 women included in the sample were interviewed more than once.

Results of the Narrative Analysis

The 26 interviews analyzed, including the one quoted at the beginning of this article, have a coherent narrative structure. They all begin with a discussion of the origin of symptoms and move chronologically to recount events that occurred relevant to the disorder. Interestingly, unlike illness narratives analyzed in other studies [20, 21, 22], these accounts devote relatively little consideration to the cause of the disorder and direct much more attention to arriving at some label and defining a set of features for it. Indeed, many of the breast narratives end with a statement about diagnosis. These narratives, moreover, contain very little commentary on the social roles played by others in the illness, most probably because others are excluded as much as possible from knowing about the condition, and individual women seldom use talk about their symptoms with others outside of the medical system as a way to arrive at a diagnostic label.

The accounts given by the breast cancer patients can thus be seen to mix two types of discourse labeled by Linde [23] as narrative and explanation. They have a narrative structure which begins with an orientation to symptoms and builds to a decision about labeling but with much explanatory justification included along the way. In this sense, they resemble in many respects the stories Farmer collected from rural Haitians when they were initially confronted with the new disease of AIDS [24].

For the majority of these women patients, the concept of breast cancer was fairly new. Although they were familiar with much of the popular discussion on breast cancer, many reported not having heard of it until recently and not having known any one who died from it. As one woman stated, "maybe it was around in the old days but no one knew it, or maybe it's just getting stronger now so they say more are getting it." These women were, in many respects, coming to terms with a novel disorder, and all 26 began their stories in much the same way as did the Haitians when AIDS first became a problem—by attempting to relate their symptoms to an indigenous or "folk" theory of disease based on an imbalance in the blood.

Over time, after receiving an official diagnosis of cancer, these women often struggled to evaluate how popular conceptions of the disease (including, for example, the belief that cancer is always ultimately fatal, medical treatment is degrading and hopeless, and that there is nothing a person can do to prevent cancer), disseminated in the media through television and magazine accounts of personal experiences of cancer and reinforced in general conversations with friends and neighbors about cancer experiences, fit with the indigenous or "folk" definition of the disorder. Finally, for those women who did go through the process of conventional medical treatment for the disease, a third layer of specific biomedical information about breast cancer as well as physician ideas about the need for a therapeutic partnership and positive, fighting spirit during the treatment process began to affect their interpretations of the disorder. Yet despite the similar progression of experience for many of these women, they often varied greatly in the ways in which they handled the contradictions that emerged between these three very different ways of conceptualizing breast disease.

All 14 of the black women with advanced disease interviewed prior to diagnosis began their narratives by discussing a host of symptoms connected, they believed, to the presence of a condition known as "dirty" or "bad" blood. The theme of blood figured significantly as well in 10 of the 12 narratives recounted retrospectively by patients with advanced disease. Moreover, segments of the blood model could also be found in about half of the narratives recounted by black women categorized as presenting with early and middle stage disease, but were absent from all of the accounts given by white patients, regardless of stage at time of presentation.

The symptoms they identified included knots or lumps that would "come and go" or move around the body; boils on the skin known as "risens" or "whiteheads," said to be impurities in the blood coming up to get out; aches and pains in the arm and side; and general flushed, feverish feelings coupled with weakness and dizzy or "falling out" spells; and occasionally, flashes of light in the head. For example, Sallie, age 53, reported "It all started with a whitehead I had on my breast. But then it disappeared. But it was a sign of that bad blood trying to get out. So it was there all the time. And then it formed a lump that was there too, but it wasn't coming up." Alternately, Frances, age 76, reported "I had this knot on my stomach. And I went to the doctor and told him about it. But he told me not to worry it was nothing. This was oh, about 1974. But then it moved up to my breast and it began to grow. But it wasn't bothering me. Only it was getting bigger and bigger." Finally, Thelma, age 41, noted, "It was a real bad time. I was hot and flushed one day, and when I was doing the dishes I started seeing these flashes of light in my head. And that night my arm and my side started hurting and I rubbed the ache out and noticed that lump there had gotten larger. But it wasn't bothering me any."

The reference to bad or dirty blood refers directly to a more inclusive system of beliefs about health and disease common to many black Americans in the South and found, in various forms, in widely distributed African and Afro-Caribbean groups [25]. This belief system attributes good health to the maintenance of balance in the blood. Weidman has labeled this theory found among Haitians as the "blood paradigm" [26]. This paradigm, as documented for the Southeast [27] and in other parts of the United States [28], posits different qualities to blood that is out of balance. It can variously be too high or low, too bitter or sweet, too thick or thin, or too dirty. Any of these conditions is itself seen to be a disorder or to cause other folk illnesses related to the different organs of the body. Treatment usually involves the application of opposites. In the discussion of breast knots and lumps, the women presenting with late stage disease are drawing on a particular notion of bad blood as blood with "impurities" in it. These impurities are believed to circulate throughout the system and are often talked about as something that is "trying to come out" of the body.

Many women draw connections in their narratives between impurities circulating in the blood and lumps and knots in the body. These lumps are said to be triggered by a bump or blow to the body which causes the impurities in the blood to "clump together in one place." Indeed, 16 of the 26 women with advanced disease described their breast lumps as resulting from bumps or blows bruising the body. For example, in two of the less well elaborated accounts, May and Jean respectively give responses that suggest this connection: "I noticed a knot in my breast in 1989, but it didn't hurt. It just came from bumping into the bed so I put it out of my mind"; "I had a sore spot on my breast that came from bumping into the car door with my groceries. A lump came up there but it never bothered me."

The narratives that make the causal links explicit are more detailed. For example, 66-year-old Clara outlines the connection:

> I had a pain in my arm for five years. It was the arthritis jumping on me so I paid it no mind. I also had a knot in my breast all that time, but it would come and go. It wasn't nothing. But then I noticed a few months ago that there was a big knot on my right breast where Mr. Jones [an Alzheimer's patient she sits for] had been hitting me on the side. You know, if you get a hard enough blow, it makes some kind of blood clot, and if it stays there long enough it's going to form something else.

Lucille, age 75, linked the impurities circulating in dirty blood to the knots formed by a blow or bruise:

> That knot I had came and went. If you have dirty blood, the impurities have to go somewhere. And once I passed the change, that blood just stayed in me all the time. It was mounting up. When I fell down that day in the garden, they all came up to that bruise and they made a lump. That's what made it so big.

This chain of logic holds that blood can become dirty either because a person has a tendency that way; has engaged in unclean, unsanitary habits or excessive sexual encounters; or has no way for impurities in the blood to leave the system after menopause. These impurities are circulating in the blood and when they become too numerous or "strong," or when the person is weak with low resistance or has an accident of some kind, the impurities may "come up" into swollen areas, skin sores, or lumps formed under the surface.

In and of themselves, lumps are not bad. They are a normal part of the system as evinced by the fact that if left alone, they tend to come and go. As 57-year-old Olivia put it, "I've had lumps all my life. Sometimes they come on you when things happen. But if a lump is not hurting you then it's nothing to bother with. I believe that if a lump ain't bothering you, you shouldn't bother it. It will probably go away."

However, as Clara indicates in her statement above, sometimes changes occur in these lumps if they stay in one place long enough. This change is usually described in patient narratives as a fundamental alteration in the character of the lump—it goes from being a static, almost non-living entity that causes no bother or pain, to something animated that begins to take on a life of its own, growing rapidly and becoming bothersome. This transition can happen for several reasons—either a blow or bruise can trigger the growth, an ever-increasing number of impurities in the blood with no other outlet can begin to "move up" or "grow out," or it can just be in one place too long and "take root."

The metaphor, either directly stated or implied in the characterization of lumps in 24 of these 26 narratives, is of a living thing, sometimes explicitly equated to a plant, as when patients refer to lumps as: "a *kernel* under my arm," or "a knot *rooted* in my breast" or a "*growth* that has taken hold in my side." In a very real sense, to borrow Clara's phrase, a lump that stays in one place long enough may become "rooted" to the spot and begin to grow taking on a life of its own that may become bothersome to the woman experiencing it.

Lakoff [29] reports that metaphors serve an important mapping function in cognition by introducing information from physical-world source domains into target domains in the nonphysical world which, according to Quinn and Holland [30], enables image-schematic thought. By drawing analogies from physical experience, metaphors assist people in conceptualizing non-physical processes in a concrete, visual way that makes these experiences more tangible and thus accessible to mental processing. For example, when women use the metaphor of a plant to characterize a breast lump which they cannot physically see or necessarily feel, they create a set of images and characteristics that can be used to conceptualize their illness experience in a concrete way and to predict likely entailments. Once a seed begins to root and grow, therefore, it can be expected to get larger. A breast lump growing uncontrollably creates a problem for women because it may "burst through the skin," "make the breast bleed," "take over the breast," or interfere with normal functions and cause pain. Just as plants require nourishment to survive, these lumps may also "keep growing and growing, taking more and more out of me." By logical extension, seeds that are dormant, that have not taken root as evinced by beginning to grow, are not a problem. Consequently, lumps that do not noticeably grow or become bothersome are best left alone.

Many aspects of this view coincide with what women hear generally and are sometimes told explicitly by physicians—i.e., that breast lumps that grow uncontrollably are dangerous because they may spread to other parts of the body and that cancer is a disease that eats you up from the inside out. Similarly, they can also understand the logic of surgery to remove the "growth" from the body. However, the notion of surgery presents a problem for many since it also calls up other, more frightening entailments of the plant metaphor.

Surgery was thought by 20 of the women interviewed to be dangerous because, "cutting on a cancer will make it spread," and "once air gets to a lump it will make it grow." The logic relating these statements to the plant metaphor is usually implied in the narrative accounts but is occasionally elaborated in some detail. Marjorie, age 78, said "I believe, I don't care what kind of lump it is, I believe that if they cut it, it spreads. It might take five years or ten, but it will come back more intensified." Alternatively, 63-year-old Pauline stated, "If you feel you haven't gotten the whole root, then it'll spread. That lump will start to grow again bigger." In both cases, the assumption is that if you want to remove a plant, you must take it out by the roots. If you don't get it all, then it will come back. But also entailed in these examples is a notion of pruning—that if you just cut it back, the lump will come back stronger and bigger than ever. Consequently, surgery or "going under the knife" is seen by these women to be very dangerous. Unless a lump or knot is extremely bothersome, surgery should be avoided. This is reflected in the desire of many patients to be given a pill that will "poison the growth" or even to undergo radiation treatment which some interpret as "using X-rays to burn up the growth."

Again, these ideas are very similar to ones that patients report hearing from physicians about "taking out the whole cancer," "getting it before it starts to spread," and "making sure to remove the whole thing." However, the notion of catching a lump early and removing it at a point before it starts to grow makes no sense to them. As Frances says: "Why would you take out a lump that isn't bothering you? If it's not growing, it should be left alone. Fooling around with it might make it start to act up. I don't hold with cutting on things that ain't bothering you." Such an attitude is also implied in Lydia's statement at the beginning of the essay when she says, "If anybody's cancer is like mine [i.e., a large cancer with lumps dripping out of it], I would remove it." She points this out because, by implication, unless it is such an abnormal type, it should not be disturbed.

The notion of air getting to cancer, discussed in 18 of the 26 narratives, is entailed in the image of plants living outdoors and drawing nourishment from the sun, air, and water. This logic suggests that lumps that are enclosed in the body have a limited amount of nourishment. But "opening them up" to the air increases the chances for them to grow and spread. Thus, as 47-year-old Mary explains, "I'm afraid to go under the knife because once that lump is opened up to the air, it will just *blossom* and grow. Even if they try and take it out, the part that's left will be stronger and it will spread."

That the concern with air follows from an entailment of the plant metaphor is made obvious when the previous examples are compared to one given in an interview with a 62-year-old, white patient with early stage disease. One of the items on the structured interview asked her to agree or disagree with the statement that air getting to a cancer will make it spread. The patient agreed that she had heard people say that was true. When asked why she thought it might be, she replied, "I don't really know but I guess, you know, it's like when a wind comes up on a wildfire and it makes it spread out of control." Obviously, this analogy provides a different but plausible mapping of a physical-world image onto the experience of tumor growth and represents a creative attempt to explain something for which the women had no explanation. Yet this analogy was unique and did not appear in any of the other interviews with white or black patients.

As Quinn and Holland determine in their review of recent studies, metaphors are not extended "willy-nilly from any one domain to any other" but rather a small number of classes of metaphors appear to be used in accounting for particular experiences. As they explain it, "The classes from which speakers select metaphors they consider to be appropriate are those that capture aspects of the simplified world and the prototypical events unfolding in this world, constituted by the cultural model" [30, p. 30]. Clearly, the plant metaphor is doubly compelling in the illness domain. The indigenous or "folk" medical beliefs of many of these black patients are heavily plant-oriented, with many traditional herbal remedies being called "root medicines."

Second, the plant image itself accounts for many aspects of the particular experiences women have with breast lumps and makes possible many logical entailments about how plants live and grow that seem to predictively account for much of the concrete experiences these women have with breast lumps. Conversely, comparing a breast lump to a wildfire may make it possible to explain how air causes it to spread, but it does not extend logically or satisfactorily to predict and account for other aspects of the experience.

The majority, 22 of the 26 black women who presented with late stage disease, delayed seeking treatment, they said, because the lumps "weren't bothering them," "did not hurt," or "weren't growing." Only when these conditions changed and the lumps began to become bothersome, painful or extremely large did many of them seek medical help. At this point, some suspected that they might receive a diagnosis of cancer. For many of them, "waiting to see" and "finding out it was cancer" was the worst part of the entire illness experience—an event whose meaning had to be understood with reference to both indigenous conceptions of lumps as well as to popular cultural beliefs about cancer in general.

Popular Knowledge about Cancer

Once these patients began to think about the possibility of cancer, they acknowledged a whole host of feelings about the disease common in popular discourse. Much of what they said paralleled Balshem's descriptions of attitudes toward cancer in Philadelphia [3]. Cancer was seen by patients to be the worst of all diseases because it is always fatal and is essentially incurable. Moreover, cancer is an extremely painful and degrading disease that "strips away your dignity." As 71-year-old Carol said:

> Letting in the idea that it might be cancer was the hardest thing in the world for me. People don't get over cancer. It will always kill you. They might do something for you, but eventually the cancer will come back and get you. It's a horrible, degrading disease that eats you up.

Paradoxically, for many of these women, cancer was seen to have no particular cause. It just, "comes on people for no reason." Much as Balshem observed, these patients reported that everything and nothing can cause cancer, and the reasons why one person and not another falls victim to it are unexplainable. Consequently, for many of the women interviewed, cancer in its whimsical aspects, resembled illnesses that did not respond to conventional categories or cures in the indigenous medical system. Thus, by extension, the only likelihood of finding a cure for cancer was "to turn it over to God." As Ethel, age 58, explained it:

> Cancer is a horrible disease. It just eats you up. The only one powerful enough to overcome it is the Lord. You just have to trust in Jesus to do battle for you and save you from this horrible affliction.

Here the battle metaphor is used to portray a struggle between God, as the all powerful force for good, and cancer as consummate evil, or as another woman put it, "that terrible, evil sickness." While Balshem's informants also embraced this view of cancer as evil, they did not seem to emphasize it as strongly as the breast patients interviewed in this study.

Indeed, many of these women proceeded, after the diagnosis of cancer was received from a physician, to redefine the disorder suffered as a supernatural one which was no longer amenable to treatment with "ordinary means," including physician-prescribed treatments. As Clara expressed it:

> When you know you have cancer, then there's nothing for it but to turn it over to God. If you have enough faith, He will heal it and you don't need no operation. Because there is nothing a doctor can do for you—only God has the power.

It follows that because cancer is a powerful and virtually unstoppable disease once it is activated, women need to be careful not to "stir it up." Balshem reports that her Philadelphia informants view cancer as a minion of fate that may punish those who notice or defy it. She writes of them that "to think about cancer, to try to prevent it, is to tempt fate. Cancer testing is 'looking for trouble' " [3, p. 161]. For her informants, even speaking the word cancer out loud was potentially dangerous as was talking about the disease openly or acknowledging that others had it. The women interviewed in this study had similar views which mapped well onto their more traditional notions about the characteristics of breast lumps. For example, Selma explained:

If you have a lump and it's not bothering you, leave it alone. You don't want to get it started. That's why I don't hold with this idea of poking around to look for lumps. Why look for trouble? When that doctor wanted me to have the X-ray on my breast, I told him he was crazy. There's no telling what those X-rays might stir up.

Just as not tempting fate by looking for cancer may protect you, so too refusing to name the disease or acknowledge that you have it is seen as protecting you in some way from suffering its full effects. Janine, age 48, explained her feelings after she went through diagnosis:

When he told me what it was, well I just couldn't hardly even think about it. To have that disease would be the end. So I just decided then and there that I wouldn't worry no more. That I would give it to God, and that I would never speak of it again. I trusted God to heal me and I believe He has. That's all I need to know.

Once having made this decision, Janine refused surgery and abandoned her radiation treatments. Her condition deteriorated, and she was eventually hospitalized for fluid accumulation in the lungs due to the spread of the cancer. Her lungs were drained, and in an interview that day, she stated that she had been suffering from pneumonia but was feeling much better. When she was rehospitalized two weeks later, she maintained just before her death that pneumonia was killing her. She had not mentioned the word cancer since the day that she received the diagnosis.

Phase Three—Encountering Biomedical Notions of Breast Cancer

In a recent study of American oncology, Good et al. [31] have documented a major shift in physicians' attitudes since the 1950s when most felt that a diagnosis of cancer should not be revealed to the patient. Today there is virtual unanimity that diagnoses should be revealed. However, physicians vary in their notions about just when and what should be disclosed to patients in part because they perceive their mission to be one of instilling, not dashing, patients' hopes [31, p. 61]. Many oncologists embrace this mission, not because they believe as some Americans do that the mind can really influence disease, but rather because they believe that hope helps patients adopt a positive attitude which makes forging a "partnership" with them in the healing process easier. As Good et al. explain:

The construction of a partnership is understood as a necessary component of treatment, of getting patients to accept chemotherapy or radiation, and of making patients "work" or be "responsible" for eating well, taking their medication, keeping treatment appointments, and participating in a therapeutic endeavor which is often highly toxic [31, p. 75].

The authors also find that disclosure in oncological practice is not primarily about diagnosis, but rather is more focused on prognosis and treatment. This interest in prognosis appears to correlate directly with the desire to instill hope while the focus on treatment is likely due, as Good *et al.* suggest, to oncologists themselves deriving hope from and demonstrating caring through the treatment process. As they write, caring is conveyed "through offering therapeutic options and holding out hope for the development of new treatments on the cutting edge of biology and medicine" [31, p. 74].

Good *et al.*'s research provides illuminating background for understanding the responses of the late-stage patients interviewed in this study to the biomedical perspective. For 23 of the 26 patients interviewed, diagnosis was not a foregone conclusion. Much of what they wanted to do in their sessions with physicians was to discuss this issue. Yet their physicians were more focused on prognosis and treatment and tended, instead, to shift the talk toward outcomes. Consequently, 19 of the 26 patients with late-stage disease reported feeling "rushed to make a decision," and said that their doctors were "too pushy" or too "quick to jump into something." For others, the physicians' coupling of the dramatic diagnosis of cancer with a desire to perform immediate surgery was a complete turnoff. Of the initial 34 black women diagnosed with late-stage disease, 6 walked out of the clinic at that point and never returned. In this sense, these patients differed dramatically from those studied by Lind *et al.* [32] who were more interested in finding out from physicians about prognosis, disease process and treatment side effects and options than they were in obtaining basic information.

On the other hand, those women who did agree to have conventional treatments were constantly encouraged to be "partners in the *fight* against their disease," "to eat well and build up their strength for the coming *battle*," "to *play the game* and stick with the therapy," and "work with the doctors and nurses to *beat* the disease." Insofar as these women bought into the oncology model, they also tended to embrace the metaphors of warfare and sports used by the clinic staff to encourage them to become "part of the *team*" as partners invested in treatment and survival. Similarly, the patients' conversation began to reflect the use of more scientific terminology in reference to breast cancer. From this new vantage point, they often re-evaluated their initial interpretations about the nature of lumps based on indigenous beliefs or popular conceptions of the disease.

For example, once her treatment was over and the mastectomy completed, Sallie began to incorporate this medical attitude into her interpretations of her experience. She reported feeling like she "had just come through a long battle" and switches from a first person singular voice to the first person plural thereby demonstrating her solidarity with the medical team while shifting her references to popular notions to the third person thereby disassociating herself from them.

> When I found out about the tumor—you know that it was cancer, I didn't know what to do. I didn't see much point in doing anything because, you know, they all say cancer will kill you. There ain't no cure for it. But the people here were so good to me and they told me not to give up—that my family would want me to fight to live and that they would help me. So I took my treatments and I stuck with it. And those X-rays evaporated that tumor down to a little small lump that the doctor took out. And now that we won that fight, the cancer is over. The trick was shrinking that lump so that we could get it all. That's what makes the surgery O.K. so that the cancer won't spread. So I guess maybe I'm here to stay for a while longer.

As Sallie undergoes treatment, her perspective shifts. She does begin to enter into a "partnership" with medical personnel and adopts their language of war to describe the treatment she completed. In the process, her view shifts from a fatalistic acceptance of the inevitable outcome of death which led her to yield to God and a spiritual cure, to an active acceptance of the biomedical view of cancer. In embracing the entailments of the warfare metaphor, her self-definition shifts from someone doomed to die to that of a survivor of the battlefield—a person who, although scarred from the fight, showed the true "fighting" spirit by working hard and sacrificing to win a victory over the enemy. In the process of articulating this shift in self-image, she clarifies how the medical techniques make surgery, seen as not acceptable in the indigenous model, acceptable from another perspective.

Coming to Terms with Conflicting
Interpretations of Breast Disease

Despite the similar progression of experience for many of the women in this group, their efforts to come to terms with conflicting views of the disease varied greatly. Six of the twenty-six women interviewed stuck resolutely to initial interpretations and refused to give up their indigenous beliefs, even in the face of new and conflicting information, while four of the twenty-six completely gave them up in favor of the standard medical explanation. The remaining 16 women, however, worked out some type of accommodation along the lines identified by Strauss [33] in her study of Rhode Island working class men's views of success. Strauss discovered that her informants often held conflicting views simultaneously. In her effort to understand how they managed this, she analyzed their extended discourse and discovered three different ways in which different interpretative schemas can be learned and mentally stored. She labeled one "horizontal containment"—the maintenance of two opposing and contradictory schemas in separate, largely noninteracting cognitive compartments with each being used in a different context. She labels "vertical containment" a situation in which one interpretation is learned more as theory and is thus more easily verbalized than another. Both sets of beliefs are also held in separate, largely noninteracting, cognitive compartments and are expressed in different contexts with different voices. Finally, "integration" is characterized by the co-existence of different and sometimes conflicting ideas in a single schema or in a set of closely connected schemas expressed in a single, consistent voice across contexts [33, p. 315].

A brief examination of three more extended excerpts from narratives recorded after patients had been through the diagnosis and treatment phase illustrates how these different efforts at accommodation parallel the forms identified by Strauss. For example, interviews conducted with 69-year-old Leah both before diagnosis and after her chemotherapy treatments had begun illustrate Strauss's notion of "horizontal containment." In her first interview, Leah explained her disease this way:

> I have these lumps in my body—I've had lumps off and on in my life. They don't hurt or bother me. People say you should leave lumps like that alone because if you bother them, they will start to bother you. They say that if you cut on them they will start to spread and maybe they will turn into cancer. So if this lump does turn out to be something, then maybe I shouldn't have the operation.

In this excerpt, Leah describes the indigenous view of breast lumps. Yet the way in which she discusses these beliefs indicates that for her they are not so much part of her active worldview as they are examples of received cultural wisdom. Notice that she repeatedly accesses these beliefs by mentioning that "people say" or "they say" and does not discuss them in the first person as part of her own active belief system.

In a later interview, Leah talks about her disease differently:

> I am not scared of dying because when the Lord decides that my time has come, it will come. And I trust Him and know that He will reach out for me and take me out of this life to a brighter glory, thanks be to Jesus. And you know, I believe it was God himself who revealed this cancer to me. That day that I slipped and fell on the ice and bruised my breast—rubbing that bruise caused me to realize that I had this knot in my breast. And I honestly believe that God directed me to find the knot so that I could be cured. So I trust Him for bringing me this far, and I know that He will take care of me. And He sent me to this doctor and directed him to take the evil out of me to set me free. And I am thankful to him, praise Jesus.

In this passage, Leah describes a personal identification with God as manifested in her first person discussion of her beliefs about God's role in the treatment of her disease.

Clearly, Leah embraces two very different interpretations of her illness. Each was voiced in separate interview contexts, and in none of her sessions did she discuss the two together. They appeared to be organized and stored separately in her mind and accessed under different circumstances and seemed, moreover, to be differentially tied to her sense of personal identity, with her views about God being personally important while her indigenous notions of disease, voiced like lessons from childhood, were not integrated into her daily life. As a result, it is likely to suppose that the two have different levels of motivational intensity for Leah.

The initial receipt of a cancer diagnosis and the subsequent discussion of treatment options immediately caused Leah to fall back on the received wisdom of childhood invoking the "cutting on knots will make them spread" schema. However, the parroting of these notions did not influence her to reject biomedical treatment. She chose surgery, and once that choice was made she rationalized it by shifting to the "God as protector and healer" schema, which eventually came to dominate because it was a more active part of her adult identity and everyday practice and perhaps because it was ultimately more compatible with the biomedical model of the disease since the religious schema's emphasis on the "battle" between a righteous God and the evil enemy cancer mapped well onto the similar use of the battle analogy by the clinic staff.

Alternatively, the excerpt from the interview quoted at the beginning of this paper provides an example of vertical containment. In this passage, Lydia talks about two different interpretations. One, the traditional view, is obviously verbalized easily and in a more theoretical and organized fashion than is the medical interpretation. She begins by identifying her problem as having a "risen" caused by bad blood coming to the surface. She elaborates the cause, the actions taken, and her interpretation. In passing, she also voices the religious interpretation but not in a well-worked out way, saying only that you have to pray and give it to God. Her reference to the medical interpretation is given in a less-well verbalized or theoretically organized fashion. She reports what the doctor did, then from that perspective says that she doesn't have any thoughts about what caused it (meaning, the doctor's version of it as cancer), and ends by saying at some point that she suffered from both a risen and a cancer—a point she later contradicts by saying that the two are not the same. So even though she picked up on the medical interpretation, it was not convincing to her and she does not recount it from a theoretical point of view. Rather she makes short statements about what the doctor said and did almost as a meta-commentary on the indigenous view.

Finally, the story of 39-year-old Sharon demonstrates the attempt to come to some kind of integration—a perspective that appears in her final interview. When she first came in for treatment, Sharon reported that she had a knot that had begun to grow and she wanted the doctor to check on it. When she received the diagnosis of cancer she responded:

> I can't believe that this lump could be cancer. It wasn't really bother-ing me. I just thought that since it was growing larger, I should get it checked. I just can't make a decision about what to do now. You know, I believe that the Lord is watching over me and He will tell me what to do. I just need time to think and pray.

A few weeks later, when she came back to the clinic, Sharon, who is a minister, heard the clinic staff talking about her and calling her "the preacher." She then reported what happened:

When I went in to see the doctor, I just told him I didn't want the mastectomy—that I was going to put my faith in the Lord and trust God to cure me. And he said to me, "God can't do everything; you've got to do something for yourself." Well, that did it for me. I got up and walked right out that door because he was questioning everything I have built my life on. So I went home and prayed without ceasing. I asked the people in my church to pray for me too, and I testified to them that God had cured me.

But over time, the tumor grew out of her breast and reached the size of a grapefruit. It bled but she put pads in her bra and kept working. Her friend, an aide at the medical center, was worried and repeatedly urged her to go back to the clinic. Finally, she did return and upon her arrival was seen immediately by several physicians and nurses who gave her much support and encouragement. She explained her situation this way:

One night when I was praying, the Lord spoke to me and told me it was time now to see a doctor. He directed me to go back so that he could work through the doctors to cure me. He revealed to me that a medical doctor was needed to cure a medical problem, but that He would be directing him and so I should go along with the treatment and let them remove the knot. So I came back and the day I came, all of the people came down. Three doctors came to talk to me and they discussed what to do about my tumor in front of me, and so just like the Lord said, I was part of the healing process—they were talking to me. And the nurse came down and explained it all to me about how they would first do radiation treatments to shrink the tumor and then operate. And the lady who did the radiation said that God would be on my side and would help me be strong. And all that time while I was waiting and praying, God kept my tumor from getting any bigger, and then He sent me back so the doctors could help me. And now I know what He wants me to do. When I get well, my mission is to work with these doctors to help them talk to patients and tell them about what cancer is and to teach them not to be afraid to have the treatments.

Sharon was able to work out an integration of the religious and medical interpretations of her disease, and in the process, redefined her own self identity and role in life. She is now involved in the medical partnership but has extended this notion of partnership to include God as the team leader and herself as the go-between to bring patients and physicians into a better working relationship with God.

Clearly, the women in this study resolved conflicts brought into the open by the experience of breast disease in very different ways. What remains to be understood are the factors that might account for the different types of accommodations they made. Some clues are suggested in the interviews themselves. In Leah's case, personal experience as an ardent church member appeared to dominate her thinking about cancer to such an extent that the traditional views learned in childhood were less persuasive to her. In Lydia's case, social ties played an integral role in the treatment process. She would have continued to avoid medical attention for her breast had not her granddaughter made the appointment and personally escorted her to see a physician. In order to make the granddaughter happy, Lydia says she went to the doctor and followed through with surgery. But she never really "bought in" to the oncologist's model of breast disease perhaps because her own personal allegiance was still bound to the indigenous system. Lydia's ambivalence is reflected in her refusal to agree with the biomedical definition of her disorder.

Sharon, on the other hand, had a combination of pressures acting on her. She had a bad personal experience with the medical staff when she sought treatment because they made fun of the very core concept in her identity—her role as a minister. Consequently, she rejected the medical system and its interpretation of the disease. But later, after repeated urging from a close friend who worked at the medical center, she did return, although on her own terms and guided by God. Fortunately, she received a more positive reception the second time and was made to feel like an important part of the treatment process by the medical staff. She embraced this identity melding it with her own sense of religious purpose to arrive at an integrated explanation for why she delayed as well as for why she finally sought treatment.

Equally complex is the way in which these varying interpretations affected behavior. In some cases, patients made choices consistent with their expressed views of the disease; in others, they did not. A full account of the meaning of these narratives must eventually attempt to relate them to the broader social context in which the patients operate in order to try and untangle the factors involved in their decisions to accept, reject, or accommodate to new sources of knowledge and in order to more fully understand the complex relationships that exist between mental models and social actions.

Conclusion

This preliminary analysis of a small segment of the total interviews completed raises as many questions as it answers. Although anthropologists have written recently about indigenous etiologies of cancer in French-speaking Canada [34] and northern Italy [35], there has been very little work, with the exception of Balshem's recent article, designed to explore the variation in cancer beliefs within the United States. As a result, it is not surprising that popular medical knowledge, as Saillant writes, has virtually no recognition in the clinic or in oncology [34, p. 100]. This analysis focused specifically on the factors that may contribute to the tendency of some black women in eastern North Carolina to delay seeking treatment for breast cancer until they have an advanced stage of the disease. The limited generalizability of this study must be noted since the beliefs and behaviors of women with advanced stage disease are not necessarily relevant to the behaviors of the majority of women with breast cancer. Nonetheless, a major factor consistently implicated in the continuing disparity in mortality rates for breast cancer between black and white women is the fact that significantly more black than white women present for treatment with late stage disease. Any attempt to promote early detection and treatment seeking behavior in this population must be based on a more complete understanding of the reasons accounting for delay if they are to succeed.

Too often in the past we have assumed that patients who delay seeking treatment for cancer or who fail to utilize the screening services available, are either lacking in knowledge, too poor to access services, denying reality or excessively fatalistic. The labeling of patients as fatalistic is, as Balshem writes, particularly pernicious because fatalism in medical circles is seen as being situated within the individual as a diagnosable pathology [3, p. 164]. Thus efforts at combating delay often focus on eradicating fatalism by supplying individuals with appropriate medical knowledge. Such a stance, as Balshem notes, obviates the need for health practitioners to develop a critical understanding of beliefs held by patients. For as she writes, "If fatalism is a disease, there is no need to look further at an indigenous etiology that is merely a symptom of this disease" [3, p. 164]. Consequently, dialog and discussion are stymied, and physicians often resent and usually dismiss the attempts of patients to come to terms with the cancer diagnosis by telling stories that seem to the physician to be at best irrational and at worst adversarial [3, p. 164].

While fatalism and the other attitudinal variables mentioned above may be part of the complex of behaviors leading to presentation with advanced stage disease, we cannot afford to ignore the fact that these patients also have well-worked out ideas about their own health and about disease—ideas that must be considered if oncologists truly hope to forge a therapeutic partnership with them.

Notes

1   Pseudonyms are used in the text to protect informant confidentiality.

2   Laird, C. *Webster's New World Thesaurus*, p. 448. Warner Books, New York, 1974.

3   Balshem, M. Cancer, control and causality: Talking about cancer in a working-class community. *Am. Ethnolog.* 18, 162, 1991.

4   These data were collected as part of a study entitled "Psychosocial Factors Delaying Breast Cancer Presentation," Donald Lannin, with Jim Mitchell and Holly Mathews, and funded by The American Cancer Society, Grant No. PBR-37. Special assistance was provided by Frances Swanson as project manager.

5   Feldman, J. *et al.* The effects of patient delay and symptoms other than a lump on survival in breast cancer. *Cancer* 51, 1226, 1983.

6   Elwood, J. M. and Moorehead, W. P. Delay in diagnosis and long-term survival in breast cancer. *Br. Med. J.* 280, 1291, 1980.

7   Sheridan, B., Fleming, J., Atkinson, L., and Scott, G. The effects of delay in treatment on survival rates in carcinoma of the breast. *Med. J. Aust.* 1, 262, 1971.

8   Briel, H. A. *et al.* Results of treatment of stage I–III breast cancer in black Americans: the Cook County Hospital Experience, 1973–1987. *Cancer*, 65, 1062, 1990.

9   Freeman, H. P. and Wasfie, T. J. Cancer of the breast in poor black women. *Cancer* 63, 2562, 1989.

10 Natarajan, N. *et al.* Race-related differences in breast cancer patients. *JNCI* 56, 1704, 1984.

11 Nemoto, T. *et al.* Management and survival of female breast cancer: Results of a national survey by the American College of Surgeons. *Cancer* 45, 2917, 1980.

12 Wilson, R. E. *et al.* The 1982 national survey of carcinoma of the breast in the United States by the American College of Surgeons. *Surg. Gynecol. Obstet.* 159, 309, 1984.

13 Natarajan, N., Nemoto, T., Mettlin, C. and Murphy, G. P. Race-related differences in breast cancer patients: Results of the 1982 national survey of breast cancer by the American College of Surgeons. *Cancer* 56, 1704, 1985.

14 Baquet, C. R. *et al.* Cancer among blacks and other minorities: Statistical profiles. DHHS Publication No. (NIH) 86–2785 (published by NCI, Bethesda, MD), 1, 1986.

15 The first study period ended on 30 June, 1991, but a subsequent renewal grant from American Cancer Society (No. PRB-64532) has enabled ongoing data collection. As of 30 June, 1992, data had been collected on 530 patients from 30 counties. An additional component of the five-year study has been to collect structured interview data with an identical number of female controls without breast disease randomly selected from the region and matched to patients on the basis of age, race and place of residence. Finally, each patient has been asked to name her confidant—the person she has relied upon most for advice

during her experience with breast disease. Structured interviews have also been completed with these individuals.

16 Mathews, H. F. Introduction: a regional approach and a multidisciplinary perspective. In *Herbal and Magical Medicine: Traditional Healing Today* (Edited by Kirkland, J. *et al.*), p. 1. Duke University Press, Durham, 1992.

17 This latter component of the sample was included to ensure adequate representation of the patient pool seen by private physicians, the majority of whom are white middle- and upper-income women.

18 Lannin, D. R., Mitchell, J. P. and Mathews, H. F. Progress report on American Cancer Society grant No. PBR-37, pp. 25–46. Department of Surgery, East Carolina University School of Medicine, Greenville, NC, 1990.

19 American Joint Committee on Cancer. *Manual for Staging of Cancer*, 2nd ed., pp. 127–133. J. B. Lippincott, Philadelphia, 1983.

20 Riggs, R. S. and Noland, M. P. Factors related to the health knowledge and health behavior of disadvantaged black youth. *JOSH* 54, 431, 1984.

21 Price, L. Ecuadorian illness stories: cultural knowledge in natural discourse. In *Cultural Models in Language and Thought* (Edited by Holland, D. and Quinn, N.), p. 313. Cambridge University Press, London, 1987.

22 Early, E. A. The logic of well being: therapeutic narratives in Cairo, Egypt. *Soc. Sci. Med.* 16, 1491, 1982.

23 Linde, C. Explanatory systems in oral life stories. In *Cultural Models in Language and Thought* (Edited by Holland, D. and Quinn, N.), p. 343. Cambridge University Press, London, 1987.

24 Farmer, P. Sending sickness: sorcery, politics and changing concepts of AIDS in rural Haiti. *Med. Anthrop. Q.* 4, 6, 1990.

25 See for example, Ingstad, B. The cultural construction of AIDS and its consequences for prevention. *Med. Anthrop. Q.* 4, 28, 1990; Laguerre, M. *Afro-Caribbean Folk Medicine.* Bergin and Garvey, Granby, MA, 1987; Mathews, H. and Hill, C. E. Applying cognitive decision theory to the study of regional patterns of illness treatment choice. *Am. Anthrop.* 92, 155, 1990.

26 Weidman, H. *Miami Health Ecology Project Report: A Statement on Ethnicity and Health.* University of Miami, Miami.

27 Mathews, H. F. Rootwork: Description of an ethnomedical system in the American South. *South. Med. J.* 8, 885, 1987.

28 Snow, L. F. Traditional health beliefs and practices among lower class black Americans. *Western J. Med.* 139, 820, 1983.

29 Lakoff, G. Classifiers as a reflection of mind: a cognitive model approach to prototype theory. *Berkeley Cognitive Science Report* 19, 10, 1984.

30 Quinn, N. and Holland, D. Culture and cognition. In *Cultural Models in Language and Thought* (Edited by Holland, D. and Quinn, N.), p. 3. Cambridge University Press, London, 1987.

31 Good, M. J. D., Good, B. J., Schaffer, C. and Lind, S. E. American Oncology and the discourse on hope. *Cult. Med. Psychiat.* 14, 59, 1990.

32 Lind, S. E., Good, M. J. D., Seidel, S., Csordas, T. and Good, B. J. Telling the diagnosis of cancer. *J. Clin. Oncol.* 7, 583, 1989.

33 Strauss, C. Who gets ahead? Cognitive responses to heteroglossia in American political culture. *Am. Ethnolog.* 71, 312, 1990.

34 Saillant, F. Discourse, knowledge and experience of cancer: a life story. *Cult. Med. Psychiat.* 14, 81, 1990.

35 Gordon, D. R. Embodying illness, embodying cancer. *Cult. Med. Psychiat.* 14, 275, 1990.

Women Get Sicker, but Men Die Quicker
Judith Lorber

> In any gender-dichotomized society, the fact that we are born biologically female or male means that our environments will be different: we will live different lives. Because our biology and how we live are dialectically related and build on one another, we cannot vary gender and hold the environment constant. (Hubbard 1990:128)

There is a saying in epidemiology—"Women get sicker, but men die quicker." It is a succinct way of summing up the illness and death rates of women and men in modern industrialized societies. In industrialized countries, in the early years of the 20th century, women outlived men only by two to three years; today, women live almost seven years longer (Stillion 1995). Racial differences increase these gender differences. In the United States, although life expectancy for a white infant born in the early 1990s is almost seven years longer for a girl than for a boy, for black infants, the difference is nine years (Kranczer 1995). The combined racial and sex difference between the longest life expectancy (white girls) and the shortest (black boys) is almost 15 years (see table 1). Black women and men not only die earlier but are prone to more illnesses and physical traumas throughout their lives than white women and men. Paradoxically, although white women have the longest life expectancy, they have more illnesses than white men do throughout their adult lives (Verbrugge 1985, 1989a, 1989b). Although women as well as men are subject to heart diseases, cancers, and other life-threatening physical problems, on the whole, women live longer than men in industrialized countries because men get the killer diseases earlier (Verbrugge 1990).

Table 1. 1993 Life Expectancy (in years) at Birth in the United States, by Sex and Race

Race	Sex		Sex Difference
	Female	Male	
All	78.9	72.1	6.8
White	79.5	73.0	6.5
Black	73.7	64.7	9.0
Racial Difference	5.8	8.3	14.8

Source: Kranczer 1995, table 2, based on data from the National Center for Health Statistics.

In societies where women's social status is very low, their life expectancy is lower than in industrialized countries because of a combination of social factors: eating last and eating less, complications of frequent childbearing and sexually transmitted diseases because they have no power to demand abstinence or condom use, infections and hemorrhages following genital mutilation, neglect of symptoms of illness until severe, and restricted access to modern health care (Santow 1995; see table 2). The relationship between women's health and their social status is starkly demonstrated by how care is allocated within the family in many traditional societies: "A lower-status individual, such as a young female, was likely to be treated only with home remedies; when assistance was sought outside the household it was more likely to be from a traditional than a modern therapist. A higher-status individual, such as a male of almost any age or an adult mother of sons, was likely to be taken directly to a private medical practitioner" (Santow 1995:154).

Illness and death rates are not linear or uniformly progressive. Because of a combination of social and environmental factors, life expectancy rates for Russian men have declined from 65.5 years in 1991 to 57.3 years in 1995 (Specter 1995). When a women moves to another country, her risk of dying of breast cancer gradually changes, for the better or worse, to match the risk in her new place of residence (Kliewer and Smith 1995; Ziegler 1993).

The social epidemiologist's task is to explain these variances in *morbidity* (rates of illness) and *mortality* (rates of death) and to tease out the fundamental causes that produce persistent group differences. Some of these are genetic and physiological and some are social. For example, sickle cell anemia and breast cancer cluster in different racial ethnic groups, but access to knowledge, healthy environments, and up-to-date treatment

Table 2. Male-Female Life Expectancy Rates (in years)
for Developed and Developing Countries, 1990–1995

Region	Male Life Expectancy	Female Life Expectancy	Female-Male Ratio
World	62.7	66.7	106.4
Developed	71.0	78.0	109.9
Developing	61.1	63.9	104.6
Africa	51.4	54.6	106.2
North America	72.7	79.4	109.2
Latin America[a]	65.2	70.9	108.2
Asia[b]	63.6	66.1	103.9
Europe	71.9	78.5	109.2
Former USSR	65.7	74.7	113.7
Oceania[c]	69.9	75.6	108.2

Source: World Health Organization 1995:60.
a. Includes Mexico. b. Excludes Japan. c. Excludes Australia and New Zealand.

cluster by social class: "The reason is that resources like knowledge, money, power, prestige, and social connectedness are transportable from one situation to another, and as health-related situations change, those who command the most resources are best able to avoid risks, diseases, and consequences of disease" (Link and Phelan 1995:87). Morbidity and mortality rates are useful for policy recommendations only when accompanied by data on social factors, such as economic resources, access to health services, community supports, and cultural values. What Nancy Krieger (1996) calls "ecosocial theory" "asks how we literally incorporate, biologically, social relations (such as those of social class, race/ethnicity, and gender) into our bodies, thereby focusing on who and what drives population patterns of health, disease, and well-being" (p. 135).

The rates of illness and death that are used to assess the health of groups of people are themselves influenced by social factors. For example, reports of sudden infant death syndrome (SIDS) are more common where mothers are poor, have little education, and are from disadvantaged racial ethnic groups. Biological or medical models predict a random distribution over social classes. The high death rates for children of lower socioeconomic status can be interpreted two ways—either (a) social factors, such as poverty, are more important than biological causes, or (b) deaths to poor infants are attributed to SIDS more often than with children from more affluent families (Nam, Eberstein, and Deeb 1989). In either case, social factors are significant, but their effects are quite different. SIDS may be more prevalent among lower socioeconomic classes because of social factors, or it may be just as prevalent among middle and upper classes but be more often reported as a cause of death for a child in a poor family because no one investigates further for other causes.

Still another social epidemiological issue is immediate and proximate cause of death. The most immediate cause for an 85-year-old woman may be pneumonia, a frequent cause of death in the elderly, but long-term causes may be just as significant. These might be poor nutrition, poor housing, and no support services. Or the causes of death might be multiple. Drinking and smoking combined with high blood pressure, which are frequently reactions to poverty and lack of opportunities for advancement, can precipitate a fatal stroke or heart attack. According to Robert Staples (1995), "Black men suffer a disproportionate burden of illness. The drug and alcoholism rate for blacks, for example, is about four times higher than whites. Whereas black men suffer higher rates of diabetes, strokes and a variety of chronic illnesses, they are also at the mercy of public hospitals, and, therefore, are the first victims of government cutbacks. When they do go to a hospital, they are more likely to receive inadequate treatment" (p. 123). So what did a particular black man die from?

Social factors are not easily teased apart for any group.[1] Women tend to have more non-life-threatening illnesses because of the stresses of routinized jobs, child care, the care of elderly parents, and the "double day" of work and housework (Bird and Fremont 1991; Muller 1990; Ross and Bird 1994; Verbrugge 1986). Men are more prone to chronic and life-threatening diseases, such as heart attacks, because of their lifestyle and, to a lesser extent, their occupations (Helgeson 1995; Waldron 1995). They are also more at risk for traumas, accidents, and homicide because they are more likely to get into dangerous situations (Stillion 1995; Veevers and Gee 1986). Women are more likely to attempt suicide, but men are more likely to succeed at it because they use deadlier methods (Canetto 1992; World Health Organization 1995). Married men tend to be healthier mentally and physically than married women, but they have a worse time physically and mentally for about six months after a divorce, separation, or being widowed (Farberow et al. 1992; Gove 1984) or until they find another woman to look after their physical and emotional needs.

The statistical patterns of morbidity and mortality—who gets sick with what and who dies when from what—are outcomes of individual behavior shaped by cultural and social factors, such as availability of clean water and good food, access to medical knowledge and technology, and protection from environmental pollution, occupational traumas, and social hazards like war, violent crime, rape, battering, and genital mutilation. For the individual, health is as much affected by combined social statuses (gender, race, ethnic group, social class, occupation, and place of residence) as by personal choices (Calnan 1986; Staples 1995; Stillion 1995; Waldron 1995). Indeed, individual behavior is heavily circumscribed by social statuses—not everyone chooses health risks; for some people, health risks are built into their daily lives.[2] On a broader social system level, rates of illness and death are significantly affected by the behavior of health care providers, the policies of health care institutions and agencies, and the financial support of state and national governments for research and treatment (McKinlay 1996).

Because social factors are so intertwined, gender cannot be separated out from class, race and ethnicity, or age group.

Birthing and Getting Born: Have Money or Be a Boy

For mothers, economic resources can spell the difference between life and death for their infants. In poor countries that favor men, all the advantages go to boys. The physical hazards that produce infertility are evenly incurred by men and women, but the social effects and treatments are much harder on women.

Childbirth and Infancy

One of the important contributors to women's longer life expectancy in the 20th century is the reduction of illness and death in childbirth.[3] The use of antibiotics for puerperal infections ("childbed fevers") and surgical interventions to prevent heavy blood loss has made dying in childbirth a rare occurrence in many countries. However, because of uneven access to prenatal care and safe abortions and inadequate treatment of childbirth complications, women in the childbearing years still suffer from high mortality and morbidity rates in many parts of the world, including the United States (Dixon-Mueller 1994; Sundari 1994). The health of the mother directly affects the health of the infant. In industrialized countries, "the condition that enables us to predict with the greatest accuracy whether or not a baby will be stillborn, sick, malformed, premature, or will die in the first year of life, is the mother's socioeconomic status. If she

Table 3. Health Care and Maternal and Infant Mortality
Rates for Developed and Developing Countries

Region	% Prenatal Care 1990	% Attended by Trained Personnel	Maternal Mortality 1988[a]	Infant Mortality 1990–1995[a]
World	64	60	370	68
Developed	98	99	26	12
Developing	59	55	420	69
Africa	59	42	630	95
North America	95	99	12	8
Latin America[b]	72	76	200	47
Asia[c]	57	56	380	62
Europe	99	99	23	10
Former USSR	100	100	45	20
Oceania[d]	70	50	600	22

Source: World Health Organization 1995:60.
a. Deaths per 100,000 births. b. Includes Mexico. c. Excludes Japan. d. Excludes Australia and New Zealand.

belongs to a disadvantaged social class this means, among other things, low income, poor health, hard domestic and extra-domestic work, low educational level, and bad housing" (Romito and Hovelaque 1987:254).[4]

The more economic resources a country has, the better the health care and the lower the death rate of women in childbirth and their newborns in their first year.[5] Physiologically, girl babies are stronger at birth, and the female hormones generated at puberty are protective until menopause. However, women's longer life expectancy in developed countries, compared to men, reflects the effects of a healthier environment, better health care, and good nutrition, which are indicative of enough economic resources to feed women and girls as well as men and boys and to give pregnant women good health care (see table 3). Another related set of statistics is whether or not girls and women are taught to read and write and the number of children they have. Educated women are good earners and too valuable to keep at home having children; hence, they have fewer and more widely spaced children and their maternal mortality rates drop.

In countries that put a high premium on having sons, neglect and infanticide of baby girls and deliberate abortions of female fetuses after prenatal sex testing has resulted in an imbalanced sex ratio (proportion of boys to girls or men to women) (Renteln 1992). Africa, Europe, and North America have a sex ratio of 95 girls to 100 boys, considered balanced because more boys than girls are born to compensate for the higher natural death rate of male children. In China, India, Bangladesh, and West Asia, the sex ratio is 94 girls to 100 boys, and in Pakistan it is 90 girls to 100 boys. Given the number of men, there should have been about 30 million more women in India today, and 38 million more women in China (Sen 1990).

Adolescence and Young Adulthood:
Good and Bad Social Pressures

Poor teenage girls in the United States are like women in poor countries—if they get good prenatal care and have social supports after the birth, they and their children thrive. But if they are stigmatized and therefore put off getting prenatal care, they are likely to have premature births and low–birth weight babies, with accompanying health hazards. Even without childbirth, the lives of poor young men of color are the most endangered of all groups in the United States, exposing them to a host of physical and emotional traumas. Young women in college are prone to eating disorders, but in general, their health behaviors tend to be more protective than those of young men in college. The situation for young girls in non-Western countries, particularly in Africa, is starkly different. Genital mutilation is a gender-specific health issue in many countries of the world.[6]

Teenage Pregnancy

Teenage childbearing is a social problem that can be viewed from a health perspective (the effect on the body of a growing girl of having a baby in the teen years and the health of the infant) and from a social perspective (why teenage boys and girls want to have babies and what happens to those girls who do get pregnant). The data from recent research show that social conditions are more crucial than age or racial ethnic identity in predicting whether young, unmarried girls will have a pregnancy and what the physical and emotional outcome will be for the mother and the child (Luker 1996).

According to the providers in 200 randomly selected reproductive health and other service programs in New York City, girls of Puerto Rican and Dominican background got pregnant in their teen years because they lacked information about sexual relationships, procreation, and birth control (Fennelly 1993). But the reason why they couldn't acquire this knowledge was the contradictory attitudes of the Hispanic culture, attitudes that condemned sexuality outside of marriage but valued pregnancy and having children no matter when it occurred. The positive attitudes toward fatherhood among young men in many cultures and their intentions to play a significant role in the lives of their children and their children's mothers also make it difficult for teenage girls to practice birth control or have an abortion (Anderson 1989; Marsiglio 1988; Redmond 1985).

Once sexual activity begins, black teenage girls from high-risk social environments are 8.3 times more likely to become pregnant than black girls from low-risk social environments (Hogan and Kitagawa 1985). The data were based on a random sample of over 1,000 black girls aged 13–19 who lived in Chicago in 1979. High risks in this study were being poor, living in an impoverished neighborhood with a non-nuclear family and many siblings, and having a sister who had also been a teenage mother. Another study interviewed 268 Canadian teenagers during pregnancy and four weeks after delivery and found that those who had strong support from their families were less likely to have low–birth weight babies or postpartum depression (Turner, Grindstaff, and Phillips 1990).

Pregnancy soon after menarche is considered the norm in all but highly industrialized societies, and in most cultures, having a child, not marriage, is the mark of adulthood. In industrialized countries, the incidence of teenage pregnancy is low where sex education is part of the school curriculum and contraceptives and early abortions are widely available (Jones and Forrest 1985). Teenage pregnancy and childbirth may result in frequent premature births, which seems to be a more serious problem than low birthweight (Fraser 1995; Wilcox, Skjaerven, and Buekens 1995). Among black women, premature births are high when there is a combination of related factors: teenage, single, no high school graduation, and welfare support (Lieberman et al. 1987). The major *social* (not physiological) problem for the teenage mother is the risk of ending up in poverty if she is not already poor or staying poor if she is (Chilman 1989; Forsyth and Palmer 1990; Luker 1996).

Endangered Species

Even with childbearing, young women are less vulnerable to early death than the young men of their racial ethnic groups. Because of multiple risk factors, young black men living in disadvantaged environments are the most likely to die before they reach adulthood. Young black men have been called an endangered species because of their early death rates, with homicides, suicides, and accidents the leading causes of death of those between 15 and 24 years old (Gibbs 1988; Staples 1995). For black and white men between 15 and 19 years old, the annual homicide rate rose 154% from 1985 to 1991, with almost all of the increase due to the use of guns (Butterfield 1994). HIV infection and AIDS also have a high incidence in young black and Hispanic men, especially when they are intravenous drug users. However, the consequent illnesses and deaths occur later, between the ages of 29 and 41 (Kranczer 1995).

Young men's "taste for risk" has been attributed to sociobiological factors (Wilson and Daly 1985), but more plausible explanations are the seductiveness of danger, displays of masculinity, and, for black men, despair over the future (Staples 1995). Another social factor is the recruitment into often violent sports (Messner 1992). Although a path to upward mobility for poor and working-class boys, few boys become successful professional athletes. Those who break into professional teams have only a few years to make it, and they cannot afford to be sidelined by injuries. "Playing hurt" and repeated orthopedic surgeries have a high physical toll. Injuries, alcoholism, drug abuse, obesity, and heart disease take about 15 years off the life expectancy of professional football players in the United States (Messner 1992:71).

Responses to Social Pressures

Health-threatening behavior, such as smoking, drinking, and illegal drug use, is influenced by a variety of social factors, but peer group pressure is among the most significant for young men and women of all racial ethnic groups (Coombs, Paulson, and Richardson 1991; Johnson and Marcos 1988; Johnson 1988; van Roosmalen and McDaniel 1992). Drinking in college is declining among men and women, but college men still drink more often and more heavily than college women and are much more likely to get into fights, hurt others, drive while drunk, and damage property (Perkins 1992). Women as well as men who drink heavily are likely to hurt themselves physically and others emotionally and to do poorly in school.

Young women tend to adopt a somewhat healthier lifestyle than young men on such measures as using seat belts, getting adequate amounts of sleep and exercise, eating a healthy diet, taking care of their teeth, and managing stress (Donovan, Jessor, and Costa 1993; Oleckno and Blacconiere 1990). However, young middle-class women are vulnerable to eating disorders, especially in the college years (Hesse-Biber 1989).

Anorexia (self-starvation) and bulimia (binge eating and induced vomiting) are extreme ways to lose weight in order to meet today's Western cultural standards of beauty and to maintain control over one's body (Bordo 1993; Brumberg 1988). The importance of society's views of femininity in eating disorders is highlighted by research comparing heterosexual women, who are subject to pressure from the media and the significant men in their lives to stay thin to be sexually attractive, and lesbians, whose views of beauty are not influenced by men's opinions. Lesbians are heavier than comparable heterosexual women, more satisfied with their bodies, and less likely to have eating disorders (Herzog et al. 1992). Men also have an idealized body image, which may encourage anorexia and bulimia, especially among those with sexual conflicts or who identify as homosexual (Herzog, Bradburn, and Newman 1990; Herzog et al. 1984; Kearney-Cooke and Steichen-Asch 1990).

A different rationale for eating problems was found in intensive interviews with 18 women who were heterogenous on race, class, and sexual orientation (Thompson 1992). For these African American, Latina, and white women, binge eating and purging were ways of coping with the traumas of their lives—sexual abuse, poverty, racism, and prejudice against lesbians. Eating offered the same comfort as drinking but was cheaper and more controllable. Rather than a response to the culture of thinness, anorexia and bulimia were for these women "serious responses to injustices" (Thompson 1992:558).

College athletes are prone to anorexia and bulimia when they have to diet to stay in a weight class (Andersen 1990; Black 1991). A study of 695 athletes in 15 college sports found that 1.6% of the men and 4.2% of the women met the American Psychiatric Association's criteria for anorexia, and 14.2% of the men and 39.2% of the women met the criteria for bulimia (Burckes-Miller and Black 1991). The researchers argue that the reasons for strict weight control are not standards of beauty but the pressures of competition, to meet weight category requirements, to increase speed and height, and to be able to be lifted and carried easily in performances. Eating disorders here are an occupational risk taken not only by young athletes but by dancers, models, jockeys, and fitness instructors as well as professional gymnasts, figure skaters, runners, swimmers, and wrestlers.

For some young girls, being able to control the shape of your body by what you eat might look like paradise—not just to those who don't have enough to eat but to those girls aged 3 to 18 whose families insist on having their genitals amputated so that they can be properly married. Hanny Lightfoot-Klein (1989) estimated that 94 million women living in Africa in the 1980s had their clitorises and vaginal lips cut off (p. 31). In Egypt, an estimated 80–97% of girls have mutilated genitals (MacFarquhar 1996). These procedures are done on 90% of young girls in the Sudan and in Mali on 93% (Dugger 1996b). In 1996, the United States passed a law making all these procedures illegal, and other countries with large immigrant populations have also done so (Dugger 1996c).

For more than 2,000 years, in a broad belt across the middle of Africa, clitoridectomies and infibulation (scarring of the labia to create adhesions that keep most of the vaginal opening closed until marriage) have been used to ensure women's virginity until marriage and to inhibit wives' appetites for sexual relations after marriage. Ironically, these mutilating practices do neither but result in the infliction of pain as part of normal sexuality. Childbirth is more dangerous because of tearing and bleeding, and the risks of infection throughout life are high.

The procedures range from mild sunna (removing the prepuce of the clitoris) to modified sunna (partial or total clitoridectomy) to infibulation or pharaonic circumcision, which involves clitoridectomy and excision of the labia minora and the inner layers of the labia majora and suturing the raw edges together to form a bridge of scar tissue over the vaginal opening, leaving so small an opening that normal bladder emptying takes 15 minutes and menstrual blood backs up (see descriptions in Lightfoot-Klein 1989:32–36). Many women have reinfibulation after childbirth and go through the process over and over again. It is called *adlat el rujal* (men's circumcision) because it is designed to create greater sexual pleasure for men, not unlike the rationale for episiotomy and tight suturing in Western obstetrical practice (Rothman 1982:58–59).

In Lightfoot-Klein's (1989) interviews with women throughout the Sudan who had clitoridectomies and infibulation, 90% described experiencing full orgasms during intercourse once the period of excruciatingly painful opening through penile penetration was over. However, Asma El Dareer's (1982) surgery of 2,375 women, almost all of whom had had full infibulation, found that only 25% experienced sexual pleasure all or some of the time (p. 48). One of the Sudanese men Lightfoot-Klein (1989) interviewed said that his wife's evident suffering was preferable to no reaction at all (p. 8).

Circumcision of boys is much more common and occurs in societies throughout the world, where it is done for both religious and health reasons. Although there is some debate over whether sensitivity is reduced or enhanced, male circumcision does not seem to diminish either the man's or the woman's pleasure (Gregersen 1983). Removal of the prepuce lowers the risk of HIV infection in circumcised men and cervical cancer in their women sexual partners. Another practice, subincision, where the penis is cut through and flattened and urination is subsequently done squatting, occurs in only a few places in the world.

Adulthood: Health by Choice or by Circumstance?

Many of the risky health behaviors in adulthood, such as drinking and smoking cigarettes, seem to be a matter of individual choice. But a closer look reveals that social factors linked to gender, race and ethnicity, and economic class produce the situational circumstances that influence health-related behaviors.

A comparison of 654 African American and 474 white women aged 19 to over 70 living in upstate New York found that poorer, older, religious African American women were most likely to abstain from alcohol (Darrow et al. 1992). A study of 4,099 white women and men and 888 black women and men living in New York State also found that black women were most likely to abstain from drinking (Barr et al. 1993). Black men in this study were more likely than white men to abstain but also most likely, of all four groups, to be heavy drinkers when they did drink. A study of gendered styles of drinking showed that women of all racial ethnic groups who drank were less likely than men to become visibly intoxicated and to abandon control, behavior that would be considered unfeminine (Robbins and Martin 1993). When economic status was added to the analysis, it was found that the poorest and least educated black men had significantly higher rates of alcohol and illicit drug consumption and alcohol-related problems, such as accidents and run-ins with the police, bosses, fellow workers, and family members. They are, as a result, more likely to suffer from high blood pressure and die early of coronary artery disease, especially if they also smoke (Staples 1995; Waldron 1995). The New York State study found that the more education a black man had, the fewer alcohol-related problems he experienced, but that black men with college degrees experienced such problems on an average of one a month, while their white counterparts averaged only 3.4 alcohol-related problems per year. Educated black men are likely to be under increased stress because the stakes for success are so high.

Both legal and illegal drugs are commonly used by professional athletes (Messner 1992). Team doctors routinely inject painkillers and cortisone so injured players can "play hurt" and supply amphetamines to enhance performance and anabolic steroids to increase muscle mass. Steroid use among women and men bodybuilders who enter competitions is endemic, despite their virilizing effects in women and feminizing effects in men (Fussell 1993; Mansfield and McGinn 1993).

Among laypeople, women are more than twice as likely as men to be prescribed psychotropic drugs (tranquilizers and sleeping pills) for anxiety, but men often obtain such medications from women—their wives, sisters, or friends—when they are under stress because of their job or lack of one (Ettorre et al. 1994). Women and men physicians prescribe these medications to women more than they do to men with similar difficulties, but men physicians are significantly more likely to do so (Taggart et al. 1993). Elizabeth Ettorre and Elianne Riska (1995) argue that both the gendered use patterns and the prescribing patterns reflect powerlessness: Prescribing tranquilizers for women stressed out by their triple duties as wives, mothers, and paid workers treats the symptoms, not the causes, which women physicians are more likely to recognize. When men in difficult social situations ask sympathetic women they know rather than their men physicians for tranquilizers, the same gender dynamics of status and powerlessness seem to be at issue.

Homicide rates are greater for disadvantaged men but paradoxically, higher for educated women in the labor force (Gartner 1990). A cross-national, longitudinal comparison of 18 industrialized countries found that as women's lives between 1950 and 1985 moved away from traditional roles, they were more likely to be murdered (Gartner, Baker, and Pampel 1990). The researchers argue that, although women confined to the home are subject to violence from husbands and other men relatives, women who work for pay, especially in nontraditional occupations, and single women living on their own are also vulnerable to being killed by acquaintances and strangers.

The one place women maintain their life expectancy advantage despite risk behavior is with smoking—they outlive men even if they smoke heavily, leading to the conclusion that other factors provide protective health benefits for women (Rogers and Powell-Griner 1991).

Work and Family: Protection and Danger

Jobs and families are complex variables with good and bad effects on the physical and mental health of women and men. Both are arenas for social support, which is beneficial to health; both are sometimes hazardous environments with detrimental physical effects; and both produce stresses.[7]

Work-Family Demands and Rewards

Although having a paid job outside the home usually enhances women's physical and mental health, jobs can be physically hazardous to women as well as men. Many of women's jobs are as physically dangerous as some men's jobs (Chavkin 1994; Fox 1991). Nursing, for example, can be highly stressful emotionally; hospitals also expose the nurse to infections, radiation, and dangerous chemicals (Coleman and Dickinson 1984; Kemp and Jenkins 1992). Full-time housewives are not protected either: the home is a similarly stressful and dangerous work environment full of toxic chemicals and potential allergens (Rosenberg 1984).

The job and the home can also produce high levels of psychological stress for women and men, and workplace and family stresses can spill over into each other (Eckenrode and Gore 1990). For women especially, the boundaries between work and family are permeable because even when they have full-time jobs they usually have the main responsibility for child care, household maintenance, and providing help to kin outside the household (Gerstel and Gallagher 1994; Lai 1995; Lennon and Rosenfeld 1992). In dual-career marriages, women often resent having a "double shift"—paid work plus housework—and men in turn feel that demands are made on them in the home that husbands in traditional marriages don't have (Glass and Fujimoto 1994). However, marriage extends men's and women's life spans but through different means, as suggested by Lillard and Waite (1995): " 'His' marriage seems to consist of a settled life, improved perhaps by the household management skills and labors of his wife. . . . 'Her' marriage seems to offer primarily the benefits of improved financial well-being" (p. 1154).

The effects of workplace and family stress, role conflict, depression, and negative feelings on vulnerability to illness are hard to document. The connection between stress and heart attacks, for example, has not yet been proved (Waldron 1995). Moreover, some "hardy personalities" thrive under stress, according to a study of men executives (Maddi and Kobasa 1984; also see Ouellette 1993). A study of the effects of combined roles (work, marriage, and motherhood) in a sample of 1,473 black and 1,301 white women found that work was significantly associated with lower blood pressure only for educated black women (Orden et al. 1995). Being married was correlated with raised blood pressure for white women but with lower blood pressure during motherhood, even for single mothers. As an example of work's beneficial physical effects, separate studies found that older black women and men had better health if they were employed (Coleman et al. 1987; Rushing, Ritter, and Burton 1992). This finding is not surprising, for employment usually means a higher income, which in turn means better nutrition and greater access to health care. Generally, people with health problems are not as able to hold down jobs as their healthier counterparts are.

The gender differences related to paid jobs and family demands are minimized when women and men live and work in similar unpressured environments. A comparison of the health status of 230 women and men on two Israeli kibbutzes, where work and family life are communal and health care is free, found that they were alike in their health status and illness behavior and that the men had life expectancies as long as those of the women (Anson, Levenson, and Bonneh 1990).

Battering

The home is not only a place of potential environmental hazards and stress; it can also be the site of physical violence. The average yearly number of recorded acts of violence against women in the United States from 1979 to 1987 was 56,900 by husbands, 216,100 by divorced or separated husbands, and 198,800 by boyfriends (Harlow 1991:1).

Men whose masculinity is tied to norms of dominance but who do not have the economic status to back up a dominant stance are likely to be abusive to women either psychologically or physically and often both (Walker 1984; Yllö 1984). James Ptacek's (1988) interviews with 18 men in a counseling program for husbands who battered found that they felt they had a right to beat their wives: "There is a pattern of finding fault with the woman for not being good at cooking, for not being sexually responsive, for not being deferential enough . . . , for not knowing when she is 'supposed' to be silent, and for not being faithful. In short, for not being a 'good wife'" (p. 147).

Wife beating was once approved in most communities and is still condoned today where there is an ideology of men's authority over their wives. Marital rape has only recently been accorded recognition as a genuine sexual assault (Finkelhor and Yllö 1985). The response of doctors, nurses, and the police to battering reflects these mores. In general, neither the medical nor the legal system has given battered women much attention or protection (Blackman 1989; Kurz 1987; Warshaw 1989).

Women who stay in such relationships are likely to have been well socialized into the emotionally supportive feminine role but to be socially or economically superior to the men who batter them (Walker 1984). Beth Richie (1996) found that the 26 African American battered women she interviewed had had girlhoods of relative privilege and thought they could be ideal wives and mothers. They felt they could not admit to their families that they had failed to live up to their early promise as "good girls." They could not go to the police because their batterers had embroiled them in illegal activities. Julie Blackman's (1989) interviews with 172 battered women found that they did not have a sense of injustice over what was happening to them because they could not see any alternatives outside the situation. Even women who had acted on alternatives, such as calling the police or going to shelters for battered women, did not feel that they had severed the relationship.

Old Age: Women Live Longer but Not Better

Although the physiological aspects of old age seem to override social factors, in that women of every racial ethnic group in industrial societies outlive the men of their group, the quality of their lives in old age can suffer because of poverty and few social supports.

The later years of life present women and men with sex-specific health risks. The older men get, the more likely they are to develop prostate cancer, especially among blacks (Weitz 1996). It can be cured by surgery, but the operation often has side effects, such as impotence and urinary incontinence. After menopause, women are faced with the question of whether to use estrogen replacement therapy, which carries the risk of breast cancer (Bush 1992). Without it, they may suffer from bone fragility and increased risk of heart disease (Bilezikian and Silverberg 1992; Jonas and Manolio 1996; Nachtigall and Nachtigall 1995).

In addition to these sex-specific physiological risks, social factors make getting older and dying different experiences for women and men. With longer life expectancy, many women in industrialized countries can expect to outlive their husbands or long-term male companions (Verbrugge 1989b). Most patients in places with Western medical systems go to a hospital for acute illnesses, surgery, and medical crises in chronic conditions, but hospitals in the United States now routinely send even very sick patients home within a week. Many more surgical procedures are done on an outpatient or one-night basis. With the shift of care from hospitals to home, someone needs to give medications and injections and change wound dressings (Glazer 1990). Even if home health care givers are hired, someone needs to supervise and fill in; this "someone" is usually a wife or other woman relative.

Shopping, cleaning, laundry, bedmaking, and paying bills are additional chores that women relatives do for sick and frail elderly persons living at home (Graham 1985). The question is, who takes care of elderly widows and those who have never married? Women 85 years and older are more likely than same-age men to be poor and living with relatives or in nursing homes (Longino 1988). Thus, for many women, the advantage of long life may not look like such a dividend after all.

Dying: Gendered Death Dips

One area in which social factors and physiological outcomes intertwine dramatically are "death dips." These are statistical drops in the expected rate of death in the weeks or days before a socially meaningful event followed by a statistical rise a week or two later. Since social meanings are gendered, one would expect that death dips would be, too—and so they are.

In his 1970 Princeton University doctoral dissertation, "Dying as a Form of Social Behavior," David P. Phillips documented an intriguing epidemiological statistic: that famous people were less likely to die in the month preceding their birthday than in the month after. He argued that they postponed death so as to participate in their public birthday celebrations. He also found, examining official tables of dates of death, that ordinary people postponed dying until after important local occasions, such as presidential elections in the United States, and among Jews, until after the holiest day of the year, the Day of Atonement (Yom Kippur), and

Passover, the popular celebration of liberation from Egyptian slavery (Phillips and Feldman 1973; Phillips and King 1988).

This and subsequent research reveal that the death-dip phenomenon during major religious holidays is quite gendered because of the different meanings of these events for women and men (Idler and Kasl 1992; Phillips and King 1988; Phillips and Smith 1990; Reunanen 1993). The Passover death dip, for example, occurs only among men. There was a 25.8% rise in deaths in the week after Passover among white men with unambiguously Jewish names who died in California between 1966 and 1984; for women, there was no such difference in deaths immediately before and after Passover (Phillips and King 1988). Statistical analysis of the death rates in a different population found the same gender pattern for all the major Jewish holidays (Idler and Kasl 1992). These researchers' explanation is that Jewish men's involvement in religious observances is more central to their lives than it is to Jewish women, whose death patterns are similar to all nonobservant Jews: They are more likely to die in the month preceding a major holiday than in the month after, whereas Jewish men and all observant Jews are more likely to die in the month after (Idler and Kasl 1992: table 4).[8]

The opposite pattern is true for black and white Catholics and Protestants—women and men, observant and nonobservant, postpone death until after Christmas and Easter (Idler and Kasl 1992: table 3). In fact, women are more likely to postpone dying until after these events, which tend to be family-oriented rather than purely religious celebrations. A Finnish analysis of 60,000 deaths for the 1966–1986 period found that only women postponed dying until after Christmas, a family-centered holiday where the senior woman cooks the celebratory meal (Reunanen 1993).[9] A similar gendered phenomenon occurs around the Harvest Moon Festival among Chinese women aged 75 and older; their mortality rate is lower in the week before the holiday than in any other six-month period studied (Phillips and Smith 1990). Older women play the central part in the Harvest Moon Festival; the senior woman of the household supervises daughters and daughters-in-law in the preparation of an elaborate meal. The shift in dying does not occur among elderly Chinese men.

The dip in expected deaths the week before a major religious festival and the concomitant rise the week after has been documented for Chinese women with cerebrovascular and cardiac diseases and for Jewish men with these diseases and also with malignant tumors (Phillips and Smith

1990). Such psychosomatic and gendered effects of social beliefs are even starker among Chinese Americans born in a year considered ill fated in Chinese astrology who have a disease considered particularly detrimental for that birth year (Phillips, Ruth, and Wagner 1993). Their average age of death occurs almost two years earlier than among non-Chinese and those born in more advantageous years who have the same illnesses. Women with the ill-fated combination of birth year and disease lose more years of life than men. The gender pattern, Phillips et al. (1993) speculate, is due to greater traditionalism among Chinese American women. However, the researchers argue that the crucial factors involve behavior as well as beliefs: "Patients with ill-fated combinations of birth year and disease may refuse to change unhealthy habits because they believe their deaths are inevitable and thereby reduce their longevity. For example, earth patients with cancer may be less likely to quit smoking and fire patients with heart disease may be less likely to change their diets or exercise habits" (p. 1144). How should a social epidemiologist classify these early deaths? Is the cause individual behavior, cultural beliefs, community practices, gender, race, or social class? Or all the above?

Notes

The essay has been abridged for this edition.

1 On the problems of constructing categories of race and ethnicity, see Jones, Snider, and Warren 1996.

2 A substantial proportion of some morbidity rates are not explained by well-known risk factors. In breast cancer, for instance, only half of the cases in the United States are related to early menarche, having a family history of breast cancer or a personal history of benign breast disease, having a baby after the age of 19 or not having children, and being in the upper two-thirds in income (Madigan et al. 1995). Note that these factors are both physiological and social and that the social factors are circumstances over which a woman may have little control. Breast cancer genes account for only 10% of all breast cancer cases (Biesecker and Brody, 1997).

3 For the detrimental effects of extensive technology in childbirth, see Rothman 1982, 1986, 1989.

4 In her editorial preface to the September/October 1995 issue of the *Journal of the American Medical Women's Association*, which is devoted to prenatal care and women's health, Wendy Chavkin notes that "the common thread woven throughout these articles is that improvements in pregnancy outcome require care for women before and after pregnancy" (p. 143). See also Lazarus 1988a and Lieberman et al. 1987.

5 For a detailed and harrowing account of how mothers in the poorest area of Brazil choose which of their infants to feed and which to let die, see Scheper-Hughes 1992.

6 Immigration and asylum seekers have brought genital mutilation to the attention of West-

ern countries (see Crossette 1995; Dugger 1996a, 1996b, 1996c; MacFarquhar 1996; Rosenthal 1996; Walker 1992).

7 For reviews and research, see Bird and Fremont 1991; Farrell and Markides 1985; Gove 1984; Lennon 1994; Loscosso and Spitze 1990; Muller 1990; Pugliesi 1995; Roxburgh 1996; Sorensen and Verbrugge 1987; and Waldron 1995.

8 Idler and Kasl did not break down their observant versus nonobservant data by gender.

9 I am indebted to Elianne Riska for bringing this paper to my attention and for supplying me with an English summary and a description of Finnish Christmas customs.

References

Abbey, Antonia, Frank M. Andrews, and Jill L. Halman. 1991. "Gender's Role in Responses to Infertility." *Psychology of Women Quarterly* 15:295–316.

Andersen, Arnold E., ed. 1990. *Males with Eating Disorders*. New York: Brunner/Mazel.

Anderson, Elijah. 1989. "Sex Codes and Family Life among Poor Inner-City Youths." *Annuals of the American Academy of Political and Social Science* 501:59–78.

Anson, Ofra, Arieh Levenson, and Dan Y. Bonneh. 1990. "Gender and Health on the Kibbutz." *Sex Roles* 22:213–35.

Bair, Barbara, and Susan E. Cayleff, eds. 1993. *Wings of Gauze: Women of Color and the Experience of Health and Illness*. Detroit: Wayne State University Press.

Barr, Kellie E. M., Michael P. Farrell, Grace M. Barnes, and John W. Welte. 1993. "Race, Class and Gender Differences in Substance Abuse: Evidence of Middle-Class/Underclass Polarization among Black Males." *Social Problems* 40:314–27.

Biesecker, Barbara Bowles, and Lawrence C. Brody. 1997. "Genetic Susceptibility Testing for Breast and Ovarian Cancer: A Progress Report." *Journal of the American Medical Women's Association* 52:22–27.

Bilezikian, John P., and Shonni J. Silverberg. 1992. "Osteoporosis: A Practical Approach to the Perimenopausal Woman." *Journal of Women's Health* 1:21–27.

Bird, Chloe E., and Allen M. Fremont. 1991. "Gender, Time Use, and Health." *Journal of Health and Social Behavior* 32:114–29.

Black, David R., ed. 1991. *Eating Disorders among Athletes*. Reston, VA: American Alliance for Health, Physical Education, Recreation and Dance.

Blackman, Julie. 1989. *Intimate Violence: A Study of Injustice*. New York: Columbia University Press.

Bordo, Susan R. 1993. *Unbearable Weight: Feminism, Western Culture, and the Body*. Berkeley: University of California Press.

Brumberg, Joan Jacobs. 1988. *Fasting Girls: The Emergence of Anorexia Nervosa as a Modern Disease*. Cambridge, MA: Harvard University Press.

Burckes-Miller, Mardie E., and David R. Black. 1991. "College Athletes and Eating Disorders: A Theoretical Context." Pp. 11–26 in Black.

Bush, Trudy L. 1992. "Feminine Forever Revisited: Menopausal Hormone Therapy in the 1990s." *Journal of Women's Health* 1:1–4.

Butterfield, Fox. 1994. "Teen-Age Homicide Rate Has Soared." *New York Times*, October 14, p. A22.

Callan, Victor J., Belinda Kloske, Yoshihisa Kashima, and John F. Hennessey. 1988. "Toward

Understanding Women's Decisions to Continue or to Stop *In Vitro* Fertilization: The Role of Social, Psychological, and Background Factors." *Journal of In Vitro Fertilization and Embryo Transfer* 5:363–69.

Calnan, Michael. 1986. "Maintaining Health and Preventing Illness: A Comparison of the Perceptions of Women from Different Social Classes." *Health Promotion* 1:167–77.

Canetto, Silvia Sara. 1992. "Gender and Suicide in the Elderly." *Suicide and Life Threatening Behavior* 22:80–97.

Chavkin, Wendy, ed. 1994. *Double Exposure: Women's Health Hazards on the Job and at Home.* New York: Monthly Review Press.

Chilman, Catherine S. 1989. "Some Major Issues Regarding Adolescent Sexuality and Child-bearing in the United States." *Journal of Social Work and Human Sexuality* 8:3–25.

Coleman, Lerita M., Toni C. Antonucci, Pamela K. Adelmann, and Susan E. Chrohan. 1987. "Social Roles in the Lives of Middle-Aged and Older Black Women." *Journal of Marriage and the Family* 49:761–71.

Coleman, Linda, and Cindy Dickinson. 1984. "The Risks of Healing: The Hazards of the Nursing Profession." Pp. 37–56 in Chavkin.

Coombs, Robert H., Morris J. Paulson, and Mark A. Richardson. 1991. "Peer vs. Parental Influence in Substance Use among Hispanic and Anglo Children and Adolescents." *Journal of Youth and Adolescence* 20:73–88.

Crossette, Barbara. 1995. "Female Genital Mutilation by Immigrants Is Becoming a Cause for Concern in the U.S." *New York Times*, December 10, Sunday news section, p. 18.

Crowe, Christine. 1985. " 'Women Want It': *In Vitro* Fertilization and Women's Motivations for Participation." *Women's Studies International Forum* 8:57–62.

Darrow, Sherri L., Marcia Russell, M. Lynne Cooper, et al. 1992. "Sociodemographic Correlates of Alcohol Consumption among African-American and White Women." *Women and Health* 18:35–51.

Dixon-Mueller, Ruth. 1994. "Abortion Policy and Women's Health in Developing Countries." Pp. 191–210 in Fee and Krieger.

Donovan, John E., Richard Jessor, and Frances M. Costa. 1993. "Structure of Health-Enhancing Behavior in Adolescence: A Latent-Variable Approach." *Journal of Health and Social Behavior* 34:346–62.

Dugger, Celia W. 1996a. "A Refugee's Body is Intact but Her Family Is Torn." *New York Times*, September 11, pp. A1, B6–B7.

Dugger, Celia W. 1996b. "Genital Ritual is Unyielding in Africa." *New York Times*, October 5, Saturday news section, pp. 1, 6.

Dugger, Celia W. 1996c. "New Law Bans Genital Cutting in the United States." *New York Times*, October 12, Saturday news section, pp. 1, 28.

Eckenrode, John, and Susan Gore, eds. 1990. *Stress Between Work and Family.* New York: Plenum.

El Dareer, Asma. 1982. *Women, Why Do You Weep? Circumcision and Its Consequences.* London: Zed Books.

Ettorre, Elizabeth, Timo Klaukka, and Elianne Riska. 1994. "Psychotrophic Drugs: Long-Term Use, Dependency and the Gender Factor." *Social Science and Medicine* 12:1667–73.

Farberow, Norman L., Delores Gallagher-Thompson, Michael Gilewski, and Larry Thompson. 1992. "The Role of Social Supports in the Bereavement Process of Surviving Spouses of Suicide and Natural Deaths." *Suicide and Life-Threatening Behavior* 22:107–24.

Farrell, Janice, and Kyriakos S. Markides. 1985. "Marriage and Health: A Three-Generation Study of Mexican Americans." *Journal of Marriage and the Family* 47:1029–36.

Fee, Elizabeth, and Nancy Krieger, eds. 1994. *Women's Health, Politics, and Power.* Amityville, NY: Baywood.

Fennelly, Katherine. 1993. "Barriers to Birth Control Use among Hispanic Teenagers: Providers' Perspectives." Pp. 300–11 in Bair and Cayleff.

Finkelhor, David and Kersti Yllö. 1985. *License to Rape: Sexual Abuse of Wives.* New York: Holt, Rinehart & Winston.

Forsyth, Craig J., and Eddie C. Palmer. 1990. "Teenage Pregnancy: Health, Moral and Economic Issues." *International Journal of Sociology of the Family* 20:79–95.

Fox, Steve. 1991. *Toxic Work: Women Workers at GTE Lenkurt.* Philadelphia: Temple University Press.

Franklin, Sara. 1990. "Deconstructing 'Desperateness': The Social Construction of Infertility in Popular Representations of New Reproductive Technologies." Pp. 200–29 in *The New Reproductive Technologies*, edited by M. McNeil, I. Varcoe, and S. Yearley. London: Macmillan.

Fraser, Alison M. 1995. "Association of Young Maternal Age with Adverse Reproductive Outcomes." *New England Journal of Medicine* 332:1113–17.

Fussell, Sam. 1993. "Body Builder Americanus." *Michigan Quarterly Review* 32:577–96.

Gartner, Rosemary. 1990. "The Victims of Homicide: A Temporal and Cross-National Comparison." *American Sociological Review* 55:92–106.

Gartner, Rosemary, Kathryn Baker, and Fred C. Pampel. 1990. "Gender Stratification and the Gender Gap in Homicide Victimization." *Social Problems* 37:593–612.

Gerstel, Naomi, and Sally Gallagher. 1994. "Caring for Kith and Kin: Gender, Employment, and the Privatization of Care." *Social Problems* 41:519–39.

Gibbs, Jewelle Taylor, ed. 1988. *Young, Black and Male in America: An Endangered Species.* Dover, MA: Auburn House.

Glass, Jennifer, and Tetsushi Fujimoto. 1994. "Housework, Paid Work, and Depression among Husbands and Wives." *Journal of Health and Social Behavior* 35:179–91.

Glazer, Nona. 1990. "The Home as Workshop: Women as Amateur Nurses and Medical Care Providers." *Gender & Society* 4:479–99.

Gove, Walter R. 1984. "Gender Differences in Mental and Physical Illness: The Effects of Fixed Roles and Nurturant Roles." *Social Science and Medicine* 19:77–91.

Graham, Hilary. 1985. "Providers, Negotiators, and Mediators: Women as the Hidden Carers." Pp. 25–52 in *Women, Health, and Healing*, edited by Ellen Lewin and Virginia Oleson. New York: Tavistock.

Gregersen, Edgar. 1983. *Sexual Practices: The Story of Human Sexuality.* New York: Franklin Watts.

Greil, Arthur L. 1991. *Not Yet Pregnant: Infertile Couples in Contemporary America.* New Brunswick, NJ: Rutgers University Press.

Harlow, Carolina Wolf. 1991. *Female Victims of Violent Crime.* Washington: U.S. Department of Justice, Bureau of Justice Statistics.

Helgeson, Vickie. 1995. "Masculinity, Men's Roles, and Coronary Heart Disease." Pp. 68–104 in Sabo and Gordon.

Herzog, David B., Isabel Bradburn, and Kerry Newman. 1990. "Sexuality in Males with Eating Disorders." Pp. 40–53 in Andersen.

Herzog, David B., Kerry L. Newman, C. J. Yeh, and Meredith Warshaw. 1992. "Body Image

Satisfaction in Homosexual and Heterosexual Women." *International Journal of Eating Disorders* 11:391–96.

Herzog, David B., Dennis K. Norman, Christopher Gordon, and Maura Pepose. 1984. "Sexual Conflict and Eating Disorders in 27 Males." *American Journal of Psychiatry* 141:989–90.

Hesse-Biber, Sharlene J. 1989. "Eating Patterns and Disorders in a College Population: Are College Women's Eating Problems a New Phenomenon?" *Sex Roles* 20:71–89.

Hogan, Dennis P., and Evelyn M. Kitagawa. 1985. "The Impact of Social Status, Family Structure, and Neighborhood on the Fertility of Black Adolescent." *American Journal of Sociology* 90:825–55.

Hubbard, Ruth. 1990. *The Politics of Women's Biology.* New Brunswick, NJ: Rutgers University Press.

Idler, Ellen L., and Stanislav V. Kasl. 1992. "Religion, Disability, Depression, and the Timing of Death." *American Journal of Sociology* 97:1052–79.

Johnson, Richard E., and Anastasios C. Marcos. 1988. "Correlates of Adolescent Drug Use by Gender and Geographic Location." *American Journal of Drug and Alcohol Abuse* 14:51–63.

Johnson, Valerie. 1988. "Adolescent Alcohol and Marijuana Use: A Longitudinal Assessment of a Social Learning Perspective." *American Journal of Drug and Alcohol Abuse* 14:419–39.

Jonas, Helen A., and Teri A. Manolio. 1996. "Hormone Replacement and Cardiovascular Disease in Older Women." *Journal of Women's Health* 5:351–61.

Jones, Elise, and Jacqueline Darroch Forrest. 1985. "Teenage Pregnancy in Developed Countries: Determinants and Policy Implications." *Family Planning Perspectives* 17:53–63.

Jones, Wanda, Dixie E. Snider, and Rueben C. Warren. 1996. "Deciphering the Data: Race, Ethnicity, and Gender as Critical Variables." *Journal of the American Medical Women's Association* 51:137–38.

Kearney-Cooke, Ann, and Paule Steichen-Asch. 1990. "Men, Body Image, and Eating Disorders." Pp. 54–74 in Andersen.

Kemp, Alice Abel, and Pamela Jenkins. 1992. "Gender and Technological Hazards: Women at Risk in Hospital Setting." *Industrial Crisis Quarterly* 6:137–52.

Kliewer, Erich V., and Ken R. Smith. 1995. "Breast Cancer Mortality among Immigrants in Australia and Canada." *Journal of the National Cancer Institute* 87:1154–61.

Koch, Lene. 1990. "IVF-An Irrational Choice?" *Issues in Reproductive and Genetic Engineering* 3:235–42.

Kranczer, Stanley. 1995. "U.S. Longevity Unchanged." *Statistical Bulleting* 76(3): 12–20.

Krieger, Nancy. 1996. "Inequality, Diversity, and Health: Thoughts on 'Race/Ethnicity' and 'Gender.'" *Journal of the American Medical Women's Association* 51:133–36.

Kurz, Demie. 1987. "Emergency Department Response to Battered Women: A Case of Resistance." *Social Problems* 34:501–13.

Lai, Gina. 1995. "Work and Family Roles and Psychological Well-Being in Urban China." *Journal of Health and Social Behavior* 36:11–37.

Lasker, Judith N., and Shirley Borg. 1995. *In Search of Parenthood: Coping with Infertility and High-Tech Conception.* Philadelphia: Temple University Press.

Lazarus, Ellen. 1988a. "Poor Women, Poor Outcomes: Social Class and Reproductive Health." Pp. 39–54 in *Childbirth in America*, edited by Karen L. Michaelson. South Hadley, MA: Bergin & Garvey.

Lennon, Mary Clare. 1994. "Women, Work, and Well-Being: The Importance of Work Conditions." *Journal of Health and Social Behavior* 35:235–47.

Lennon, Mary Clare, and Sara Rosenfeld. 1992. "Women and Mental Health: The Interaction of Job and Family Conditions." *Journal of Health and Social Behavior* 33:316–27.

Lieberman, Ellice, Kenneth J. Ryan, Richard R. Monson, and Stephen C. Schoenbaum. 1987. "Risk Factors Accounting for Racial Differences in the Rate of Premature Birth." *New England Journal of Medicine* 317:743–48.

Lightfoot-Klein, Hanny. 1989. *Prisoners of Ritual: An Odyssey into Female Circumcision in Africa*. New York: Harrington Park Press.

Lillard, Leea A., and Linda J. Waite. 1995. "'Till Death Do Us Part: Marital Disruption and Mortality." *American Journal of Sociology* 100:1131–56.

Link, Bruce G., and Jo Phelan. 1995. "Social Conditions as Fundamental Causes of Disease." *Journal of Health and Social Behavior* (Extra issue):80–94.

Longino, Charles F., Jr. 1988. "A Population Profile of Very Old Men and Women in the United States." *Sociological Quarterly* 29:559–64.

Loscosso, Karyn A., and Glenna Spitze. 1990. "Working Conditions, Social Support, and the Well-Being of Female and Male Factory Workers." *Journal of Health and Social Behavior* 31:313–27.

Luker, Kristin. 1996. *Dubious Conceptions: The Politics of Teen Pregnancy*. Cambridge, MA: Harvard University Press.

MacFarqhar, Neil. 1996. "Mutilation of Egyptian Girls: Despite Ban, It Goes On." *New York Times*, August 8, p. A3.

Maddi, Salvatore R., and Suzanne C. Kobassa. 1984. *The Hardy Executive: Health under Stress*. Homewood, IL: Dow Jones-Irwin.

Madigan, M. Patricia, Reginia G. Ziegler, Jacques Benichou, et. al. 1995. "Proportion of Breast Cancer Cases in the United States Explained by Well-Established Risk Factors." *Journal of the National Cancer Institute* 87:1681–85.

Mansfield, Alan, and Barbara McGinn. 1993. "Pumping Irony: The Muscular and the Feminine." Pp. 49–68 in *Body Matters: Essays on the Sociology of the Body*, edited by Sue Scott and David Morgan. London: Falmer.

Marsiglio, William. 1988. "Commitment to Social Fatherhood: Predicting Adolescent Males' Intentions to Live with Their Child and Partner." *Journal of Marriage and the Family* 50:427–41.

McKinlay, John B. 1996. "Some Contributions from the Social System to Gender Inequalities in Heart Disease." *Journal of Health and Social Behavior* 37:1–26.

Merrick, Janna C., and Robert H. Blank. 1993. *The Politics of Pregnancy: Policy Dilemmas in the Maternal-Fetal Relationship*. New York: Haworth.

Messner, Michael. 1992. *Power at Play: Sports and the Problem of Masculinity*. Boston: Beacon.

Miall, Charlene E. 1986. "The Stigma of Involuntary Childlessness." *Social Problems* 33:268–82.

Muller, Charlotte. 1990. *Health Care and Gender*. New York: Russell Sage.

Nachtigall, Lila E., and Lisa B. Nachtigall. 1995. "Estrogen Issues in Relation to Cardiovascular Disease." *Journal of the American Medical Women's Association* 50:7–10.

Nam, Charles B., Isaac W. Eberstein, and Larry C. Deeb. 1989. "Sudden Infant Death Syndrome as a Socially Determined Cause of Death." *Social Biology* 36:1–8.

Oleckno, William A., and Michael J. Blacconiere. 1990. "Wellness of College Students and Differences by Gender, Race, and Class Standing." *College Student Journal* 24:421–29.

Orden, Susan R., Kiang Liu, Karen J. Ruth, David R. Jacobs, Jr., et. al. 1995. "Multiple Social Roles and Blood Pressure of Black and White Women: The CARDIA Study." *Journal of Women's Health* 4:281–91.

Ouellette, Susanne K. 1993. "Inquiries into Hardiness." Pp. 77–100 in *Handbook of Stress: Theoretical and Clinical Aspects*, 2nd ed., edited by L. Goldberger and S. Breznit. New York: Free Press.

Perkins, H. Wesley. 1992. "Gender Patterns in Consequences of Collegiate Alcohol Abuse: A 10-Year Study of Trends in an Undergraduate Population." *Journal of Studies on Alcohol* 53:458–62.

Pfeffer, Naomi. 1987. "Artificial Insemination, *In Vitro* Fertilization and the Stigma of Infertility." Pp. 81–97 in *Reproductive Technologies: Gender, Motherhood and Medicine*, edited by Michelle Stanworth. Minneapolis: University of Minnesota Press.

Phillips, David P., and Kenneth A. Feldman. 1973. "A Dip in Deaths Before Ceremonial Occasions: Some New Relationships between Social Integration and Mortality." *American Sociological Review* 38:678–96.

Phillips, David P., and Elliot W. King. 1988. "Death Takes a Holiday: Mortality Surrounding Major Social Occasions." *Lancet* 337:728–32.

Phillips, David P., Todd E. Ruth, and Lisa M. Wagner. 1993. "Psychology and Survival." *Lancet* 342:1142–45.

Phillips, David P., and Daniel G. Smith. 1990. "Postponement of Death Until Symbolically Meaningful Occasions." *Journal of the American Medical Association* 263:1947–51.

Ptacek, James. 1988. "Why Do Men Batter Their Wives?" Pp. 133–57 in *Feminist Perspectives on Wife Abuse*, edited by Kersti Yllö and Michele Bograd. Newbury Park, CA: Sage.

Pugliesi, Karen. 1995. "Work and Well-Being: Gender Differences in the Psychological Consequences of Employment." *Journal of Health and Social Behavior* 36:57–71.

Redmond, Marcia A. 1985. "Attitudes of Adolescent Males toward Adolescent Pregnancy and Fatherhood." *Family Relations* 34:337–42.

Renteln, Alison Dundes. 1992. "Sex Selection and Reproductive Freedom." *Women's Studies International Forum* 15:405–26.

Reunanen, Antti. 1993. "Juhlan Aika Ja Tuonen Hetki" (The Time of Celebration and the Time of Death). *Duodecim* 109:2098–103.

Richie, Beth E. 1996. *Compelled to Crime: The Gender Entrapment of Battered Black Women*. New York: Routledge.

Riska, Elianne. 1993. Introduction. Pp. 1–12 in *Gender, Work and Medicine: Women and the Medical Division of Labor*, edited by Elianne Riska and Katarina Wegar. Newbury Park, CA: Sage.

Robbins, Cynthia A., and Steven S. Martin. 1993. "Gender, Styles of Deviance, and Drinking Problems." *Journal of Health and Social Behavior* 34:302–21.

Rogers, Richard G., and Eve Powell-Griner. 1991. "Life Expectancies of Cigarette Smokers and Nonsmokers in the United States." *Social Science and Medicine* 32:1151–59.

Romito, Patrizia, and François Hovelaque. 1987. "Changing Approaches in Women's Health: New Insights and New Pitfalls in Prenatal Preventive Care." *International Journal of Health Services* 17:241–58.

Rosenberg, Harriet G. 1984. "The Home Is the Workplace: Hazards, Stress, and Pollutants in the Household." Pp. 219–45 in Chavkin.

Rosenthal, A. M. 1996. "Fighting Female Mutilation." *New York Times*, April 12, p. A31.

Ross, Catherine E., and Chloe E. Bird. 1994. "Sex Stratification and Health Lifestyle: Consequences for Men's and Women's Perceived Health." *Journal of Health and Social Behavior* 35:161–78.

Rothman, Barbara Katz. 1982. *In Labor: Women and Power in the Birthplace.* New York: Norton.

Roth, Barbara Katz. 1989. *Recreating Motherhood: Ideology and Technology in a Patriarchal Society.* New York: Norton.

Roth, Barbara Katz. 1986. *The Tentative Pregnancy.* New York: Viking.

Roxburgh, Susan. 1996. "Gender Differences in Work and Well-Being: Effects of Exposure and Vulnerability." *Journal of Health and Social Behavior* 37:265–77.

Rushing, Beth, Christian Ritter, and Russell P.D. Burton. 1992. "Race Differences in the Effects of Multiple Roles on Health: Longitudinal Evidence from a National Sample of Older Men." *Journal of Health and Social Behavior* 33:126–39.

Sabo, Don, and David Frederick Gordon, eds. 1995. *Men's Health and Illness: Gender, Power and the Body.* Thousand Oaks, CA: Sage.

Sandelowski, Margarete. 1993. *With Child in Mind: Studies of the Personal Encounter with Infertility.* Philadelphia: University of Pennsylvania Press.

Santow, Gigi. 1995. "Social Roles and Physical Health: The Case of Female Disadvantage in Poor Countries." *Social Science and Medicine* 40:147–61.

Scheper-Hughes, Nancy, and Margaret M. Lock. 1987. "The Mindful Body: A Prolegomenon to Future Work in Medical Anthropology." *Medical Anthropology Quarterly* n.s. 1:6–41.

Sen, Amartya K. 1990. "Gender and Cooperative Conflicts." Pp. 123–49 in *Persistent Inequalities: Women and World Development*, edited by Irene Tinker. New York: Oxford University Press.

Sorensen, Gloria, and Lois M. Berbrugge. 1987. "Women, Work, and Health." *American Review of Public Health* 8:235–51.

Spark, Richard F. 1988. *The Infertile Male: The Clinician's Guide to Diagnosis and Treatment.* New York: Plenum.

Specter, Michael. 1995. "Plunging Life Expectancy Puzzles Russians." *New York Times*, August 2, p. A1.

Staples, Robert. 1995. "Health among Afro-American Males." Pp. 121–38 in Sabo and Gordon.

Stillion, Judith. 1995. "Premature Death among Males: Extending the Bottom Line of Men's Health." Pp. 46–67 in Sabo and Gordon.

Sundari, T. K. 1994. "The Untold Story: How the Health Care Systems in Developing Countries Contribute to Maternal Mortality." Pp. 173–90 in Fee and Krieger.

Taggart, Lee Ann, Susan L. McCammon, Linda J. Allred, et al. 1993. "Effect of Patient and Physician Gender on Prescriptions for Psychotropic Drugs." *Journal of Women's Health* 2:353–57.

Teresi, Dick. 1994. "How to Get a Man Pregnant: My (True) Adventures on the Frontiers of Science." *New York Times Magazine*, November 27, pp. 6, 54.

Thompson, Becky Wansgaard. 1992. "'A Way Outa No Way': Eating Problems among African-American, Latina, and White Women." *Gender and Society* 6:546–61.

Turner, R. Jay, Carl F. Grindstaff, and Norma Phillips. 1990. "Social Support and Outcome in Teenage Pregnancy." *Journal of Health and Social Behavior* 31:43–57.

Van Roosmalen, Erica H., and Susan A. McDaniel. 1992. "Adolescent Smoking Intentions: Gender Differences in Peer Context." *Adolescence* 27:87–105.

Veevers, Jean E., and Ellen M. Gee. 1986. "Playing It Safe: Accident Mortality and Gender Roles." *Sociological Focus* 19:349–60.

Verbrugge, Lois M. 1985. "Gender and Health: An Update on Hypotheses and Evidence." *Journal of Health and Social Behavior* 26:156–82.

Verbrugge, Lois M. 1986. "Role Burdens and Physical Health of Women and Men." *Women and Health* 11:47–77.

Verbrugge, Lois M. 1989a. "The Twain Meet: Empirical Explanations of Sex Differences in Health and Mortality." *Journal of Health and Social Behavior* 30:282–304.

Verbrugge, Lois M. 1989b. "Gender, Aging, and Health." Pp. 23–78 in *Aging and Health: Perspectives on Gender, Race Ethnicity, and Class,* edited by Kyriakos S. Markides. Newbury Park, CA: Sage.

Verbrugge, Lois M. 1990. "Pathways of Health and Death." Pp. 41–49 in *Women, Health and Medicine in America,* edited by Rima D. Apple. New York: Garland.

Waldron, Ingrid. 1995. "Contributions of Changing Gender Differences in Behavior and Social Roles to Changing Gender Differences in Mortality." Pp. 22–45 in Sabo and Gordon.

Walker, Alice. 1992. *Possessing the Secret of Joy.* New York: Harcourt, Brace, Jovanovich.

Walker, Lenore E. 1984. *The Battered Woman Syndrome.* New York: Springer.

Warsaw, Carole. 1989. "Limitations of the Medical Model in the Case of Battered Women." *Gender & Society* 3:506–17.

Weitz, Rose. 1992. *Life with AIDS.* New Brunswick, NJ: Rutgers University Press.

Wilcox, Allen, Rolv Skjaerven, and Pierre Buekens. 1995. "Birth Weight and Perinatal Mortality: A Comparison of the United States and Norway." *Journal of the American Medical Association* 273:709–11.

Williams, Linda S. 1988. "'It's Going to Work for Me.' Responses to Failures of IVF." *Birth* 15:153–56.

Wilson, Margo, and Martin Daly. 1985. "Competitiveness, Risk Taking, and Violence: The Young Male Syndrome." *Ethology and Sociobiology* 6:59–73.

World Health Organization. 1995. *Women's Health: Improve Our Health, Improve the World.* Position paper, Fourth World Conference on Women, Beijing, China.

Wright, Lawrence. 1996. "Silent Sperm." *The New Yorker,* January 15, pp. 42–55.

Yllö, Kersti. 1984. "The Status of Women, Martial Equality, and Violence Against Wives. *Journal of Family Issues* 5:307–20.

Ziegler, R. G. 1993. "Migration Patterns and Breast Cancer Risk in Asian-American Women." *Journal of the National Cancer Institute* 85:1819–27.

Hormones for Men: Is Male Menopause a Question of Medicine or of Marketing?

Jerome Groopman

It goes by many names. "Male menopause" is perhaps the most popular, but "andropause" is the term that many doctors favor, and PADAM ("partial androgen deficiency in aging men") has its partisans, too. The condition may afflict millions of Americans, and, if they do not yet recognize the symptoms, a public-awareness campaign has been launched to help them. A two-page ad that ran in *Time* not long ago showed a car's gas gauge pointing to Empty and beside it the words "Fatigued? Depressed mood? Low sex drive? Could be your testosterone is running on empty." The ad explains that "as some men grow older, their testosterone levels decline," and that such men should consult their doctors about testosterone therapy. At the bottom of the page, the gas gauge points to Full.

Physicians have been targeted with similar ads. One that appeared in a recent issue of a primary-care journal calls on them to "identify the men in your practice with low testosterone who may benefit from clinical performance in a packet." The photographs are eye-catching: there's a well-built fellow in his middle years beside the words "improved sexual function"; a smiling man in shorts and a T-shirt who is standing next to a mountain bike ("improved mood"); a policeman directing traffic ("increased bone mineral density"). Doctors are told to "screen for symptoms of low testosterone" and "restore normal testosterone levels."

These ads were paid for by Unimed, a division of the Belgian conglomerate Solvay. Unimed makes AndroGel, a drug that was approved by the F.D.A. two years ago, and is the fastest-growing form of testosterone-replacement therapy for men. Pills, introduced in the sixties, often caused liver damage. Intramuscular injections, particularly favored by body-builders and competitive athletes, produce a sharp spike of the hormone, and then a fall, and these fluctuations are often accompanied by swings in mood, libido, and energy. In the late eighties, a transdermal patch was developed, and its use is still widespread. The patch provides safer and steadier dosing, but often causes skin irritation, and sometimes falls off during exercise. AndroGel, by contrast, delivers testosterone in a color-less, drying gel that is simply rubbed on an area of the body—usually the shoulders—once a day. It has thus made testosterone available in a form that almost any man can use conveniently.

If hormone-replacement therapy for andropause becomes as common as such therapies have been for menopause—and this seems to be the ambi-tion of some drug companies—the consequences, both medical and finan-cial, could be dramatic. Given the popular desire to reverse human aging with a simple nostrum and the growing intimacy between commercial and clinical concerns, the trend may prove to be irresistible. The phar-maceutical industry is, of course, in the business of inventing treatments. Some people wonder whether it may help invent diseases, too.

To be treated for andropause, you first need physicians who can con-fidently make the diagnosis. One of them is Dr. Abraham Morgentaler, the director of Men's Health Boston. He is forty-six years old, with thick black hair and deep-set eyes. Trained as a urologist, he specializes in male sexual dysfunction and infertility. He views testosterone deficiency in older men as a silent epidemic, and worries that, of the perhaps five mil-lion American men who suffer from it, 95 percent go undiagnosed. Re-placing missing testosterone, he believes, will help restore youthful mus-cle tone, body strength, potency, and general vigor. He recently put an ad in the Boston *Globe* urging men who were experiencing "low sex drive" or "low energy" to have their testosterone level tested at his clinic. The costs of both the ad and the tests were underwritten by a Unimed educa-tional grant.

Men's Health Boston is in a modern brick-and-glass office building at a busy intersection in Brookline. It has a well-appointed waiting room with soft lighting and upholstered chairs; photographs of famous local athletes adorn the walls. The men who came to see Morgentaler on a recent after-noon had all been given a questionnaire provided by Unimed:

1. Do you have a decrease in libido (sex drive)?
2. Do you have a lack of energy?

3. Do you have a decrease in strength and/or endurance?

4. Have you lost height?

5. Have you noticed a decreased "enjoyment of life"?

6. Are you sad and/or grumpy?

7. Are your erections less strong?

8. Have you noticed a recent deterioration in your ability to play sports?

9. Are you falling asleep after dinner?

10. Has there been a recent deterioration in your work performance?

Among the patients was a real-estate broker in his late fifties. He had answered "Yes" to questions 1, 2, 3, 5, 7, and 10. "I'm just exhausted by the end of the afternoon," he said, after Morgentaler gave him a physical. "And my brain often feels foggy." He likes to shoot pool, and he remarked that his game wasn't what it used to be.

"Have you noticed any change in sexual performance?" Dr. Morgentaler asked.

"Well, I'm not a kid anymore," the patient said, but he had no real complaints.

Morgentaler then showed the man the results from his blood assay. His testosterone levels were "somewhat low," Morgentaler said. "Now, if I had a magic wand and I could do anything for you, what would it be?"

"Fix the energy thing."

"I have good news for you," Dr. Morgentaler said. "There is an excellent chance that giving you testosterone will help to restore your energy. And, in terms of being foggy, I can't promise, but I have several men in my practice who are professors. They take testosterone, and they say it makes their brains much sharper."

Dr. Morgentaler explained that, while testosterone would not cause prostate cancer, if the patient had a hidden tumor the hormone would "act like food, nourishing the cancer." For that reason, his P.S.A. (prostate-specific antigen) level would be checked, and Morgentaler would take six biopsy samples of the prostate gland to make sure that there was no malignancy.

"I'll give you a prescription now, and you can get started once we complete these tests," Dr. Morgentaler said. "When I give men back testosterone, some say, 'Whoa!'"

The patient liked the sound of that. "Maybe I'll be a stallion again," he said.

Testosterone, an androgen, is a steroid hormone derived from cholesterol. It is produced primarily by the testes, but the signal to produce it comes from the pituitary gland, in the form of two other hormones, which arrive in pulses at certain times of the day. As men age, the response of the testes becomes more muted; for men over the age of forty, the levels of testosterone in the bloodstream decline, on average, by about 1.2 percent each year.

Morgentaler's next patient was a construction worker in his forties. The man was on cardiac medication and had an implanted defibrillator, because he was prone to life-threatening arrhythmias, and occasionally he received electric jolts from the device. His wife had died some three years before, but in the previous six months he had been in a stable relationship. He had come to the clinic because he had difficulty reaching orgasm.

Morgentaler asked about other symptoms.

"I used to be able to play racquetball non-stop, but I'm tired now after four games."

Morgentaler nodded. "We caught it just at the right time."

"But my primary-care doctor checked my testosterone and said it was 800, which is normal. He told me he couldn't do anything about my problem."

Morgentaler looked at the results of the man's blood assay. Total testosterone was in the normal range, at 509 nanograms per decilitre. But his free testosterone, Morgentaler told him, was another matter. At any moment, about 2 percent of circulating testosterone is "free"—unbound to any protein—and thus biologically active. The patient's free testosterone was a little under the lower limit of normal. ("Normal" testosterone levels refer to what's normal for men in their twenties.)

"If I had a magic wand and I could do anything for you, what would it be?" Morgentaler asked.

"Get rid of the problem with orgasm."

"Well, I believe we have a very good chance of helping you." Morgentaler wrote out a prescription for AndroGel. "We'll check your P.S.A. today, but we don't need to do biopsies of your prostate gland until after the age of fifty. So you can get started right away."

"I can't thank you enough," the patient said.

When the F.D.A. decides to permit the sale of a new drug, it specifies a list of "indications"—particular medical conditions for which the drug has been approved. "The F.D.A. never approved AndroGel for andropause," says Dr. Dan Shames, the director of the Division of Reproductive and

Urological Drug Products at the F.D.A. "We're not sure what 'andropause' is. The intention was that AndroGel would be for people with conditions like Klinefelter's and pituitary dysfunction." Klinefelter's syndrome is a congenital disorder in which men have an extra X chromosome and underdeveloped testes. Other suitable candidates for therapy are men whose testes have been scarred by viral inflammation. Still others have had a tumor that damaged the hypothalamus or the pituitary gland, so the brain no longer sends activating signals to the testes. In such men, muscle strength, libido, and bone density are diminished, and testosterone replacement is an effective treatment.

The trouble is that there aren't very many of these people—they number only in the tens of thousands. But there are some thirty-five million men in the United States over the age of fifty, and if the andropause movement takes off, annual revenues for the producers of testosterone-replacement drugs could reach billions of dollars. Estrogen-replacement therapy in menopausal women—a comparable market—has generated more than two billion dollars a year in revenue, largely for Wyeth, the maker of Premarin, the most popular estrogen-replacement drug.

This is where marketing and medical science may part ways. Pharmaceutical companies often obtain F.D.A. approval of a new product for a niche population with a relatively rare disease, hoping to expand later to a larger and more profitable market. Once a drug is approved for sale, a physician can legally prescribe it for any clinical condition he thinks would benefit from it. The F.D.A. prohibits drug companies from advertising "off label" uses—those other than the approved indications—but they can pursue alternative strategies. They can run adds that "raise awareness" of a condition without mentioning the proprietary therapy by name. And they can align themselves with so-called "opinion leaders," well-known physicians whose views are thought to have influence among their peers, by financing their research, say, or offering them consulting agreements.

If you're hoping to expand the medical "indications" for a drug regimen, there are few greater boons than the endorsement of a major medical society. Unimed's andropause campaign won a considerable victory when the Endocrine Society—a prestigious organization of hormone specialists—convened its First Annual Andropause Consensus Conference, in April of 2000, just six weeks before AndroGel came on the market. The conference, which was held in Beverly Hills, set out to define andropause and decide how it should be treated. The chair was Dr. Ronald Swerdloff, an endocrinologist at Harbor-U.C.L.A. Medical Center, and he assembled a panel whose task was to come up with recommendations for clinical practice. These recommendations were distributed at this year's annual meeting of the Endocrine Society, in June, and undoubtedly they will have considerable influence in the medical community.

The panel acknowledged that the benefits of testosterone replacement in aging men hadn't been established, but it nonetheless recommended that all men over the age of fifty be screened for testosterone deficiency. Screening should start with a questionnaire, like the one that Unimed had provided for Morgentaler. Patients who had symptoms, whose morning testosterone levels were under the lower limit of normal, specified as 300, and who had no conditions that would rule out testosterone replacement, like prostate cancer, "would likely benefit from treatment," the panel stated. A table accompanying the recommendations suggested that low testosterone levels would be found in more than ten percent of men over fifty, and nearly 30 percent of men over seventy—in perhaps as many as seven million Americans.

There's no doubt that the panel reached its conclusions in good faith; the androgen enthusiasts are nothing if not sincere. But it's also the case that a Unimed/Solvay educational grant was the sole source of funding for the Beverly Hills conference. According to Scott Hunt, the Endocrine Society's executive director, Unimed even suggested some of the panel's members. And, of the thirteen panelists in the final group, at least nine, including Swerdloff and his co-chair, had significant financial ties to the drug company, in the form of research grants, consulting arrangements, or speaking fees. The recommendations made reference to the educational grant but not to the panelists' ties to Unimed.

The bid to medicalize middle age may be well supported by the pharmaceutical industry, but it remains poorly supported by scientific research. Is the decline in testosterone levels really responsible for most of the symptoms of aging in men? What levels of testosterone are, in fact, "normal"? Does andropause even exist? The limits of medical knowledge are starkly evident when you visit a research center like the one run by Dr. William Crowley, the chief of the Reproductive Endocrine Unit at Massachusetts General Hospital, and his associate Dr. Frances Hayes. In a laboratory crowded with centrifuges, chemical hoods, and spectrophotometers, they and their team spend hours double-checking sensitive chemical assays for hormones produced by the hypothalamus and the testes, as well as the pituitary and adrenal glands. In an adjoining clinical-research center, volunteer human subjects are hooked up to I.V.s and insulin clamps.

Several years ago, Dr. Crowley realized that, in order to study hypogonadal men, he needed a clear definition of normal testosterone levels. So he inserted catheters into the veins of healthy young subjects in their twenties and drew blood samples every ten minutes in the course of twenty-four hours. He still sounds amazed by what he found.

"We measured the size of their testes, evaluated body hair, erectile function, sperm count, muscle mass, bone density, pituitary function," Crowley recalls. "These men were completely normal from every parameter. And it was incredible: 15 percent had testosterone levels during the day that were well below what is set as the lower limit of normal—more than 50 percent below the cutoff."

Why do testosterone levels among healthy men vary so much? Hayes speculates that some men may have highly efficient testosterone receptors—cellular traps that grab the free hormone in the blood—so that what appears to be an abnormally low testosterone level is all the hormone they need. But even an individual's testosterone levels can be markedly different at different times. One factor may be stress, which seems to reduce levels of sex steroids. Drug interactions, too, might alter testosterone levels in unpredictable ways. And much of the variation simply eludes explanation. Crowley studied several young men whose initial test results showed testosterone levels ranging from 150 to 200—well below the 300 cutoff—over twenty-four hours. "They had a perfectly normal testosterone profile," Crowley says. "There can be a funny disconnect between one measurement and a later one"—which means that testosterone deficiency may be easily overdiagnosed.

"This variability in testosterone levels was really a physiological curiosity until AndroGel was approved," Crowley continues. "Now every time the testosterone level is below 300 the question of prescription is raised." As for the often quoted figure of four or five million "andropausal" men—the figure touted in the Unimed ads—Hayes says, "Frankly, I don't know where that number comes from or how real it is."

What makes things more confusing is that the usual commercial tests that physicians use to measure testosterone levels are notoriously unreliable. The andropause movement has made laboratory assays a lucrative business, and all kinds of patented kits have come on the market. But, as Swerdloff's panel discovered, the results tend to be inconsistent. "It's really a big problem," Swerdloff says. "Practicing doctors have a great belief in the numbers, but in the past few years the assays have deteriorated." If you assayed blood samples from normal men with one proprietary test, you might find values between 300 and 900, while another test would give values between 160 and 700. So men whose tests report low total testosterone levels—like the real-estate broker Morgentaler saw—might actually have normal levels. The tests for free testosterone seem to be even less accurate.

Not every practitioner finds reason for concern. "The tests aren't as reliable as we want them to be, but it doesn't matter," says Morgentaler, who sometimes even prescribes AndroGel "preventatively" for middle-aged men whose testosterone levels are in the lower quarter of the normal range. "It's not credible that we aren't helping these men by giving them testosterone. The truth is, there's a deep emotional issue in some people who oppose hormone-replacement therapy, because it asks the question 'Is there hope of achieving eternal youth?' There are those who don't want to oppose Mother Nature."

And there are those who don't want to wait for scientific validation. Last year, a panel organized by the National Institutes of Health—maybe the closest thing we have to a voice of independent scientific consensus—released a paper concluding that the andropause hypothesis is unproved. The report that Swerdloff's group released at the Endocrine Society meeting in June contains references to sixty-two relevant publications, but omits any reference to the N.I.H. report.

Swerdloff and his colleagues reviewed the half-dozen controlled studies available on giving testosterone to healthy aging men, and were evidently impressed by those which found that it increased lean muscle mass, strength, and bone-mineral density in the spine. Unfortunately, most of these studies were small, involving forty or fifty men. The reported improvements were far from dramatic, and different studies have had contradictory findings. In fact, the largest and longest-term study, of 108 men over three years, showed no improvements in energy level, sexual performance, or strength.

So there's a lot of uncertainty about the effects of the age-related lowering of testosterone. "There appears to be a threshold level of testosterone below which libido and sexual function are impaired," Hayes says. "Boosting above this threshold doesn't seem to enhance sexual performance." The role that testosterone plays in maintaining strong bones in healthy elderly men is highly controversial, too. Dan Shames, of the F.D.A., says, "Just because you are increasing bone density doesn't mean you prevent fractures." Even in studies that found a positive correlation between testosterone levels and bone strength, the hormone accounted for only about 5 percent of age- and weight-adjusted differences. Men with severely low testosterone levels showed improvement in the spine, but no change was observed in the hips—and it is mainly hip fractures that debilitate the elderly.

"Each pharmaceutical company wants to get up and say, 'This is the magic bullet for aging,' " Crowley says. "But it's overly simplistic to attribute such a complex process as aging to the change in the level of a single hormone like estrogen or testosterone."

If the benefits of treating "andropause" are in doubt, so, more worrisomely, is the safety. The known side effects of testosterone therapy include gynecomastia (abnormal enlargement of the breasts) and testicular shrinkage (as gonads compensate by making less of the hormone). Testosterone also raises the level of circulating red blood cells; if this level is excessive, the blood becomes viscous, which can lead to congestive heart failure or stroke. And among men who received a 100-milligram daily dose of AndroGel over a year, nearly 20 percent developed some sort of prostate disorder, such as prostatic hyperplasia.

More troubling is how testosterone accelerates the growth of prostate cancer. The majority of men over the age of sixty-five have clusters of cancer cells in their prostate glands which are both "occult" and "indolent": they're hard to find, and they grow so slowly that they're unlikely to create any trouble by themselves. Here the perils are twofold. On the one hand, unnecessary biopsies can lead to unnecessary surgery, aimed at eradicating cancers that might have remained inactive. On the other hand, biopsies can easily miss cancers that, under a regimen of testosterone replacement, become more aggressive than they otherwise would be. Not surprisingly, Dr. Shames says that the F.D.A. has "issues of concern over the safety" of prescribing testosterone-replacement therapy for men whose hormone levels fall as part of normal aging.

Even Dr. Swerdloff acknowledges these uncertainties. "I agree that currently there are insufficient data on the long-term effects of testosterone-replacement therapy on the heart or on the development of prostate cancer, but the benefits seem considerable," he says. The andropause panel he chaired was aware that the N.I.H. is thinking of doing rigorous, placebo-controlled clinical studies that would span six or more years. "If the answer is yes, that replacement therapy causes heart damage or sparks emergence of prostate cancer, then you will know in six years or so," he says. "But older people in this age group won't wait six to ten years to have solid answers. Clinical practice will move at one rate, and the data will trail."

This is precisely what concerns many scientists. "Pharmaceutical marketing is the driver, not physiology," Crowley complains of the andropause movement. "Maybe we're *meant* to lower our testosterone levels—maybe it's healthy and protects us from developing prostate cancer. Of course, that's pure conjecture, but it's something that needs to be carefully addressed." When you elevate the testosterone levels in a seventy-year-old man to those he had at twenty, are you really returning him to "normal"? Crowley says, "I worry that this widespread prescription of testosterone for aging men is going to precipitate an epidemic of prostate cancer."

Of course, it will not be the first time that hormones have been heavily marketed—in advance of the scientific evidence—as a way to recapture youth. In the late sixties, estrogens were touted to women as their chance to be "feminine forever." And initial data from small or uncontrolled studies were encouraging. Estrogen therapy was believed to help sustain sexual health, and mood, while protecting bones from osteoporosis and the heart from arteriosclerosis. The media were flooded with ads for estrogen therapy, and publishers churned out books celebrating its benefits. Nearly 40 percent of postmenopausal women have been prescribed hormone-replacement therapy.

As we now know, conventional H.R.T. not only increases the risk of breast cancer but can lead to heart attacks, strokes, and blood clots. A nationwide trial of sixteen thousand women—part of the Women's Health Initiative—was recently terminated when the therapy was linked to a 26 percent increase in invasive breast cancer and a significant increase in cardiovascular disease as well. A hormone regimen meant to reverse the effects of aging has proved to accelerate serious disease. As Dr. Swerdloff put it, the data trailed clinical practice.

Meanwhile, testosterone-replacement therapy is becoming increasingly popular. Last year alone, sales of transdermal testosterone doubled. An estimated quarter of a million American men are now taking the hormone. If the current rates continue, that number will rise to nearly a million within two years—and, with the newly conferred imprimatur of the Endocrine Society, the rates could surge.

To date, the best published safety data we have on AndroGel as a treatment for andropause comes from a study of sixty-seven men who took the drug for an average of twenty-nine months. An accurate assessment of its effects on the heart, blood vessels, and prostate would require many years of observing many thousands of men—a male counterpart to the Women's Health Initiative. Until then, the attempt to reverse the gradual decline in testosterone levels in aging men can't be considered the treatment of a disorder: it amounts to a vast, uncontrolled experiment, whose consequences remain uncertain. As Hayes says, "It would be a shame to make the same mistakes again."

The Five Sexes, Revisited

Anne Fausto-Sterling

The emerging recognition that people come in bewildering
sexual varieties is testing medical values and social norms.

As Cheryl Chase stepped to the front of the packed meeting room in the Sheraton Boston Hotel, nervous coughs made the tension audible. Chase, an activist for intersexual rights, had been invited to address the May 2000 meeting of the Lawson Wilkins Pediatric Endocrine Society (LWPES), the largest organization in the United States for specialists in children's hormones. Her talk would be the grand finale to a four-hour symposium on the treatment of genital ambiguity in newborns, infants born with a mixture of both male and female anatomy, or genitals that appear to differ from their chromosomal sex. The topic was hardly a novel one to the assembled physicians.

Yet Chase's appearance before the group was remarkable. Three and a half years earlier, the American Academy of Pediatrics had refused her request for a chance to present the patients' viewpoint on the treatment of genital ambiguity, dismissing Chase and her supporters as "zealots." About two dozen intersex people had responded by throwing up a picket line. The Intersex Society of North America (ISNA) even issued a press release: "Hermaphrodites Target Kiddie Docs."

It has done my 1960s street-activist heart good. In the short run, I said to Chase at the time, the picketing would make people angry. But eventually, I assured her, the doors then closed would open. Now, as Chase began to address the physicians at their own convention, that prediction was coming true. Her talk, titled "Sexual Ambiguity: The Patient-Centered Ap-

Anne Fausto-Sterling, "The Five Sexes, Revisited," from *Science*, July/August 2000, 18–23. © 2000 by the New York Academy of Sciences in association with The Gale Group and Look-Smart. Reprinted by permission of the publisher.

proach," was a measured critique of the near universal practice of performing immediate, "corrective" surgery on thousands of infants born each year with ambiguous genitalia. Chase herself lives with the consequences of such surgery. Yet her audience, the very endocrinologists and surgeons Chase was accusing of reacting with "surgery and shame," received her with respect. Even more remarkably, many of the speakers who preceded her at the session had already spoken of the need to scrap current practices in favor of treatments more centered on psychological counseling.

What led to such a dramatic reversal of fortune? Certainly, Chase's talk at the LWPES symposium was a vindication of her persistence in seeking attention for her cause. But her invitation to speak was also a watershed in the evolving discussion about how to treat children with ambiguous genitalia. And that discussion, in turn, is the tip of a biocultural iceberg—the gender iceberg—that continues to rock both medicine and our culture at large.

Chase made her first national appearance in 1993, in these very pages [Science], announcing the formation of ISNA in a letter responding to an essay I had written for The Sciences, titled "The Five Sexes" [March/April 1993]. In that article I argued that the two-sex system embedded in our society is not adequate to encompass the full spectrum of human sexuality. In its place, I suggested a five-sex system. In addition to males and females, I included "herms" (named after true hermaphrodites, people born with both a testis and an ovary); "merms" (male pseudohermaphrodites, who are born with testes and some aspect of female genitalia); and "ferms" (female pseudohermaphrodites, who have ovaries combined with some aspect of male genitalia).

I had intended to be provocative, but I had also written with tongue firmly in cheek. So I was surprised by the extent of the controversy the article unleashed. Right-wing Christians were outraged, and connected my idea of five sexes with the United Nations–sponsored Fourth World Conference on Women, held in Beijing in September 1995. At the same time, the article delighted others who felt constrained by the current sex and gender system.

Clearly, I had struck a nerve. The fact that so many people could get riled up by my proposal to revamp our sex and gender system suggested that change—as well as resistance to it—might be in the offing. Indeed, a lot has changed since 1993, and I like to think that my article was an important stimulus. As if from nowhere, intersexuals are materializing before our very eyes. Like Chase, many have become political organizers, who lobby physicians and politicians to change current treatment practices. But more generally, though perhaps no less provocatively, the boundaries separating masculine and feminine seem harder than ever to define.

Some find the changes under way deeply disturbing. Others find them liberating.

Who is an intersexual—and how many intersexuals are there? The concept of intersexuality is rooted in the very ideas of male and female. In the idealized, Platonic, biological world, human beings are divided into two kinds: a perfectly dimorphic species. Males have an X and a Y chromosome, testes, a penis, and all of the appropriate internal plumbing for delivering urine and semen to the outside world. They also have well-known secondary sexual characteristics, including a muscular build and facial hair. Women have two X chromosomes, ovaries, all of the internal plumbing to transport urine and ova to the outside world, a system to support pregnancy and fetal development, as well as a variety of recognizable secondary sexual characteristics.

That idealized story papers over many obvious caveats: some women have facial hair, some men have none; some women speak with deep voices, some men veritably squeak. Less well known is the fact that, on close inspection, absolute dimorphism disintegrates even at the level of basic biology. Chromosomes, hormones, the internal sex structures, the gonads, and the external genitalia all vary more than most people realize. Those born outside of the Platonic dimorphic mold are called intersexuals.

In "The Five Sexes" I reported an estimate by a psychologist expert in the treatment of intersexuals, suggesting that some 4% of all live births are intersexual. Then, together with a group of Brown University undergraduates, I set out to conduct the first systematic assessment of the available data on intersexual birthrates. We scoured the medical literature for estimates of the frequency of various categories of intersexuality, from additional chromosomes to mixed gonads, hormones, and genitalia. For some conditions we could find only anecdotal evidence; for most, however, numbers exist. On the basis of that evidence, we calculated that for every 1,000 children born, 17 are intersexual in some form. That number—1.7%—is a ballpark estimate, not a precise count, though we believe it is more accurate than the 4% I reported.

Our figure represents all chromosomal, anatomical, and hormonal exceptions to the dimorphic ideal; the number of intersexuals who might, potentially, be subject to surgery as infants is smaller—probably between 1 in 1,000 and 1 in 2,000 live births. Furthermore, because some populations possess the relevant genes at high frequency, the intersexual birthrate is not uniform throughout the world.

Consider, for instance, the gene for congenital adrenal hyperplasia (CAH). When the CAH gene is inherited from both parents, it leads to a baby with masculinized external genitalia who possesses two X chromosomes and the internal reproductive organs of a potentially fertile woman. The frequency of the gene varies widely around the world: in New Zealand it occurs in only 43 children per million; among the Yupik Eskimo of southwestern Alaska, its frequency is 3,500 per million.

Intersexuality has always been to some extent a matter of definition. And in the past century physicians have been the ones who defined children as intersexual—and provided the remedies. When only the chromosomes are unusual, but the external genitalia and gonads clearly indicate either a male or a female, physicians do not advocate intervention. Indeed, it is not clear what kind of intervention could be advocated in such cases. But the story is quite different when infants are born with mixed genitalia, or with external genitals that seem at odds with the baby's gonads.

Most clinics now specializing in the treatment of intersex babies rely on case-management principles developed in the 1950s by the psychologist John Money and the psychiatrists Joan G. Hampson and John L. Hampson, all of Johns Hopkins University in Baltimore, Maryland. Money believed that gender identity is completely malleable for about 18 months after birth. Thus, he argued, when a treatment team is presented with an infant who has ambiguous genitalia, the team could make a gender assignment solely on the basis of what made the best surgical sense. The physicians could then simply encourage the parents to raise the child according to the surgically assigned gender. Following that course, most physicians maintained, would eliminate psychological distress for both the patient and the parents. Indeed, treatment teams were never to use such words as "intersex" or "hermaphrodite"; instead, they were to tell parents that nature intended the baby to be the boy or the girl that the physicians had determined it was. Through surgery, the physicians were merely completing nature's intention.

Although Money and the Hampsons published detailed case studies of intersex children who they said had adjusted well to their gender assignments, Money thought one case in particular proved his theory. It was a dramatic example, inasmuch as it did not involve intersexuality at all:

one of a pair of identical twin boys lost his penis as a result of a circumcision accident. Money recommended that "John" (as he came to be known in a later case study) be surgically turned into "Joan" and raised as a girl. In time, Joan grew to love wearing dresses and having her hair done. Money proudly proclaimed the sex reassignment a success.

But as recently chronicled by John Colapinto, in his book *As Nature Made Him*, Joan—now known to be an adult male named David Reimer—eventually rejected his female assignment. Even without a functioning penis and testes (which had been removed as part of the reassignment) John/Joan sought masculinizing medication, and married a woman with children (whom he adopted).

Since the full conclusion to the John/Joan story came to light, other individuals who were reassigned as males or females shortly after birth but who later rejected their early assignments have come forward. So, too, have cases in which the reassignment has worked—at least into the subject's mid-20s. But even then the aftermath of the surgery can be problematic. Genital surgery often leaves scars that reduce sexual sensitivity. Chase herself had a complete clitoridectomy, a procedure that is less frequently performed on intersexuals today. But the newer surgeries, which reduce the size of the clitoral shaft, still greatly reduce sensitivity.

The revelation of cases of failed reassignments and the emergence of intersex activism have led an increasing number of pediatric endocrinologists, urologists, and psychologists to reexamine the wisdom of early genital surgery. For example, in a talk that preceded Chase's at the LWPES meeting, the medical ethicist Laurence B. McCullough of the Center for Medical Ethics and Health Policy at Baylor College of Medicine in Houston, Texas, introduced an ethical framework for the treatment of children with ambiguous genitalia. Because sex phenotype (the manifestation of genetically and embryologically determined sexual characteristics) and gender presentation (the sex role projected by the individual in society) are highly variable, McCullough argues, the various forms of intersexuality should be defined as normal. All of them fall within the statistically expected variability of sex and gender. Furthermore, though certain disease states may accompany some forms of intersexuality, and may require medical intervention, intersexual conditions are not themselves diseases.

McCullough also contends that in the process of assigning gender, physicians should minimize what he calls irreversible assignments: taking steps such as the surgical removal or modification of gonads or genitalia that the patient may one day want to have reversed. Finally, McCullough urges physicians to abandon their practice of treating the birth of a child with genital ambiguity as a medical or social emergency. Instead, they should take the time to perform a thorough medical workup and should disclose everything to the parents, including the uncertainties about the final outcome. The treatment mantra, in other words, should be therapy, not surgery.

I believe a new treatment protocol for intersex infants, similar to the one outlined by McCullough, is close at hand. Treatment should combine some basic medical and ethical principles with a practical but less drastic approach to the birth of a mixed-sex child. As a first step, surgery on infants should be performed only to save the child's life or to substantially improve the child's physical well-being. Physicians may assign a sex—male or female—to an intersex infant on the basis of the probability that the child's particular condition will lead to the formation of a particular gender identity. At the same time, though, practitioners ought to be humble enough to recognize that as the child grows, he or she may reject the assignment—and they should be wise enough to listen to what the child has to say. Most important, parents should have access to the full range of information and options available to them.

Sex assignments made shortly after birth are only the beginning of a long journey. Consider, for instance, the life of Max Beck: Born intersexual, Max was surgically assigned as a female and consistently raised as such. Had her medical team followed her into her early 20s, they would have deemed her assignment a success because she was married to a man. (It should be noted that success in gender assignment has traditionally been defined as living in that gender as a heterosexual.) Within a few years, however, Beck had come out as a butch lesbian; now in her mid-30s, Beck has become a man and married his lesbian partner, who (through the miracles of modern reproductive technology) recently gave birth to a girl.

Transsexuals, people who have an emotional gender at odds with their physical sex, once described themselves in terms of dimorphic absolutes—males trapped in female bodies, or vice versa. As such, they sought psychological relief through surgery. Although many still do, some so-called transgendered people today are content to inhabit a more ambiguous zone. A male-to-female transsexual, for instance, may come out as a lesbian. Jane, born a physiological male, is now in her late 30s and living with her wife, whom she married when her name was still John. Jane takes hormones to feminize herself, but they have not yet interfered with her ability to engage in intercourse as a man. In her mind Jane has a lesbian relationship with her wife, though she views their intimate moments as a cross between lesbian and heterosexual sex.

It might seem natural to regard intersexuals and transgendered people as living midway between the poles of male and female. But male and female, masculine and feminine, cannot be parsed as some kind of continuum. Rather, sex and gender are best conceptualized as points in a multidimensional space. For some time, experts on gender development have distinguished between sex at the genetic level and at the cellular level (sex-specific gene expression, X and Y chromosomes); at the hormonal level (in the fetus, during childhood and after puberty); and at the anatomical level (genitals and secondary sexual characteristics). Gender identity presumably emerges from all of those corporeal aspects via some poorly understood interaction with environment and experience. What has become increasingly clear is that one can find levels of masculinity and femininity in almost every possible permutation. A chromosomal, hormonal, and genital male (or female) may emerge with a female (or male) gender identity. Or a chromosomal female with male fetal hormones and masculinized genitalia—but with female pubertal hormones—may develop a female gender identity.

The medical and scientific communities have yet to adopt a language that is capable of describing such diversity. In her book *Hermaphrodites and the Medical Invention of Sex*, the historian and medical ethicist Alice Domurat Dreger of Michigan State University in East Lansing documents the emergence of current medical systems for classifying gender ambiguity. The current usage remains rooted in the Victorian approach to sex. The logical structure of the commonly used terms "true hermaphrodite," "male pseudohermaphrodite," and "female pseudohermaphrodite" indicates that only the so-called true hermaphrodite is a genuine mix of male and female. The others, no matter how confusing their body parts, are really hidden males or females. Because true hermaphrodites are rare—possibly only 1 in 100,000—such a classification system supports the idea that human beings are an absolutely dimorphic species.

At the dawn of the 21st century, when the variability of gender seems so visible, such a position is hard to maintain. And here, too, the old medical consensus has begun to crumble. Last fall the pediatric urologist Ian A. Aaronson of the Medical University of South Carolina in Charleston organized the North American Task Force on Intersexuality (NATFI) to review the clinical responses to genital ambiguity in infants. Key medical associations, such as the American Academy of Pediatrics, have endorsed NATFI. Specialists in surgery, endocrinology, psychology, ethics, psychiatry, genetics, and public health, as well as intersex patient-advocate groups, have joined its ranks.

One of the goals of NATFI is to establish a new sex nomenclature. One proposal under consideration replaces the current system with emotionally neutral terminology that emphasizes developmental processes rather than preconceived gender categories. For example, Type I intersexes develop out of anomalous virilizing influences; Type II result from some interruption of virilization; and in Type III intersexes the gonads themselves may not have developed in the expected fashion.

What is clear is that since 1993, modern society has moved beyond five sexes to a recognition that gender variation is normal and, for some people, an arena for playful exploration. Discussing my "five sexes" proposal in her book *Lessons from the Intersexed*, the psychologist Suzanne J. Kessler of the State University of New York at Purchase drives this point home with great effect: "The limitation with Fausto-Sterling's proposal is that . . . [it] still gives genitals . . . primary signifying status and ignores the fact that in the everyday world gender attributions are made without access to genital inspection. . . . What has primacy in everyday life is the gender that is performed, regardless of the flesh's configuration under the clothes."

I now agree with Kessler's assessment. It would be better for intersexuals and their supporters to turn everyone's focus away from genitals. Instead, as she suggests, one should acknowledge that people come in an even wider assortment of sexual identities and characteristics than mere genitals can distinguish. Some women may have "large clitorises or fused labia," whereas some men may have "small penises or misshapen scrota," as Kessler puts it, "phenotypes with no particular clinical or identity meaning."

As clearheaded as Kessler's program is—and despite the progress made in the 1990s—our society is still far from that ideal. The intersexual or transgendered person who projects a social gender—what Kessler calls "cultural genitals"—that conflicts with his or her physical genitals still may die for the transgression. Hence legal protection for people whose cultural and physical genitals do not match is needed during the current transition to a more gender-diverse world. One easy step would be to eliminate the category of "gender" from official documents, such as driver's licenses and passports. Surely attributes both more visible (such as height, build, and eye color) and less visible (fingerprints and genetic profiles) would be more expedient.

A more far-ranging agenda is presented in the International Bill of Gender Rights, adopted in 1995 at the fourth annual International Conference on Transgender Law and Employment Policy in Houston, Texas. It lists 10 "gender rights," including the right to define one's own gender, the right to change one's physical gender if one so chooses and the right to marry whomever one wishes. The legal bases for such rights are being hammered out in the courts as I write and, most recently, through the establishment, in the state of Vermont, of legal same-sex domestic partnerships. No one could have foreseen such changes in 1993. And the idea that I played some role, however small, in reducing the pressure—from the medical community as well as from society at large—to flatten the diversity of human sexes into two diametrically opposed camps gives me pleasure.

Sometimes people suggest to me, with not a little horror, that I am arguing for a pastel world in which androgyny reigns and men and women are boringly the same. In my vision, however, strong colors coexist with pastels. There are and will continue to be highly masculine people out there; it's just that some of them are women. And some of the most feminine people I know happen to be men.

Case Study: Culture Clash Involving Intersex
David Diamond, Sharon Sytsma, Alice Dreger, and Bruce Wilson

Parents from a Middle Eastern country bring their 13-year-old son to the hospital seeking treatment for a minor abnormality of the penis (hypospadias) and for breast development. The child has had two episodes of bleeding through the penis. The physician determines that the boy had a 46xx karyotype, both a uterus and ovaries, and severe congenital adrenal hyperplasia, which caused the child to virilize in utero. The bleeding was actually menstruation.

The physician tells the parents that a hysterectomy and an oophorectomy are necessary to prevent further bleeding. Also, one of the child's kidneys is not functioning and needs to be removed. The parents ask the pediatric urologist to perform hypospadias surgery, a bilateral mastectomy, hysterectomy, oopherectomy, and nephrectomy. Further, they want them performed all at one time (because they cannot remain in the country very long) and without involving the child in the decision making or informing him of his medical condition or of his potential female reproductive capacity. The child expresses a desire to have the mastectomies performed in order to avoid teasing.

While in the United States 46xx babies with severe masculinization have traditionally been raised as females in order to preserve fertility, there has been a shift to male sex assignment for two reasons: evidence of early androgen imprinting on behavior and identity and a desire to minimize the trauma of surgery on external genitalia. Further, given that for 13 years the child has been reared as a male and that, according to his parents, his behavior has been characteristic of his society's male gender role, he probably could not now develop a female gender identity.

The culture favors males, and the parents assert that they would have difficulty accepting their child if his gender were reassigned. They also indicate that in their society, if he turns out to be homosexual, someone would probably kill him. The physician tells the parents that the child may or may not, regardless of gender identity, develop a homosexual orientation, but that the child is too young to have a reliable opinion of his sexual orientation, especially given his ignorance of his medical condition and his culture's views about homosexuality.

The urologist consults with a psychologist knowledgeable about intersex, and both feel uncomfortable about doing the surgeries without the child's consent. The parents insist that the decision is the father's and that the father knows what is best for the child. Should the urologist comply with their wishes?

Commentary
David Diamond

The dilemma confronting the treating physicians is remarkably difficult under ordinary circumstances. In this situation it is further complicated by cultural differences.

The 13-year-old, pubertal patient is a chromosomal and gonadal female with a male appearance and male gender role. Following a thorough evaluation of his situation, it is apparent that his problems are far more complex than originally anticipated. There appear to be three management options for this boy. The first is to maintain (and enhance) his male appearance by repairing the penile abnormality, performing bilateral mastectomy, and removing all discordant female reproductive organs. Given the patient's age, exogenous male hormones should be started to enhance secondary sexual characteristics. This course of treatment would most closely approximate what the family had in all likelihood anticipated before the diagnosis of congenital adrenal hyperplasia with a 46xx karyotype. The second option is to assign the patient to a female gender role, convert the external genitalia to a female phenotype, and maintain the female reproductive organs. This approach would preserve the patient's fertility, whereas the first would certainly sacrifice it. A third option is to acknowledge that the patient's situation has turned out to be far more complex than anticipated and for the parents to defer treatment until the child can make the decision personally on the preferred management.

The father, assuming the responsibility of decision maker, has selected the first option. In so doing, he has preserved the child's gender role, thereby preserving his established status within the family and within his community. The father thereby rejects the considerable uncertainty of a gender reassignment, with its attendant risks for his child's role within the family and community. While we can appreciate such a risk in our own culture, the extent of the risk for this boy within his own culture is impossible for us to comprehend.

One might argue that the father's decision is supported by a "family-centered model" of autonomous decision making. In this context, a higher priority is placed on harmonious functioning of the family than on autonomy of its individual members. One could imagine that a son's gender reassignment to female might well make it impossible for the family to return to its original community, making the price of such a decision for the family prohibitive.

On the other hand, the son's autonomy is sacrificed by the father's approach. He has been denied an explanation of his diagnosis and a discussion of the alternatives. The extent to which the father's approach is culturally driven is difficult to ascertain. In a previous era, such a secretive and paternalistic approach to intersex disorders was commonplace in this country, and it was justified on the basis of beneficence. However, long-term feedback from many patients has demonstrated that the veil of secrecy heightened anxiety and undermined the physician-patient relationship. Such practices would be regarded as improper today in the context of enlightened American medicine.

So what is the proper posture of the treating urologist? Given the significant cultural divide, the parents' own value system must be the guide. Such an approach would seem to combine the family-centered model of autonomous decision making with a patient's best interest standard of surrogate decision making by the father. As a result, a determination would be made of the net benefits among available options, incorporating quality-of-life criteria for the patient and the family. The urologist must believe that the selected treatment will benefit the child and justify the associated surgical and anesthetic risks. Without such conviction, surgical treatment by the practitioner would be inappropriate.

Commentary
Sharon Sytsma

The doctors in this case face a heart-rending quandary, caught as they are in a culture clash that places their patient in a precarious situation. Acceding to the parents' wishes places the child at greater risk from the multiple surgeries performed, fails to respect the child's autonomy, irreversibly deprives the child of all procreative capacity, and puts the child at significant psychological risk. On the other hand, not performing the surgery means that the child will continue to be taunted and suffer almost certain disenfranchisement and rejection and that he quite possibly will be murdered.

Balancing the advantages against the disadvantages of performing the surgeries would seem to indicate that the physicians should agree to the parents' requests. We now know that those who have been assigned to a certain gender because of intersex conditions usually do not express a desire to change their gender as they mature. Because the child has maintained a firm male identity throughout his childhood and seems to enjoy participating in male pattern behavior, he is even less likely to assume a female gender identity and to resent the loss of his female reproductive capacity. Given the cultural bias toward males, the parental attitudes, and the apparently consistent male gender identity and behavior, the child would probably choose not only the mastectomies and kidney removal, but the other surgeries and treatment as well. Changing the boy is certainly more within our power than changing his culture, and the surgeries will make it easier for him to thrive in that culture.

However, we have learned that withholding information about intersex from children is more likely to be damaging than not. Children who are kept in the dark are made to feel freakish, alone, and fearful that they must be dying. They think of their parents as coconspirators with the doctors, causing a deep feeling of alienation. Children's trust in their parents and in the medical profession is thus often irretrievably lost. The experience of not being unconditionally loved causes lifelong psychological difficulties. Allowing the child to make the decisions to accept the greater risk of the combined surgeries is more respectful of the child's intrinsic worth; and should the child actually come to identify as female and regret the decision, at least he would not experience resentment toward his parents and the doctors. Nevertheless, this child has not been prepared for learning the truth about his condition and could very well be traumatized by it, and trauma increases the risks of any surgery. Because he must leave the country soon, he would not be able to receive sufficient counseling to enable him to recover psychologically.

Insisting that the child participate in the decision might seem to fail to recognize the right of parental autonomy and to display a lack of respect for the values of another culture. The concern is compelling, but problematic. Surely, not all cultural values are worthy of respect. We should not be morally required to set aside our own moral judgments, especially when they are backed by experience, scientific study, and ethical principles. Allowing the values of other cultures to override our own would be appropriate only when those values are morally or epistemically on par or superior to our own. In other cases, doing so would be a matter of moral abdication. A duty to respect the values of another culture cannot consist in simply deferring to those values, but only the duty to try to understand why a culture values what it values, to withhold wholesale condemnation of individuals belonging to that culture for holding such values, to be open-minded to the possibility that the values of another culture may be either equally tenable or morally superior to our own, and to refrain from imposing our own values on a culture whose circumstances are such that doing so would lead to harm.

Clearly, the physicians here face a conflict of duties. Refusal puts the child's well-being in greater jeopardy, but performing the surgeries involves going against what we have come to see as morally required and might lead to more such requests. The physicians should deliberate with the parents and explain the advantages of allowing the child to participate in decisions about his medical treatment. The physicians involved should also attempt to educate our own public—citizens and doctors—about the importance of open communication and informed consent. The importance of full disclosure should be included in pediatric urology textbooks and should be posted on the Internet. Doing so could have the effect of dissuading parents from other cultures seeking surgery for their children without their participation.

Commentary
Alice Dreger and Bruce Wilson

From our own extensive contact with people born with intersex conditions, and from emerging follow-up reports on the care of people with intersex conditions, this is what we know: the gender identities and sexual orientations of children with (or without) intersex conditions cannot be engineered with medicine, nor can they be easily diagnosed or predicted. Surgeries designed to make children with sexual ambiguity look "normal" carry with them substantial uncertainty: they often do not achieve the aim, and they frequently result in lifelong detrimental "side effects," physical and psychological.

We also know that for decades people with intersex conditions have been exempted from the moral rules employed to protect others. A standard practice in medicine has been to actively deceive people with intersex conditions about their diagnoses and medical histories. Many have been subjected to extensive cosmetic genital surgeries while being led to believe that the surgeries were necessary for their physical survival. This unjustified double standard has harmed many people with intersex. More to the point, it is just that—a double standard—where none ought to exist. Just because intersex makes most of us uncomfortable does not mean that people with intersex should be treated with care we would otherwise consider substandard. We therefore begin and end our commentary on this case of intersex with the assertion that people with intersex are entitled to the same decency in health care as others. Even as children, they are entitled to know the truth about what is happening to them, to whatever extent they are capable of understanding, and they are entitled to make critical decisions about their bodies when they are able, particularly when there is no medical urgency.

A fundamental but common mistake has been made in the treatment of this family. The case has been understood primarily as a surgical problem, and the question is, "Should the surgeries be done?" But that is the wrong way to approach intersex. Because intersex poses a multifaceted problem, when a case is uncovered, a team approach should be implemented, with the participation of a pediatric psychiatrist or psychologist and a social worker as the keystone. Ideally, the team would also include an endocrinologist, a surgeon, a geneticist, and a primary care physician.

In the case at hand, a team could help the child and parents explore the data, the risks, and the options—many of which are not presented here because the case has been framed by a surgical mindset. A psychiatrist or psychologist would already have seen the child repeatedly and would be able to advise about his competency to participate in making decisions about the nonurgent surgeries. If the child is not ready to decide whether he wants hypospadias surgery, bilateral mastectomy, hysterectomy, and oopherectomy, then the endocrinologist could prescribe leuprolide, a once-a-month injectable hormone which would essentially stall puberty, halting the menstruation (if that's what the bleeding is), preventing further breast development, and so on. Regardless of which surgeries are done, this patient is going to need regular medical care. The case description implies that, if the surgeries are done, the patient might go on in life "cured," never having been the wiser. But in fact, this patient will need lifelong endocrinological management, regardless of the surgeries. (An oopherectomy will only increase that need.) Now is the time to start enlisting the *knowing* cooperation of this patient in his lifelong medical care.

It is more important to get it right than to be fast. There is no compelling reason to override the right to self-determination of this child, and there are many reasons not to override it. Some might argue that the cultural differences justify following the father's wishes. Nevertheless, we are unsympathetic to the idea that children's sexual anatomies are an acceptable locale for cultural relativism. In 1996, federal legislation was enacted to protect girls from a set of cultural practices known as female genital mutilation, female circumcision, or female genital cutting. The central premise of that legislation was that every minor girl is entitled to legal protection from adults who seek to surgically alter her genitals for social reasons—regardless of her family's cultural background—because, according to the law, "the practice of female genital mutilation often results in the occurrence of physical and psychological health effects that harm the women involved." People with intersex bear the same sorts of risks and deserve the same protections.

In the case before us, if even with sensitive team care the parents refuse to allow the child to be consulted about his condition and treatment, the physicians should refuse to cooperate in the deception and should, if they feel the child's well-being is at serious risk, seek legal help in protecting this child from what might amount to neglect or abuse.

The Meanings of "Race" in the New Genomics: Implications for Health Disparities Research

Sandra Soo-Jin Lee, Joanna Mountain,
and Barbara A. Koenig

The challenge is then to analyze the causes of racism while avoiding the implication that race exists.—Steven Miles, 1993

A foolish consistency is the hobgoblin of little minds, adored by little statesmen and philosophers and divines.—Ralph Waldo Emerson, "Self-Reliance," 1841

Eliminating the well-documented health disparities found within the United States population is a laudable public policy goal. Social justice demands that we understand the sources of health inequality in order to eliminate them. A central dilemma is, to what extent are health disparities the result of unequal distribution of resources, and thus a consequence of varied socioeconomic status (or blatant racism), and to what extent are inequities in health status the result of inherent characteristics of individuals defined as ethnically or racially different? How we conceptualize and talk about race when we ask these questions has profound moral consequences.

Prior to the Human Genome Project (HGP), scientific efforts to understand the nature of biological differences were unsophisticated. The new technologies for genomic analysis will likely transform our thinking about human disease and difference, offering the promise of in-depth studies of disease incidence and its variations across human populations. In her opening remarks at a meeting of the President's Cancer Panel, which focused on health disparities in cancer treatment in the United States, Dr. Karen Antman noted that racial differences in cancer rates have been

Sandra Soo-Jin Lee, Joanna Mountain, and Barbara Koenig, "The Meanings of 'Race' in the New Genomics: Implications for Health Disparities Research," from *Yale Journal of Health Policy, Law and Ethics*, vol. 1, 33–73. © 2001 by Yale Schools of Law, Medicine, Epidemiology and Public Health, and Nursing. Reprinted by permission of the publisher.

reported for decades, "but for the first time, science now has the opportunity to quantify such differences genetically."[1] Will the light refracted through the prism of genomic knowledge illuminate straightforward explanations of disease etiology, offering simple solutions to health inequalities? Or are there consequences, currently hidden in the shadows, that require our attention?

Protesting that their genes are being singled out as "mutant," individuals of Ashkenazi Jewish descent fear being targeted for genetic testing for breast cancer.[2] They ask if targeted testing might not lead ultimately to stigmatization and discrimination. The genetic variation in question, BRCA-1, is believed to be more prevalent among Ashkenazi Jewish women and has resulted in the identification of this population as "high risk." Researchers report that the frequency of BRCA-1 mutations in the general population is 1 in 1,666,[3] compared to 1 in 107[4] among Jewish women of Eastern European origin. No one has a definitive explanation for this higher incidence among Ashkenazi Jewish women, although geneticists hypothesize a "founder's effect." Discord among Jewish groups has become pronounced, as the benefits and risks associated with targeted genetic testing and research are considered. While many scientists of Ashkenazi Jewish descent have supported testing as critical to the prevention and treatment of unsuspecting women who carry the breast cancer gene mutations, others, fearful of the potential harm of stigmatization, have discouraged participation. The issue is further complicated by the fact that breast cancer can be neither definitively cured, even if diagnosed early, nor prevented with certainty, although drastic measures, such as surgical removal of the breasts, are possible.

Increasing ability to detect genetic mutations linked to disease susceptibility has not been paralleled by therapeutic discoveries. This disjuncture has contributed to the conflict about population-based testing and disagreement about the calculus of the largely known risks and benefits to individuals and populations. Knowing one has a BRCA mutation does not mean that one will ultimately develop cancer. Individuals must interpret complex, uncertain information to make sense of their cancer risk, and are often confused as to how to make sense of genetic information. The additional burden of contemplating the ramifications of targeted testing of their community, including the possibility of categorical discrimination and prejudice, is a daunting challenge. The mutations found most commonly among those of Ashkenazi ancestry were identified by chance. Blood stored for other purposes, notably screening for Tay-Sachs, a heritable disease, was available for research. Other mutations in the BRCA-1 and BRCA-2 genes are specific to certain groups, generally isolated populations such as those in Iceland or Finland. How will knowledge that common diseases are associated with socially identifiable populations affect the treatment of those individuals? But more important, how will an increasingly sophisticated knowledge of molecular genetics affect our understanding of the nature of "difference" among human groups?

The discovery of genetic mutations associated with breast cancer has been heralded as one of the initial, and most dramatic successes of the HGP.[5] For the first time a common adult onset disorder was linked with a genetic abnormality. Ironically, this discovery also reveals a potentially dangerous, although unintended, consequence of genomic technology— the association of disease with an identifiable human population, in this instance, Ashkenazi Jews. Unfortunately, the lessons of history provide strong evidence that scientific research on the relationship of "race" to disease may have negative outcomes, in spite of good intentions. Sickle cell anemia provides the best-studied example. Indeed, it was the first "racialized" disease.[6] The association of sickle cell anemia with the black "race" was complete, a one-to-one correspondence; it took decades to recognize that the illness was not a marker of race. Treatment initiatives, in particular mandated screening programs, reflected existing social bias and prejudice.[7] Given the consequences of 20th-century Nazi racial science, individuals of Ashkenazi descent have particular reason to fear the notion that they are somehow biologically distinct. As we discuss in detail below, there is widespread agreement that *Homo sapiens* consists of a single population; that biologically distinct races do not exist. Will the tools of the new genomics, allowing us to map biological variation precisely, reinforce the idea that the human population can be divided into discrete biological entities? What policies might avert this end?

Medicine through a Genomic Prism

Recent announcements celebrating the completion of the full sequencing of the human genome trumpeted the emergence of a "new genomic medicine."[8] Having the full human gene sequence available will quicken the pace of genetic discovery, and many believe it will transform all domains of medicine, including our understanding of the etiology of illness (and the meaning of health), disease prevention, diagnostics, treatment, and the development of targeted drugs, through the emergence of pharmacogenomics.[9] Indeed, for the foreseeable future, our scientific investigations—and basic understanding—of disease and illness will be conducted within a genomic paradigm.

The high-throughput genetic technologies now available, including high-speed sequencing machines and micro-array technologies, allow scientists to correlate specific genetic mutations with disease (or other "traits") much faster than in the past. We believe that the advent of genomic medicine has coincided with the resurrection of a genetic epistemology of difference among human groups that is predicated on the existence of "race," through which populations are conceptualized as having inherent, immutable biological differences. Three social and scientific trends have refocused attention on the meaning and significance of difference at the level of biology.

The first is the U.S. government's health disparities initiative—the national public health goal of eliminating health inequality among racially and ethnically identified populations by the year 2010.[10] The second is the recent announcement of the earlier than anticipated completion of the HGP. The joint public and private effort has produced expectations that gene-sequencing research will lead to important discoveries, such as solutions for diabetes, cancer, and other major diseases. It has also created a paradox. Public announcements of the genome have highlighted the news that human beings from throughout the world share a virtually identical genome; proclamations about the mapping and sequencing of the genome included conspicuous attention to the fact that human beings share 99.9% of their DNA.[11] The cover of *Science*, announcing the completion of the HGP, included an array of human faces of all ages—young and old—and individuals of varying phenotypes: African, Asian, and so on. Hence the paradox. Although the political message of the unity of the human species was highlighted, the third force contributing to the salience of race in genomic medicine is the increasing body of genetic research focused on variation among populations. Although the vast majority of the human population shares the same genes, it is the minute differences between individuals and among groups that researchers focus on as they seek to explain the incidence and severity of disease at the molecular level, through the examination of single nucleotide polymorphisms, or SNPS.

In light of these trends, it is of critical importance to examine the deployment of the race concept in health disparities research as the tools of the new genomic medicine come into widespread use. Increased funding for health-related genomics research, including the creation of new DNA repositories to serve as resources for genetic analyses, presents an opportunity to consider how existing understandings of racial and ethnic difference might shape the trajectory of research and the form of health care policies. We approach the issues from the broad disciplinary perspective of anthropology, including anthropological genetics, cultural anthropology, and medical anthropology.

Interrogating the Concept of "Race"

Why have we enclosed race in "scare quotes"? The power of race, or racial thinking, is derived from the supposition that race is biological and hence, immutable—inextricable from the essential character of individuals. Historically, race has been identified through physiological characteristics such as skull size, skin color, facial features, and other qualities readily available for scrutiny by the passing observer. The first classificatory system dividing human beings into distinct races is credited to French naturalist Georges-Louis Leclerc (comte de Buffon) in 1479.[12] In his *Systema Naturae* (1758), botanist Carolus Linnaeus identified four racial groups: *Americanus rubescus* (American red)—reddish, obstinate, and regulated by custom; *Europaeus albus* (Europeans white)—white, gentle, and governed by law; *Asiaticus luridus* (Asians yellow)—sallow, severe, and ruled by opinion; and *Afer niger* (Africans black)—black, crafty, and governed by caprice.

Linnaeus's classificatory scheme is an amalgam of physical features and behavioral traits that reflect the social attitudes and political relations of the times, although presented in seemingly neutral, scientific terms. These racial distinctions arrange groups in a hierarchical fashion that reflect particular social values. This results in an ideology of race that is used to explain, predict, and control social behavior. Historians point out that the concept of immutable, biologically based human races developed in concert with Western exploration and colonialism, providing a scientific justification for economic exploitation and practices such as slavery.[13] Prior to that time, the idea of distinct human subspecies whose differences were attributed to biology did not exist. The Greek term "barbarian," for example, reflects a hierarchical ranking according to one's closeness to civilization, and particularly to language, not a biologically based scheme.

When considering the relationship of "race" to health, one needs to pay attention to the conceptual underpinnings of race and racial thinking, not simply the terminology used. Other deployments of racial concepts elide social, behavioral, and environmental factors that contribute to the onset of disease. The conceptual problem—conflating biology with group identity—is not solved simply by a change in vocabulary. Emerging historically in response to the anthropological critique of race and racial thinking, the concept of "ethnicity" emphasizes the cultural, socioeconomic, religious, and political qualities of human groups, including language, diet, dress, customs, kinship systems, and historical or territorial identity.[14] In contrast to race, ethnicity has been conceptualized as socially articulated, reflecting common political interests and perspectives of individuals.[15] However, the appropriation of ethnicity in health research often belies this distinction. Ethnicity, as well as "culture," has been used as a surrogate for biological difference in epidemiological and health services research. We argue that this confusion in terminology is potentially dangerous and requires serious attention. How we define difference has moral consequences.

A recent edition of *Webster's Medical Dictionary* defines race as "a division of mankind possessing traits that are transmissible by descent and sufficient to characterize it as a distinct human type."[16] This usage of the term "race" reflects an outmoded concept that attempts to convey biological difference among human population groups as the defining feature of seemingly distinct human subpopulations. The definition is unfortunately characteristic of the careless approach to definition found within much of biomedical discourse and writing. A definition found in a key dictionary of epidemiology reflects a similar bias, defining race as "persons who are relatively homogenous with respect to biological inheritance (see also ethnic group)."[17] By contrast, the fields of physical or biological anthropology and population genetics have long held that the idea that distinct human races exist is scientifically incorrect, as well as harmful.

The widely accepted consensus among evolutionary biologists and genetic anthropologists is that biologically identifiable human races do not exist; *Homo sapiens* constitutes a single species, and has been so since the evolution of humans in Africa and throughout their migration around the world.[18] Population genetics provides the best evidence for this conclusion: the genetic variation within a socially recognized human population is greater than the genetic variation between population groups.

In evolutionary biology the idea of race, although rarely used because of its fundamental ambiguity, is considered a synonym for subspecies. The term "subspecies" refers to a geographically circumscribed, genetically differentiated population. As Alan Templeton describes in a review in the *American Anthropologist*, "Genetic surveys and the analyses of DNA haplotype trees show that human 'races' are not distinct lineages, and that this is not due to recent admixture; human 'races' are not and never were 'pure.' Instead, human evolution has been and is characterized by many locally differentiated populations coexisting at any given time, but with sufficient genetic contact to make all of humanity a single lineage sharing a common evolutionary fate."[19]

Of course this does not mean that human populations long exposed to climatic variation or geographic isolation have not acquired health-related biological differences. Clearly such features exist, generally the result of random events, such as genetic drift or population bottlenecks. The point is that meaningful genetic and biological differences do not always map clearly onto social categories of human difference, whether defined as race, ethnicity, or culture. Population geneticists use the concept of "clinal variation"—which specifies deviation across a geographic gradient—when analyzing meaningful subdivisions of *Homo sapiens.* Sometimes genetically meaningful population differences correlate with social categories of difference; the populations of Iceland and parts of Finland provide examples. However, in a population as diverse as the United States this is often not the case. The political categories of difference used in much health research, for example, "Hispanic," are biologically and genetically meaningless.

Before proceeding, we need to make one point clear. Arguing against the legitimacy of race as a category in biomedical research is not meant to suggest that the social category of race is not real, or that race as a key dimension of stratified societies does not exist. On the contrary, racial divisions have been a defining feature—some would say the defining feature—of U.S. history. Race is socially, not biologically, meaningful; it is "real" because we have acted as if certain people, at certain points in time, were inferior based on innate or "essentialized" characteristics.

Our preferred language when discussing human populations that have been categorized by race is to describe them as "racialized" groups. Although we use words such as "race" and "ethnicity" in this essay, in general we prefer to use race as an adjective ("racialized") rather than a noun ("race"). This terminology allows us to grant legitimacy to the social aspects of race while at the same time calling into question the idea that distinct human races exist. It also recognizes that who is defined as racially and ethnically different changes over time, a point to which we return below.

Terminology matters. We will argue against using race as a biological category in health research. However, we do not deny that health status varies among U.S. racialized populations. Genetic and biological differences should be studied directly, not through the distorting lens of a previous era's racial thinking. There may, however, be one exception in health disparities research: Studies of the health effects of racism per se may be one arena where using traditional political categories of race is justified.[20]

Elimination of Health Disparities as a National Priority

The National Institutes of Health (NIH), following the political leadership of the surgeon general David Satcher, published the nation's blueprint for improved health in *Healthy People 2010*.[21] A main objective of the plan is the elimination of glaring health disparities among segments of the population, particularly those identified as members of minority racial and/ or ethnic groups. The report states that current information about the biological and genetic characteristics of African Americans, Hispanics, American Indians, Alaska Natives, Asians, Native Hawaiians, and Pacific Islanders does not explain the health disparities experienced by these groups compared with the white, non-Hispanic population in the United States. Although *Healthy People 2010* posits that these disparities are the result of complex interactions among genetic variation, environmental factors, and specific health behaviors, nonetheless, the categories of difference used to define the U.S. population are primarily racial categories— as opposed to other measures such as socioeconomic status, environment, or behavior.

Leaving aside for a moment the question of terminology, the statistics included in the report are alarming. Death rates due to heart disease and all cancers are more than 40% and 30% higher, respectively, for African Americans than for whites; for prostate cancer, it is more than double that for whites. African American women have a higher death rate from breast cancer despite having a mammography screening rate that is nearly the same as the rate for women identified as white. Hispanics living in the United States are almost twice as likely to die from diabetes than are non-Hispanic whites. Hispanics also have higher rates of high blood pressure and obesity than non-Hispanic whites. African Americans, American Indians, and Alaska Natives have an infant mortality rate almost double that for whites.

Asians and Pacific Islanders, on average, are reported as being one of the healthiest population groups in the United States. However, when this broad census category is divided into its many subpopulations, disparities for specific groups are quite marked. Women of Vietnamese origin, for example, suffer from cervical cancer at nearly five times the rate of white women. The case of Asian Americans, as with other groups, reflects the multiple terms, such as "race," "ethnicity," and "national origin," used to describe American populations. Although unclear, it appears that Asian and Pacific Islanders are being treated as a single racial group. What remains consistent, however, is a comparison to an implicit category of "whiteness," that while tacitly evoked in each comparison, is left largely undefined. In addition, the nature of the relationship between racialized identity and disease is left unexplained. Categorizing individuals according to race labels, which are then associated with incidence of disease, conflates many complex factors that might contribute to disease in a population.

As with other government agencies, the NIH makes use of the racial classification scheme mandated by the Office of Management and Budget (OMB). This scheme is familiar to most of us because it is used by the U.S. Census Bureau. The passage of the NIH Revitalization Act of 1993 required that NIH-funded research projects include human subjects who are women, as well as members of minority groups.[22] While these regulations were intended to correct the historical exclusion of women and minorities from participation in clinical trials, one unintended effect of the legislation has been the uncritical inclusion of one or two populations—often defined according to census categories unrelated to health outcomes—into a research design without adequate rationale for anticipated differences between populations. Such practices reinforce notions of racial difference and often come at the expense of a more nuanced study of the similarities among groups and the differences within broadly defined racial groups.

A critical review of the use of race is necessary in light of its profound effect on the production of medical knowledge. Statistics describing health differences between whites and racialized populations, such as those published in *Healthy People 2010*, are the result of epidemiological research that focuses on race as a category of inherent distinction. This research, in turn, establishes the agenda for progress in improving health status and determines the measures of success in achieving the NIH goals. The racial taxonomy used by epidemiologists impacts directly on the research design of studies examining the biological basis of difference among groups, initiating a trajectory of inquiry that is uncritical of the relationships among racialized groups, genetic characteristics, and environment.

The Mutability of Racial Categories

The taxonomy of race used in health research is primarily political. To understand fully the historical mutability of categories of race, we will discuss the evolution of census categories in the United States. Through comparison with categories used by other nations, the problematic nature of race as a scientific variable becomes evident. The U.S. Census Bureau has collected information on race since the first census in 1790. Historically, the Census Bureau has used widely varying principles and criteria in classifying the population, including national origin, tribal affiliation and membership, and physical characteristics. During the 19th century, African Americans were identified through a calculus based on percentage of African "blood." The term "mulatto" was used to describe an individual born of one black and one white parent. Although it was largely abandoned at the beginning of the 20th century, other terms measuring descent, such as "quadroon" and "octoroon," were used to refer to individuals with one-quarter and one-eighth black ancestry respectively. In the 1920s the United States extended this racial paradigm by instituting the infamous "one-drop rule," by which individuals with even one ancestor of African origin were classified as black. This framework of identifying race focused on lineage and implicitly defined "whiteness" by a standard of genetic "purity," despite physiological markers that may give the appearance of whiteness or blackness. This rule, although no longer embraced officially by the government, reflects a belief in the biological basis for group differences that continues to characterize racial thinking in the United States.

During the 20th century, 26 different schemes were used to categorize racial difference in the U.S. population.[23] Certain groups, such as Jews, who at one time were defined as nonwhite, were "deracialized" later in the century. Since 1977, the federal government has sought to standardize data on race and ethnicity among all of its agencies through the OMB's issuance of the Statistical Policy Directive Number 15, "Race and Ethnic Standards for Federal Statistics and Administrative Reporting." In these

Table 1. U.S. Census Categories, 2000

☐ White	☐ Black, African	☐ American Indian	☐ Asian Indian
☐ Chinese	American or	or Alaska Native	☐ Korean
☐ Vietnamese	Negro	☐ Japanese	☐ Samoan
☐ Other Pacific	☐ Filipino	☐ Gaumanian or	
Islander	☐ Native Hawaiian	Chamorro	
	☐ Other Asian	☐ Some Other Race	

standards, four racial categories were established: American Indian or Alaskan Native, Asian or Pacific Islander, black, and white. In addition, an "ethnicity" category was codified identifying individuals as "Of Hispanic origin" or "Not of Hispanic origin." The OMB guidelines stipulate that Hispanics may be of any racial category, although in practice, many who self-define as Hispanic check "other" when answering the race question, reflecting widespread confusion about the meaning of terms such as race and ethnicity.[24]

In 1997, in preparation for the 2000 census, the OMB revised these racial and ethnic categories, citing that they no longer reflect the diversity of the population. The reconsideration of these categories emerged in large part because of lobbying efforts by various groups seeking to broaden the choices available to respondents. As a result, the category of "Native Hawaiian or Other Pacific Islander" was added to the existing four, as well as the choice of "Some Other Race." In addition, the ethnicity category was modified to "Hispanic or Latino" and "Not Hispanic or Latino." Although testimony presented in public and congressional hearings indicated a strong desire to include the option of "multiracial" among the census categories, the OMB decided against this, but allows respondents to choose more than one of the existing racial categories in identifying themselves.[25] These new standards on racial and ethnic categorization were used in the 2000 Census and are effective immediately for data collection by federal agencies, including the NIH. The categories on the actual census questionnaire included a wide range of different groups that are then collapsed into the five racial groups and two ethnicities. These are given in table 1.

A separate question asks respondents for their ethnicity. The choices are Mexican, Mexican American, or Chicano; Puerto Rican; Cuban; and other. The taxonomy that emerges from this multitiered approach to defining difference is not readily apparent. Recognizing the plurality and diversity among populations identified as Hispanic or Latino, the OMB

Table 2. Canadian Census Categories, 2001

☐ White	☐ Chinese	☐ South Asian (East Indian, Pakistani, Sri Lankan)	☐ Black
☐ Filipino	☐ Latin American		☐ Arab
☐ West Asian (Afghan, Iranian)	☐ Southeast Asian (Cambodian, Indonesian, Laolian, Vietnamese)	☐ Japanese	☐ Aboriginal (North American Indian, Metis, Inuit)
		☐ Korean	

designated these as ethnic or social categories in which groups share common cultural history, practices, and/or beliefs. Quite similarly, the category of Asian American consists of no fewer than 25 different populations of diverse origins. What makes Asian Americans a "race" and Latinos and Hispanics an "ethnic group" is difficult to determine.

The racial categories used by the census reflect terms of group identity that have emerged historically from the shared social and political experience of particular immigrant groups, which in turn have been influenced significantly by the historical immigration policies of the U.S. government. In light of this, the use of a racial taxonomy in the arena of biological research is particularly problematic. The designation of these terms as "racial," and their adoption and use in scientific research sponsored by federal agencies such as the NIH, threatens to reconstitute these groups according to assumptions of biological connections that are not valid.

When the U.S. Census Bureau's racial categories are compared to those employed by other nation-states, the arbitrariness and historical contingency of racial taxonomies becomes evident. Table 2 shows the 2001 Canadian Census Bureau categories. Of note is the fact that Canada does not explicitly highlight the historical concept of race by asking a "race" question; nonetheless, the category seems to be implicit. As a catalog of the "visible minority population" in Canada, these categories reflect a potpourri of terms indicating skin color, nationality, regional and territorial identity, ethnicity, and political sovereignty (as in the category of "aboriginal").[26] As is the case with the U.S. Census, one's identity is not easily determined. How should an individual of Japanese descent who was born in Brazil and carries Brazilian citizenship describe herself? Is she a Latin American or Japanese? Knowing the reasons behind such questions might greatly influence how one "chooses" to identify oneself. The answer may change depending on the purpose of the question, for example:

to determine the immigration rates of specific populations, to calculate the number of foreign residents in a particular district, or to assess the incidence of genetically related disease among a population. Of interest is the fact that the Canadian subgroup known to express a unique array of rare genetic illness (due to a founder effect)—French Canadians in Quebec—is not included. Identification of this group by primary language spoken further complicates the classification dilemma when the social goal is amelioration of health status.

The absence of a universal taxonomy of race is further documented by examining the census categories utilized by the United Kingdom. Whereas "Asian" in the United States includes a broad range of populations with origins throughout the Asian continent, in the United Kingdom the term is limited to those from the Indian subcontinent. In the United States, the categorization of these individuals depends on their historical location. Early in the 20th century, individuals whose origins were South Asian were categorically identified as "Hindu," regardless of whether they actually subscribed to the Hindu religion. This was incongruous for many groups, and the policy changed to classify individuals from the Indian subcontinent as "white," in spite of the large phenotypic variation in skin color dependent on distance from the equator found throughout the world.

More recently, South Asians in the United States were added to the long laundry list of groups that constitute the category of Asian American. Table 3 indicates that, in contrast to the conventional wisdom on race in the United States, Chinese in the United Kingdom are not considered Asian, but rather are combined in a separate racial category with all "other" racial groups. While this categorization scheme may be the result of the small numbers of Chinese and other groups in the United Kingdom, combining all other nonidentified populations with Chinese further reveals the lack of scientific rigor in the classification of race.

In defining systems of classification, Geoffrey C. Bowker and Susan Leigh Star identify three properties.[27] The first is that there are "consistent, unique classificatory principles in operation."[28] The principles establish the rules of order as in, for example, genealogical descent. In the case of racial categorization, it is difficult to identify what rules are operative as they are often varied, inconsistent, and context specific. Physical appearance, geographic origin, language, and birthplace are just a few of the criteria used to determine racial identity. Despite its ubiquity, race

Table 3. United Kingdom Census Categories, 2001

☐ White (British, Irish, Other White)

☐ Black or Black British (Black Carribean, Black African, Other Black)

☐ Mixed (White and Black Caribbean, White and Black African, White and Asian, and Other Mixed)

☐ Chinese or Other Ethnic Group (Chinese, Other Ethnic Groups)

☐ Asian or Asian British (Indian, Pakistani, Bangladeshi, Other Asian)

has yet to be explicitly defined. The second property of a classification system according to Bowker and Star is that the "categories be mutually exclusive."[29] The principles must be sufficiently specific so that entities may not be put in more than one category. The reality of human diversity confounds this second criterion, as the generally disguised presupposition of "racial purity" is fundamental to racial classification. Since *Homo sapiens* consist of a single species, genetic purity is a myth. The exclusionary social functions of race exist in sharp contrast to the porosity of group boundaries, leaving this classification system ill equipped to address the reality of biological difference across the human population, which is continuous, rather than divided into discrete segments. Finally, the third criterion is that a classification system must be complete and able to absorb even those entities not yet identified.

The historical mutability of racial categories—as illustrated by the census bureaus in the United States and abroad—and the inconsistent use of terms in both defining and describing race indicate that a classification system based on race is inevitably historically contingent. The possibility of it ever becoming a rigorous system with scientific utility is questionable. This does not mean that racial categorization is an unimportant factor in studying the cause of health disparities throughout the world. Rather, the ever changing taxonomy of race is a reminder that any research utilizing the concept of race and/or ethnicity must include an interrogation of the economic, political, and cultural factors that inform the struggle over how these categories are defined and used.[30] In the new genomic medicine, the uncritical use of racial and ethnic categories by those interested in biological difference often distorts the relationship between genetics, disease, and group difference.

The Use of Genetic Technology in Ascribing Identity

The promise of genomic medicine is improved health. Perhaps medicines will be developed that target diseases found more frequently in people with a particular ancestry, or genetic epidemiological research carried out with an isolated population will identify a biological marker for schizophrenia. But might there be other consequences of the genomics prism? Will the reductionist paradigm transform, and perhaps "geneticize," our understanding of identity? The rapid production of genetic information through collaborations such as the HGP and the concomitant rise of gene-mapping technologies suggest a need to reexamine current models of human identity. Genetic epidemiological studies often compare populations defined by social categories of racial and ethnic difference. Results indicating significant genetic variation may continue a cycle of reaffirming patterns that are built a priori into the research design. This conundrum, while not unique to genomics research, is further complicated by the current trajectory of studies that attempt to locate race or ethnic identity in the genes. The technically optimistic believe that genetic "evidence" may definitively identify individuals as belonging to certain groups. We remain skeptical of such claims. That categories of race and ethnicity are always historically constructed and context driven suggests a need to carefully consider the consequences of using genetics to define ethnic or racial identity.

DNA Testing: Proof of Native American Ancestry?

The eagerness to use genetic technology and research in determining race and ethnicity has resulted in a renewed faith that genetics will be able to reveal who and what we are. Recently, House Bill 809 was presented to the Vermont legislature by the state representative Fred Maslack, which stipulated that results from genetic testing would be accepted as definitive "proof" of Native American ancestry.[31] The genetic criteria that would be used in making this determination were not explained nor were the potential uses for the genetic test described.[32] While the bill stipulated that this would be offered to individuals on a voluntary basis, one cannot contemplate the deployment of a genetic standard of race without considering the potentially discriminative and prejudicial ways this might be used, setting aside for the moment whether such testing could ever be "accurate" or what accuracy would mean. Given that humans have developed socially meaningful mechanisms for determining group membership, the central question is: Why is genetic testing necessary? If an individual has lived in a Native American community, has adopted the history and cultural practices and beliefs of her tribe, and is embedded in a nexus of social relationships that recognize her as a member, then what does a "negative" genetic test mean for her and perhaps, more importantly, to the group as a whole? By supplanting history and experience with a standard of relatedness measured by genetic similarity, human cultural identity is relegated to a simplistic biological standard.

The Role of Genetics in Defining African American Identity

It would be misleading to claim that the search for identity through genetic testing has only been proposed by those residing outside of the groups in question. Reconstructing genealogy has been of great interest to African Americans seeking to locate their ancestral homelands, lost through the social disruptions of slavery. Genes are gaining increasing attention as an alternate way to reveal connections between contemporary African Americans and current populations in Africa. Recently, a geneticist from Howard University advertised the service of DNA analysis for African Americans who wanted to determine their pre-slavery heritage by locating their point of origin in Africa. Through a Web site entitled *African Ancestry*, Rick Kittles urged African Americans to send in blood samples as a means of examining their "genetic makeup and developing a genetic fingerprint."[33] Although he abandoned his original plan of selling his services to interested individuals for $300 per test because of mounting public and scientific criticism, Kittles's endeavors represent a general embrace of genetics as a medium through which validation of identity may be achieved. Of concern are the potential negative consequences of locating African American identity in the realm of genetics. These concerns are not foregrounded; indeed, they remain unaddressed. This is surprising, given the warnings of scholars like Patricia King, who writes, "In a racist society that incorporates beliefs about the inherent inferiority of African Americans in contrast with the superior status of whites, any attention to the question of differences that may exist is likely to be pursued in a manner that burdens rather than benefits African Americans."[34]

Testing for Race/Ethnicity

Through probabilistic techniques, genetic testing of continental ancestry is technically possible. Other research efforts seek to identify genetic markers that are highly correlated, not only with populations residing in (or with origins from) geographic areas that have been racially categorized, but also with phenotypic features associated with race.[35] A particular trajectory of genetic research is reflected in linkage and association studies that attempt to detect racial and ethnic differences in cases that are physically ambiguous. An example is the effort to determine genetic linkages of individuals of mixed descent. Using statistical procedures, one such study has claimed that 70–90% of ancestry information could be "extracted" even when "admixture" had occurred up to 10 generations before.[36] The implications of this line of research are far reaching. The use of genetic technologies in directly determining race and ethnicity not only redirects identity from the social domain into the physical substrates of the body, but also, more importantly, shifts the power of defining who and what humans are into the arena of biomedicine. Testing for race/ethnicity may be justified as a means of improving the health status of minority populations, for example by targeting disease prevention programs to individuals from certain groups. This approach, however, reinforces the idea that disease results from essential characteristics within the individual.

Genetic Determinism and Reductionism

The powerful tools of molecular discovery, in concert with the promise of molecular medicine, represent a dominant cultural discourse on science and health. An unintended byproduct of the genomics revolution is a näive, almost religious faith in the power of genetics. The gene has become a powerful cultural icon;[37] genetic explanations have a pride of place in the popular imagination. Of course geneticists are well aware that genes act in concert with the environment, and that a full understanding of the genetic component of common illnesses requires sophisticated, multifactoral research. Nonetheless, the paradigm of genetic reductionism may powerfully affect health disparities research by placing undue emphasis on genetics at the expense of other explanatory mechanisms, moving attention—and funding for research—away from features of the social and political environment that lead to ill health.

Alternatives to a reductionist understanding of ethnic or racialized identity allow a different approach to health research. Recent work in the social sciences on race and ethnicity has emphasized notions of "situational ethnicity,"[38] in which identity is dependent on the specific contexts in which individuals find themselves. In addition, the concept of "plastic ethnicity"[39] highlights individual and group agency as opposed to structural inscriptions of identity. The significance of such theories for health disparities research is an understanding that racial and ethnic identities—including health-related beliefs—take on different qualities and cannot be treated as stable entities even within an individual life course. We possess "multiple identities",[40] one's gender, religion, nationality, or age may take on lesser or greater importance at different times and in different places, contributing to a number of cultural identities.

Reductionist research that locates ethnic identity in genetic variation confounds the notion of malleable identity. Such research may lead to the replacement of current concepts of identity by genetically based concepts of the individual and group. If so, identity becomes ascribed by science, with serious implications for how race and ethnicity are conceived. Critical to this process is the "appearance and allure of specificity"[41] of genetics, which makes a shift in the politics of identity more likely."

The Reification of Race in Health Research

Historically, race, genetics, and disease have been inextricably linked, producing a calculus of risk that implicates race with relative health status. Racialized groups have been associated with particular diseases. Sometimes these associations are accurate and sometimes they reflect underlying social prejudice. It is against this backdrop that investigations into health inequalities in the United States play out. Troy Duster, a sociologist who has examined these associations, has identified this process as the "prism of heritability," in which disease is uncritically linked to individuals because of racial assignment and categorically disassociated from other populations.[42] He cautions that race-based etiological theories may become hegemonic, effectively eliminating explanations of illness that take account of environmental or behavior factors associated with social class. Melbourne Tapper has studied this process with respect to the identification and management of sickle cell anemia in colonial Africa.[43] Tapper reveals that the political project of colonialism was further justified by the dominant discourse on race that identified sickle cell anemia as a "black disease" and contributed to a definition of "whiteness" that was predicated on the notion of invulnerability and health. Similarly, in the United States, prejudicial attitudes toward African Americans and immigrants from the Mediterranean region fueled racial rhetoric around sickle cell anemia and thalassemia. In the 20th century, the association of race with disease was utilized by those who were politically opposed to miscegenation and immigration of people from southern Europe.

Given this history, particular caution must be employed when using the race concept in health-related research. Some have argued that the concept should be abandoned, based on the overwhelming scientific evidence that human races do not exist. Others argue for retaining the term "race," but limiting its application to the social, as opposed to the biological, realm. Recently, the American Anthropological Association, the official professional organization of physical, biological, social, and cultural anthropologists and archeologists in the United States, released a statement emphasizing the social and historical construction of race. Reflecting a general consensus among social scientists, physical and biological scientists and other scholars, the statement contended that race could not be considered a valid biological classification:

> The "racial" worldview was invented to assign some groups to perpetual low status, while others were permitted access to privilege, power, and wealth. The tragedy in the U.S. has been that the policies and practices stemming from this worldview succeeded all too well in constructing unequal populations among Europeans, Native Americans, and people of African descent. Given what we know about the capacity of normal humans to achieve and function within any culture, we conclude that present-day inequalities between so-called "racial" groups are not consequences of their biological inheritance but products of historical and contemporary social, economic, educational, and political circumstances.[44]

Despite such proclamations, race continues to be used erroneously, even harmfully, as a scientific variable, particularly in biomedical research designed to explain health behavior. Its use is ubiquitous; from 1910 to 1990, race was used in 64% of articles appearing in the *American Journal of Epidemiology*.[45] One author suggests that historians will find our current terminology to be inherently racist, rather than scientifically useful.[46] A review of biomedical literature claiming links between race and disease reveals that researchers rarely describe their racial and ethnic measurement or classification methods. In a review of articles published in *Health Services Research*, David R. Williams noted, "Terms used for race are seldom defined and race is frequently employed in a routine and uncritical manner to represent ill-defined social and cultural factors."[47] Lack of precision—näively conflating biology and culture—makes it impossible to tease out the causes of health disparities between economically disadvantaged racialized populations and more privileged groups.

The lack of consistency in the use of terminology for concepts of race, ethnicity, ancestry, and culture is manifest in the wide variance in terms used to identify individual and group identities.[48] Terms such as "white," "Caucasian," "Anglo," and "European" are routinely used interchangeably to refer to certain groups; whereas "black," "colored," "Negro," and "African American" are used to refer to comparison groups.[49] And white-black comparisons are straightforward in contrast to the confused use of terms such as "Hispanic" and "Asian." Fundamental ambiguity in the concept of race obscures the role that genetic variation plays in our current understanding of disease. Socially defined notions of race are treated as legitimate biological variables; race itself is often used as a proxy for disease risk. Epidemiological studies employ race as shorthand for social and environmental factors that are associated with particular racialized groups.[50] When treated in this way, race is understood to have some contributory effect to particular conditions and diseases, but in a very imprecise way. For example, a report that black smokers are 10 times more likely to develop *Helicobactor pylori* infection—a cause of duodenal ulcers—than white smokers,[51] treats skin color as an independent variable, and thus circumvents an explicit engagement with the complex interaction of social, environmental, and perhaps biological factors that may have produced the statistically significant findings.

Research utilizing race serves to "naturalize" the boundaries dividing human populations, making it appear that the differences found reflect laws of nature.[52] In fact, the use of race and ethnicity in biomedical research is problematic because it is caught in a tautology, both informed by and reproducing "racialized truths."[53] We assume that racial differences exist, and then proceed to find them.

Race, Smoking, and Nicotine Metabolism

Recent research on smoking and nicotine metabolism illustrates the implications of the reification of the race concept in health research. The use of tobacco is singled out as a leading health indicator in the *Healthy People 2010* vision statement. According to the report, adolescent rates of cigarette smoking have increased in the 1990s among white, African American, and Hispanic high school students after years of declining rates during the 1970s and 1980s. A central goal of the *Healthy People 2010* mission is to decrease the rate of tobacco use through prevention programs and to focus research on treatment programs for existing smokers.

Epidemiological and behavioral research on cigarette smoking has clearly identified sociodemographic variation in smoking rates. "Race" is highlighted as a significant predictor of smoking behavior, yet its exact salience is difficult to tease out. Studies indicate that although a larger proportion of blacks[54] than whites smoke, several differences in tobacco use exist between these groups. Blacks consume fewer cigarettes[55] and begin smoking later in life than whites.[56] Blacks smoke cigarettes higher in tar and nicotine[57] and are specifically targeted by the tobacco industry as potential consumers.[58] Smoking among African Americans has been associated with a higher incidence of lung cancer, cardiovascular disease, low birth weight, and infant mortality.[59]

Research on a genetic basis for differences between African Americans and non-Hispanic European Caucasians has focused on differences in the metabolism of tobacco. The logic of such studies is founded on the notion that racial groups may have distinct genetic characteristics that result in different biochemical processes such as variations in nicotine metabolism.[60] Recently it has been reported that racial and ethnic differences may exist in the serum cotinine levels of cigarette smokers.[61] Levels of cotinine, a metabolite of nicotine, indicate relative exposure to tobacco smoke. In this study, sponsored by the National Center for Chronic Disease Prevention and Health Promotion, non-Hispanic black smokers had significantly higher levels of serum cotinine than either white or Mexican American smokers despite reporting to have smoked the same number of cigarettes a day. The study concluded that these differences may explain why blacks find it harder to quit and are more likely to experience higher rates of lung cancer than white smokers. The authors suggest that biological differences may account for the differential health status of certain groups. Studies like this contribute to a trajectory of research that links race and genetics to disease. However, by assuming a tight link between nicotine metabolism and race, researchers may overlook other biological or environmental mechanisms that could explain the elevated cotinine. They also rule out racism on the part of physicians as an explanation of excess cancer deaths among blacks. A recent study found racial differences in referral for potentially curative surgery among patients diagnosed with early-stage lung cancer associated with smoking.[62]

Research on the relative incidence of disease among racialized groups reflects a paradigm of inquiry that presumes racial differences exist. "Race biology," as described by Gary King, reflects current sociopolitical beliefs, values, and agendas regarding racial differences and is "predisposed to and rewarded for investigating 'inherent differences' rather than commonality."[63] Research findings—such as differences in nicotine metabolism—provide the promise of drug therapies based on presumed genetic differences between racialized groups. Such targeted medicines are a hallmark of the new genomic medicine.

Race and Pharmacogenomics

The emergence of the field of pharmacogenomics is based on the promise of individually tailored drugs; therapeutics will be tailored to the unique genetic makeup of specific populations. Those more likely, or less likely, to respond to a particular medicine, or those likely to have a severe adverse event, will be identified through genomic analysis. Pharmaceutical companies believe that such tests, and the medicines based on them, will be an important feature of health care in the future; intense and highly competitive research is under way.

Pharmacogenomics creates drugs for individuals by matching medicines to patients' personal genetic codes.[64] However, in practice, research targets variation within pre-defined racialized groups, not individuals. According to a recent article in the *Washington Post,* "Race influences which people are genetically predisposed to lack various enzymes needed to break down medications. Without those enzymes, the medication can have either a heightened or lessened effect."[65] In this case, race is identified as the independent variable that explains the necessary presence or absence of a biochemical agent that aids the metabolism of the drug. The use of the word "lack" redirects focus from the limitations of synthetic pharmacopoeia to the biological shortcomings associated with particular racialized groups. Who will be defined as "normal?" Racial thinking, or the belief that race is defined by biological differences between groups of individuals, informs the search for genetically tailored therapeutics intended to compensate for deviations from an unstated standard of genomic normality.

Targeted Population-Based Research and Services:
Avoiding Social Harms

The association of the BRCA-1 mutation with Ashkenazi Jews is merely one of many correlations that have been, and continue to be, drawn between a disease and a racially identified population. The search for genetic variation in concert with categories of race threatens to perpetuate the racialization of disease. Two major strategies for discovering the relationship between human disease and variations in genetic polymorphisms have become standard. The first is a search for polymorphisms through sequencing in which any variation in gene sequences from a reference sequence is by definition identified as a new polymorphism. The second is a population genetics approach in which variation is detected within and between "identified" populations. Biomedical research focused on discovering associations between allelic frequencies and the occurrence of disease produces probability statements. For most common diseases, a particular genotype does not cause a specific disease in the same manner that genes determine blood type. Rather, genes are one factor among many that contribute to illness and are best understood in terms of statistical risk assessment. While genetic testing may be able to determine the presence or absence of genes or gene complexes, it cannot determine whether associated diseases and disorders will result; testing provides a set of probabilities only.

As noted in our discussion of pharmacogenomics research, the use of race in the identification of genomic materials is the critical initial step in the chain of knowledge production that results in correlations between racialized groups and risk of disease. Racial or ethnic labeling of an individual DNA donor by cell repositories and independent researchers may affect the health and welfare not only of that individual but of the group with which that individual has been identified. Correlations that are derived from racial categorization of genomic materials used in research may result in policies regarding targeted genetic screening. Such recommendations have been made for various populations, including Europeans/Caucasians for cystic fibrosis testing, African Americans for sickle cell anemia, and Southeast Asians for beta-thalassemia. A potential benefit of such targeted testing is the early identification of disease—or pregnancy termination, depending on the timing of testing—in individuals who may not have been tested without being identified as belonging to a particular population.

However, the conflation of race with risk of disease has negative implications for both the identified population and for society at large. Public health benefits are not the only outcome. Stigma and discrimination are risks associated with the diagnosis of disease for any individual, particularly if curative measures are not available. While genetic markers are not definitive predictors of the onset of complex, common diseases—as opposed to rare Mendelian single-gene disorders—their value in determining relative risk is important in the delivery of health care. Insurance companies and managed care organizations, in particular, have economic stakes in controlling the potential costs of "high risk" clients.[66] In addition, social prejudice could arise in the identification of correlations between genes and disease. The calculus of risk may result in social consequences for individuals in the anticipation that they will fall ill.[67]

However, harm may extend beyond the individual at risk for a particular disease. When racially identified genetic markers are associated with illness, "race" itself becomes the surrogate risk factor. The potential harms associated with targeted genetic testing befall socially identifiable groups. The categorization of individuals according to race erases the individual specificity of genetic signatures. Associations become interpreted as causative relationships and race emerges as the salient scientific variable in the reporting of research findings.

Consequences are twofold: First, "race" itself becomes a source of stigma. Breast cancer becomes a "Jewish disease," and Jews become associated with high rates of cancer. Second, ideas of genetic reductionism are reinforced. The elision of economic factors such as poverty, employment, and unequal access to resources that are manifested in differences in nutrition, housing, and access to health care are subsumed within a genetics discourse that reifies notions of physiological difference. Ironically, such racial thinking renders the effects of racism on the relative health status of groups of individuals invisible. By pursuing targeted population testing in the shift to a genomic approach to health care, significant nongenetic factors will be left unaddressed. In addition, racially targeted programs may result in the neglect of individuals not identified with "at-risk" populations who may be afflicted with the diseases in question.

Abandoning Race, Recrafting the Language of Difference: Implications for Health Care Research and Policy

We have argued that the way human difference is conceptualized and used in health-disparities research has profound moral consequences—that potential ill effects abound. Yet readers have undoubtedly noticed the seemingly inconsistent use of the term "race" in our analysis. On the one hand, we have highlighted the historical contingency and lack of scientific specificity of the concept. On the other hand, we have made clear that health disparities occur more often among racialized populations. Race does not exist, but racialized groups do, and the effects of this racialization are real. As Emerson noted, "A foolish consistency is the hobgoblin of little minds."[68] It is imperative *not* to think and talk about race in the simplistic, one-dimensional way characteristic of other scientific "variables." Rather, we must use extreme care and caution when invoking categories of difference in biomedicine, moving between concepts depending on the context and the purpose of the research. In health care, we are convinced it is legitimate to use traditional categories of racial difference only when engaged in studies of the pernicious effects of racism itself. When searching for the causes of health inequality, we must carefully tailor our approach to the demands of a specific research question, not simply follow conventional rituals of population stratification. Doing so will not only avoid reinforcing the destructive notion that biological races exist; it will also lead to a fuller understanding of health disparities. Of course this will require change in law and government regulation, as well as the way we think about race.

The Dangers of Genetic Reductionism

The prism of genetic reductionism yields dangers throughout health care. The effects are subtle and not easily remedied by top-down regulatory change. One potent implication of the conflation of genotype with phenotype in the new genomic medicine is a reconceptualization of disease etiology. By adopting a genetics-based explanatory model of illness, genes—rather than symptoms—become the critical way in which illness is identified. This may result in a shift in how disease is defined, which inevitably affects treatment and prevention strategies. Geneticists are engaged in research that links single genes, or more often, gene complexes, to particular diseases and/or conditions. While these genetic characteristics do not, in and of themselves, indicate the inevitability of the onset of illness, they are portrayed as of primary significance in determining one's risk of developing a particular disease. Despite the complex interplay of environmental and genetic factors in the eventual onset of disease, increasing emphasis has been placed on the existence of "genetic markers" for disease. Such genetic reductionism undermines the lived experience of patients while privileging genetic signatures characterized by the presence or absence of "good" and "bad" genes. As a result, health will be measured less by one's condition in the present, and more through a calculus of risk for disease in the future.[69]

From such speculation, new definitions of healthy and unhealthy populations may emerge. Implicit to this new understanding of disease is a shifting boundary between normality and abnormality. Relying on a comparative and relational framework, the standard of health may be based on a human genome that is free of mutation. However, the labeling of genes as dysfunctional is complex and highly contextual, and has often been linked—without justification—to racialized populations. As noted previously, the now classic morality tale of sickle cell trait illustrates this point. The protective effect of the trait for individuals residing in areas where malaria is endemic is clear. In the United States, however, sickle cell trait serves no benefit in protecting against a disease that no longer poses a substantial threat. Rather, its deleterious effects for individuals who carry two copies of the altered gene have transformed a gene that is highly functional in malaria-ridden areas to a dangerous and dysfunctional mutation. The assignment of normality and abnormality is contingent on changing environmental conditions. As one of the first-recognized molecular diseases, sickle cell anemia clearly reveals the racialization of illness. The disease was believed to be confined to a particular racialized group, and race became the salient factor in explaining its etiology; from the outset of scientific and medical investigation it was identified as a "black disease."[70]

Our research paradigms and public policies must work to avoid the racialization of new diseases, with the associated stigmatization of populations. The legacy of mistrust created by the abuse of African American subjects in medical research, symbolized by the Tuskegee syphilis study, serves as an ironic brake on genetics research. Black participants in the large-scale National Health and Nutrition Examination Survey (NHANES) were less likely than whites to allow their blood or other specimens to be stored for future research, regardless of guarantees of anonymity and privacy.[71] Fear of stigmatization overrides confidence in medical progress. The potential benefit of studying gene-environment interaction in human populations with varied ancestry may be lost.

A further consequence of over-reliance on the paradigm of genetic reductionism is the erasure of etiological explanations of critical importance in accounting for health disparities: environment, social structure, poverty, or interactions among complex factors. When disease is "located" within the individual, strategies to ameliorate ill health tend to be similarly focused. The social dimensions of health and disease are ignored, or at best paid lip service only. Resources—both governmental and private—flow to projects that embrace genomics and offer the possibility of products marketed to individuals who are encouraged to take responsibility for their own health. We do not dispute the promise of this scientific approach; rather, we wish to point out how the light cast by genomics leaves alternative explanations of ill health in the shadows.

A final consequence of the genomic prism is the potential "rebiologization" of race as a conceptual category. Throughout the 20th century, scholars, particularly anthropologists, have fought against the "essential" explanations of racial difference inherent in Western thought since the time of Linnaeus. In previous eras fundamental biological difference was assumed but could not be directly assessed through genetic studies. The powerful technologies developed in support of the HGP are transformative, allowing the precise study of difference at the DNA level. We believe that caution is indicated in projects that employ powerful genetic technologies to study social categories of human difference. A possible, although not inevitable, outcome of the popular efforts to "prove" identity or origin through genetic research is that racial difference will once again be located in biology. Even research that focuses on disease etiology, as opposed to ethnic classification, has the potential for harm. It is possible, for example, that genetic research on breast cancer that targets individuals of Ashkenazi descent will have dual consequences: stigmatizing the population through the creation of a new racialized disease, while at the same time contributing to the idea that this population is somehow biologically distinct, that it constitutes a separate "race." We need to consider if alternative approaches to research design might avoid these dilemmas.

Avoiding Racial Classification through
"Individualized" Research and Practice

An alternative to the use of racial categories in health-related genomics research is a disciplined focus on patterns of genetic variation that are not influenced by prior racial categorization of individual research subjects or patients. SNPs research could utilize powerful genomic technologies to identify genetic signatures that are then classified according to similarity or difference, and correlated with health outcomes. In this way, variation at the genetic level might dictate new categories for making meaningful comparisons across human populations based on molecular difference. This relies on the ability to sample and make comparisons within large populations. To achieve this, it is critical that we dispense with a priori racial classifications. Such a shift in methodology saves us from the tautological quandary of searching for differences in places where they are expected, thus reifying the idea of racial difference and ignoring the true range of genetic variation across the human population. In the same way, clinical policies and public health interventions that do not rely on racial or ethnic classification can be developed. Examples include existing newborn-screening programs that are not targeted by socially defined racial categories but examine genetic variation directly. Testing only people who are identified as black for sickle cell disease reinforces the racialization of disease and misses a significant proportion of cases. Given the current climate of research and policy, such strategies will not always be easy to implement. It is difficult to disabuse researchers, pharmaceutical companies, and public health managers of the idea that one must always classify by race.

Refining the Language of Race in Health Care Policy

The intersection of the genomics revolution with the health-disparities initiative provides an opportunity to refine our language. Prompted by the HGP, Joseph Graves Jr., an evolutionary biologist, has called for a "Manhattan Project" on how we use the concept of race in the United States.[72] In fact, journal editors and editorial boards in a number of fields have recognized the need to reexamine the ritualistic use of racial and ethnic classifications in biomedical publications. Holding scientists accountable for their use of racial categories and racialized populations in their research is a promising intervention. Often populations are stratified into racialized groups in a research design without any rationale for why differences might be expected. In response to the lack of precision and potential danger of careless use of concepts such as race and ethnicity, the *British Medical Journal* took an early stand, issuing a statement in 1996.[73] More recently, *Pediatrics* issued guidelines requiring that authors explain why they chose to stratify research samples as they did, rather than rely on formulaic use of racial or ethnic categories.[74] *Nature Genetics* has also issued editorial guidelines, stating that there is no justification to use race as a proxy for genetic variation: "The laudable objective to find means to improve the health conditions for . . . specific populations must not be compromised by the use of race or ethnicity as pseudo-biological variables. *Nature Genetics* will therefore require that authors explain why they make use of particular ethnic groups or populations, and how classification was achieved."[75]

The NIH held a conference in June 2000 called "Higher Levels of Analysis," which developed consensus recommendations including a call for a comprehensive re-examination of how foundational concepts like race, ethnicity, culture, and social class are measured and implemented in biomedical research.[76] In spite of the recognized need, barriers to change are significant. Another irony is that governmental efforts to protect racialized populations from the potentially stigmatizing consequences of genetic research may play into the notion of bounded, biologically distinct groups. Care needs to be taken in how community consultation is carried out or how group consent is implemented.

We have emphasized that it is not enough simply to substitute a more "politically correct term"—such as "ethnicity" or "culture"—and continue to make use of an archaic race concept. The scientific evidence is clear that genetic variation does not neatly map onto socially meaningful groups. What alternatives exist to using the word "race"? When considering the health effects of racism, we prefer the term "racialized" group or population, to emphasize that the concept of race is historically contingent. How we speak is a direct reflection of how we think; the language of race is a nontrivial policy issue. Great care must be taken, particularly in the highly charged domain of human genetics research. In order to avoid the erroneous assumption that human races exist, one policy-making body has made a conscious decision to avoid use of the word "race" when discussing biological difference or genetic variation. Instead, the Secretary's Advisory Committee on Genetic Testing has used the concept of "ethno-cultural groups" when referring to human populations that might be adversely affected by genetic testing.[77]

The Dilemma of Difference

Finally, we recognize that a major challenge to eliminating the careless use of race in health research stems from a disjuncture between the goals of scientific investigation and those of public policy. Good science precludes the naïve use of race. Yet the policy goal of eliminating health disparities among racially and ethnically identified populations significantly influences how health research is designed and conducted. When alternative approaches to a priori racial categorization of human subjects are employed, research results must be reinterpreted in terms of political categories in order to determine progress toward the realization of the public health goal of reducing inequality. If researchers are to be held accountable for their use of race, we must develop policies that allow both scientific and policy goals to be met, using the social and political concept of race, or of racialized groups, only when salient.

Debates about the significance of race in the new genetics are in this way no different from those about public policies like affirmative action. Calling attention to race in order to ameliorate inequality has the unintended effect of perpetuating the social divisions one wishes to eliminate. Legal scholar Martha Minow has called this the "dilemma of difference."[78] Minow asks: When does treating people differently lead to the goal of equal treatment and opportunity, and when does it stigmatize or hinder them when differences are ignored? It is imperative not to conduct research in a way that conveys the idea that biologically distinct human races exist. At the same time, real health inequalities must be remedied; genuine genetic variation across the human population must be better understood. A close examination of the historical practices of racial classification reveals the complexity that has plagued the deployment of race since the concept entered modern discourse. The racialization of human groups, historically linked to the maintenance of rigid, hierarchical boundaries rooted in unequal access to resources and opportunities, stands in direct opposition to the social justice goals of *Healthy People 2010*. The advent of the HGP, and the development of genetic technologies, provide great opportunity for reducing health inequalities. Achieving that goal requires careful attention to the moral significance of "race" in health disparities research.

Notes

The original article has been abridged for this edition.

1   Harold P. Freeman, The Meaning of Race in Science—Considerations for Cancer Research: Concerns of Special Populations in the National Cancer Program, 82 *Cancer* 219, 220 (1998).

2   Patricia Wen, Jews Fear Stigma of Genetic Studies, *Boston Globe*, Aug. 15, 2000, at Fl.

3   D. Ford et al., Estimates of the Gene Frequency of BRCA-1 and Its Contribution to Breast and Ovarian Cancer Incidence, 57 *Am. J. Hum. Genetics* 1457 (1995).

4 Jeffrey P. Struewing et al., The Carrier Frequency of the BRCA1 185delAG Mutation is Approximately 1 Percent in Ashkenazi Jewish Individuals, 11 *Nature Genetics* 198 (1995).

5 Barbara A. Koenig et al., Genetic Testing for BRCA1 and BRCA2: Recommendations of the Stanford Program in Genomics, Ethics, and Society, 7 *J. Women's Health* 531 (1998).

6 Vanessa Northington Gamble, Race and the New Genetics: An Historical Perspective in The Implications of Genetics for Health Professional Education, a conference sponsored by the Josiah Macy, Jr. Foundation, Santa Fe, New Mexico, October 25–28, 1998. New York: Josiah Macy, Jr. Foundation (1999).

7 Troy Duster, *Backdoor to Eugenics* 46–57 (1990).

8 In February 2001, *Nature and Science* published special issues dedicated to genomic research.

9 Francis Collins, Shattuck Lecture—Medical and Societal Consequences of the Human Genome Project, 341 *New Eng. J. Med.* 28 (1999).

10 U.S. Dep't of Health and Human Serv. *Healthy People 2010: Understanding and Improving Health* (2d ed. 2000) [hereafter *Healthy People 2010*].

11 This figure has been widely used in reports announcing the completion of the HGP. See, e.g., Steve Mitchell, Genetics Is Not Behind Minorities' Health Discrepancies, NIH Advisory Council Stresses, *Reuters Health*, Sept. 12, 2000, available at http://www.reuters health.com (last visited May 3, 2001).

12 Gamble, *supra* note 6, at 8.

13 Anton L. Allahar, When Black First Became Worth Less, 34 *Int'l J. Comp. Soc.* 39 (1993).

14 Fredrik Barth, Introduction, in *Ethnic Groups and Boundaries: The Social Organization of Cultural Difference* 9–38 (Fredrik Barth ed., 1969).

15 Edna Bonacich, A Theory of Middleman Minorities, *38 Am. Soc. Rev.* 583 (1973).

16 *Webster's Medical Desk Dictionary* 599 (1986).

17 *A Dictionary of Epidemiology* 110 (John M. Last ed., 2d ed. 1988).

18 Luigi Luca Cavalli-Sforza, Genes, People, and Languages (2000). The nonexistence of biological race has been widely reported in the popular press. See, e.g., Natalie Angier, Do Races Differ? Not Really, Genes Show, *N.Y. Times*, Aug. 22, 2000, at F1; Steve Olson, The Genetic Archeology of Race, 287 *Atlantic Monthly* 69 (2001), at http://www.theatlan tic.com/issues/2001/04/olson.htm (last visited Apr. 21, 2001).

19 Alan R. Templeton, Human Races: A Genetic and Evolutionary Perspective, 100 *Am. Anthropologist* 632 (1998).

20 Thomas Denberg, Studying Health Disparities (Sept. 2000) (unpublished manuscript, on file with authors).

21 *Healthy People 2010*, *supra* note 10.

22 NIH Revitalization Act of 1993. Pub. L. No. 103–43, 107 Stat. 122 (1993).

23 American Anthropological Association, *Response to OMB Directive 15: Race and Ethnic Standards for Federal Statistics and Administrative Reporting*, available at http:// www.aaanet.org/gvt/ombdraft.htm (last visited Apr. 21, 2001).

24 Judith C. Barker, Cultural Diversity: Changing the Context of Medical Practice, 157 *W. J. Med.* 248 (1992).

25 U.S. Census Bureau, *Racial and Ethnic Classifications Used in Census 2000 and Beyond* (Apr. 12, 2000), available at http://www.census.gov/population/www/socdemo/race/ racefactcb.html (last visited Apr. 21, 2001).

26 Canadian Statistics Menu, available at http://www.statcan.ca/english/Pgdb/People/ popula.htm#ori/ (last visited Apr. 24, 2001).

27 Geoffrey C. Bowker & Susan Leigh Star, *Sorting Things Out: Classification and Its Consequences* 10–11 (1999).

28 *Id.*

29 *Id.*

30 Simon M. Dyson, "Race," Ethnicity, and Haemoglobin Disorders, 47 *Soc. Sci. Med.* 121 (1998); *see also* Paul Gilroy, *There Ain't No Black in the Union Jack: The Cultural Politics of Race and Nation* (1987).

31 H. D. 809, 1999–2000 Leg. Sess. (Vt. 2000).

32 Although there are genetic variations found in greater or lessor frequency among Native Americans, most geneticists would agree that no definitive genetic markers of Native-American status exist. However the relative frequency of genetic polymorphisms varies from continent to continent, and in other subpopulations separated by natural or social boundaries. As with the use of DNA analysis in forensics, if one can measure many hundreds or thousands of genetic differences, the accuracy of the technology improves. However, the ultimate accuracy of such an approach depends on the source of the initial reference samples that are selected to define the group. Hence the problem of circularity.

33 Sam Fulwood, His DNA Promise Doesn't Deliver, *L.A. Times*, May 29, 2000, at A12 (African Ancestry Web site is located at http://www.africanancestry.com).

34 Patricia A. King, The Dangers of Difference, *Hastings Center Rep.*, Nov.-Dec. 1992, at 35.

35 Mark D. Shriver et al., Ethnic-Affiliation Estimation by Use of Population-Specific DNA Markers, 60 *Am. J. Hum. Genetics* 957 (1997).

36 Paul M. McKeigue, Mapping Genes That Underlie Ethnic Differences in Disease Risk: Methods for Detecting Linkage in Admixed Populations, by Conditioning on Parental Admixture, 63 *Am. J. Hum. Genetics* 241 (1998).

37 Dorothy Nelkin & M. Susan Lindee, *The DNA Mystique: The Gene as Cultural Icon* (1995).

38 Jonathan Y. Okamura, Situational Ethnicity, 4 *Ethnic & Racial Studies* 452 (1981).

39 David Gillborn, Racism, Identity, and Modernity: Pluralism, Moral Antiracism and Plastic Ethnicity, 5 *Int'l Stud. Soc. Educ.* 3–23 (1995).

40 *Formations of Modernity* (Stuart Hall & Bram Gieben eds., 1992).

41 Peter Conrad, A Mirage of Genes, 21 *Soc. Health & Illness* 228 (1999).

42 Troy Duster, *Backdoor to Eugenics* (1990).

43 Melbourne Tapper, *In the Blood: Sickle Cell Anemia and the Politics of Race* (1999).

44 American Anthropological Association, *Statement on "Race,"* available at http://www.aaanet.org/stmts/racepp.htm (last visited Apr. 21, 2001).

45 Thomas A. LaVeist, Why We Should Continue to Study Race . . . But Do a Better Job: An Essay on Race, Racism, and Health, 6 *Ethnicity & Disease* 21–29 (1996).

46 Raj Bhopal, Is Research into Ethnicity and Health Racist, Unsound, or Important Science?, 314 *Brit. Med. J.* 1751 (1997).

47 David R. Williams, The Concept of Race in Health Services Resarch: 1966 to 1990, 29 *Health Services Res.* 261 (1994).

48 Robert A. Hahn, The State of Federal Health Statistics on Racial and Ethnic Groups, 267 *JAMA* 268 (1992).

49 Peter J. Aspinall, Describing the "White" Ethnic Group and its Composition in Medical

Research, 47 *Soc. Sci. & Med.* 1797 (1998). *See also* Ritchie Witzig, The Medicalization of Race: Scientific Legitimization of a Flawed Social Construct, 125 *Annals Internal Med.* 675 (1996).

50   Richard S. Cooper, A Case Study in the Use of Race and Ethnicity in Public Health Surveillance, 109 *Pub. Health Rep.* 46 (1994). *See also* David R. Williams, Race and Health: Basic Questions, Emerging Directions, 7 *Annals Epidemiology* 322 (1997).

51   Elizabeth T. H. Fontham et al., Determinants of Helicobacter Pylori Infection and Chronic Gastritis, 90 *Am. J. Gastroenterology* 1094, 1096 (1995).

52   David Theo Goldberg, *Racist Culture: Philosophy and the Politics of Meaning* (1993).

53   Nancy Leys Stepan & Sander L. Gilman, Appropriating the Idioms of Science: The Rejection of Scientific Racism, in *The "Racial" Economy of Science: Toward a Democratic Future* 170 (Sandra Harding ed., 1993).

54   The terms "blacks" and "whites" are borrowed from the terminology used in the studies cited.

55   Thomas E. Novotny et al., Smoking by Blacks and Whites: Socioeconomic and Demographic Differences, 78 *Am. J. Pub. Health* 1187 (1988).

56   Sandra W. Headen et al., Are the Correlates of Cigarette Smoking Initiation Different for Black and White Adolescents?, 81 *Am. J. Pub. Health* 854 (1991).

57   Karl E. Bauman & Susan E. Ennett, Tobacco Use by Black and White Adolescents: The Validity of Self-Reports, 84 *Am. J. Pub. Health* 394 (1994).

58   Paul Cotton, Tobacco Foes Attack Ads That Target Women, Minorities, Teens, and the Poor, 264 *JAMA* 1505 (1990).

59   Randall E. Harris et al., Race and Sex Differences in Lung Cancer Risk Associated with Cigarette Smoking, 22 *Int'l J. Epidemiology* 592 (1993).

60   Lynne E. Wagenknecht et al., Racial Differences in Serum Cotinine Levels among Smokers in the Coronary Artery Risk Development in (Young) Adults Study, 80 *Am. J. Pub. Health* 1053 (1990).

61   Ralph S. Caraballo et al., Racial and Ethnic Differences in Serum Cotinine Levels of Cigarette Smokers: Third National Health and Nutrition Examination Survey, 1988–1991, 280 *JAMA* 135 (1998).

62   Peter B. Bach et al., Racial Differences in the Treatment of Early-Stage Lung Cancer, 341 *New Eng. J. Med.* 1198 (1999).

63   Gary King, The "Race" Concept in Smoking: A Review of the Research on African Americans, 45 *Soc. Sci. & Med.* 1075, 1079 (1997).

64   M.T. Zühlsdorf, Relevance of Pheno and Genotyping in Clinical Drug Development, 36 *Int'l J. Clinical Pharmacology & Therapeutics* 607 (1998).

65   Rick Weiss, The Promise of Prescriptions: "Pharmacogenomics" Also Raises Issues of Race, Privacy, *Wash. Post*, June 24, 2000, at A1.

66   Karen H. Rothenberg, Genetic Information and Health Insurance: State Legislative Approaches, 23 *J.L. Med. & Ethics* 312 (1995).

67   Barbara A. Koenig & Heather Silverberg, Understanding Probabilistic Risk in Predisposition Genetic Testing for Alzheimer Disease, 3 *Genetic Testing* 55 (1999); Nancy Press et al., Collective Fear, Individualized Risk: The Social and Cultural Context of Genetic Screening for Breast Cancer, 7 *Nursing Ethics* 237 (2000).

68   Ralph Waldo Emerson, *Self-Reliance* (Gene Dekovic ed., 2d ed. Illuminations Press 1983) (1841).

69   Deborah Lupton, *The Imperative of Health: Public Health and the Regulated Body* (1995);
     Alan R. Peterson & Deborah Lupton, *The New Public Health: Health and Self in the Age
     of Risk* (1996).

70   Melbourne Tapper, Interrogating Bodies: Medico-Racial Knowledge, Politics and the Study
     of a Disease, 37 *Comp. Stud. Soc'y & Hist.* 76 (1995).

71   Todd Zwillich, African Americans Reluctant to Allow Genetic Testing, *Reuters Health*,
     Jan. 17, 2001, available at http://www.reutershealth.com (last visited May 3, 2001).

72   *See* the *Secretary's Advisory Committee on Genetic Testing*, available at http://www4.od.
     nih.gov/oba/sacgt/highlights/sacgt1025-2699.htm (last visited May 2, 2001).

73   Editorial, Ethnicity, Race and Culture: Guidelines for Research, Audit, and Publication,
     312 *Brit. Med. J.* 1094 (1996).

74   American Academy of Pediatrics: Committee on Pediatric Research, Race/Ethnicity, Gen-
     der, Socioeconomic Status—Research Exploring Their Effects on Child Health: A Subject
     Review, 105 *Pediatrics* 1349 (2000).

75   Editorial, Census, Race and Science, 24 *Nature Genetics* 97 (2000).

76   The draft report summarizing research recommendations from the NIH Office of Behav-
     ioral and Social Science Research (OBSSR)-sponsored conference, *Toward Higher Levels
     of Analysis: Progress and Promise in Research on Social and Cultural Dimensions of
     Health: A Research Agenda*, is available at http://obssr.od.nih.gov/Conf_Wkshp/higher
     level/sociocultural-draft.pdf (last visited May 1, 2001).

77   Coauthor Koenig serves on this committee, which is charged with recommending mecha-
     nisms to improve the oversight of genetic testing in the United States. *See also* the SACGT's
     report to Surgeon General David Satcher, available at http://www4.od.nih.gov/oba/sacgt/
     gtsecondary.pdf (last visited May 2, 2001).

78   Martha Minow, *Making all the Difference: Inclusion, Exclusion, and American Law*
     (1990).

White, European, Western, Caucasian, or What? Inappropriate Labeling in Research on Race, Ethnicity, and Health

Raj Bhopal and Liam Donaldson

Contemporary European and American research on race, ethnicity, and health uses poorly defined labels to describe study populations. The search for accurate terminology remains controversial, for scientific and social reasons,[1-16] as illustrated by discussions of the terms *Hispanic*[3,4] and *Asian*[5] and the changing meaning of ethnicity and race in the United Kingdom[1,10] and the United States.[2,12] Researchers should describe the study populations, define the terms used, and avoid lumping together heterogeneous populations.[3,5-7]

The controversy[2] and scholarly and political debate[12-16] have largely bypassed the label *White*. Words such as *White* and *Caucasian* have been accepted as self-evidently suitable. While, for example, the labels *Hispanic* and *South Asian* are indexed in key textbooks,[10,11] *White* is not. *White* is institutionalized in the censuses of the United States and the United Kingdom and is used freely in compiling statistics,[14] in epidemiology,[10,11] and in clinical medicine.[17]

Racial and ethnic nomenclature in the United States is dominated by the classification of the Office of Management and Budget,[14] which was devised by a subcommittee of the Federal Interagency Committee on Education.[16] It was adopted in 1977 and has been reviewed.[15] Its purpose was to collect data on groups that are discriminated against, primarily for monitoring civil rights.[16] The recent review drew little attention to the category White, although there were requests to include European American, German American, and Arab American categories.[16]

The U.S. census has 10 subcategories for Asians and Pacific Islanders

Raj Bhopal and Liam Donaldson, "White, European, Western, Caucasian, or What? Inappropriate Labeling in Research on Race, Ethnicity, and Health," from *American Journal of Public Health*, vol. 88, 1303–1307. © 1998 by the American Public Health Association. Reprinted by permission of the publisher.

but none for Whites, who accounted for 80% of the population in 1990. The British census is similar. White is effectively a category for everyone left out of specific racial and ethnic groups.[2] Researchers tend to rely on these classifications because of cost and convenience, even though they were devised for a different purpose other than research. As health and social research is an important by-product of statistics on population, this debate is relevant to future discussions on the census.

Gimenez[3] noted the problem of lumping together heterogeneous minority groups under one label but did not consider White groups. Williams et al.[18] also pointed to cultural and health variations within categories (e.g., African Americans, Asian Americans) but not within White populations. Hahn and Stroup[13] criticized the *Atlas of US Cancer among Non-Whites: 1950–1980* for combining data for all non-Whites but not for combining Whites into one group. The *British Medical Journal*'s guidance emphasizes the need to describe the populations studied and to avoid shorthand ethnic and racial labels. Examples are given for minority groups, but not for the majority population. Critical appraisal of the term *White* and similar labels is overdue.

The Term *White* in Medicine and Epidemiology

In the United States the patient's racial/ethnic group is often given in the opening of a case presentation. Caldwell and Popenoe[17] have argued that racial labeling of patients is superficial and misleading and should be abandoned in this context.

Racial labels are common in research on populations. Williams showed that in the journal *Health Services Research*, 55% of papers gave only a Black-White contrast.[19] Words for the latter group included *White, Caucasian, Anglo,* and nationalities of persons (e.g., U.S., British). Jones et al.[20] found these terms for White populations in the *American Journal of Epidemiology*: *White, predominantly White, Anglo, Caucasian.* Ahdieh and Hahn[21] made similar observations on research in the *American Journal of Public Health.*

Journal editors, the guardians of language, might be expected to take the lead in clarifying terms. The International Committee of Medical Journal Editors published its first, perfunctory statement on terminology for research on race and ethnicity in 1997: "The definition and relevance of race and ethnicity are ambiguous. Authors should be particularly careful about using these categories."[22]

In most research on race, ethnicity, and health published in English (which includes most such work in the United States and the United Kingdom), the comparison group has been the majority (White) population.[10,11] In this essay we consider the complex issue in the context of naming the population against which the health of racial and ethnic minority groups is compared. This context prompted our analysis, although the ramifications are clearly much wider. (Whether White populations are the most appropriate ones for comparison in ethnicity and health research is beyond the scope of the essay.)

The Purposes of Race, Ethnicity, and Health Research

The biological concept of race, whereby human populations were divided into subspecies, was dominant from the early 19th century until its decline with the collapse of Nazi racism at the end of the Second World War. In retrospect, the biological concept of race was ill-defined, poorly understood, and invalid,[23,24] and the science based on it needed sharper scientific criticism.[24]

The concept of ethnicity is slowly replacing the concept of race.[10,11] While race and ethnicity are separate, overlapping concepts,[10,25] they are often used synonymously. For example, in their examination of systemic lupus erythematosus by race, Hopkinson et al.[26] used census data on populations by *ethnic* group, and recent textbooks use both *race* and *ethnicity*, either in the title[10,11] or in the text,[27] without distinguishing the ideas. The points in this essay apply to both race and ethnicity.

The overriding *perceived* benefit of race, ethnicity, and health research is a better understanding of the causes of disease, particularly the relative contributions of genetic and environmental factors.[10,11,25,27,28] (Differences postulated to be due to genetic factors should, however, be demonstrated to be so by genetic studies.) Such research is also part of surveillance that helps develop a scientific basis for policy, as in the United Kingdom[29,30] and the United States.[31,32]

Studies have shown multiple differences between racial and ethnic groups in the pattern of disease and culture, which researchers and policy makers have emphasized as important to effective health service delivery. Studies have also drawn attention to communication barriers and racist attitudes. Ethnicity and health research has, therefore, a scientific purpose of elucidating the causes of diseases and the interplay between cultural factors and health, and a practical purpose of ensuring that services and policies are appropriate. While the terminology and concepts used ought to be purpose driven, in practice this does not happen, particularly with the word *White*. Despite criticism of the historical[23,24] and current[33-37] concepts and methods underpinning race, ethnicity, and health research, such work is increasing.

The Role of the Comparison Population

Ethnicity and health research, or at least the principles derived from such research must bridge geographic boundaries and time periods to be scientifically useful. The scientific paradigm, strong in epidemiology, is to seek understanding through comparison. The comparison population eases, but does not solve, the problem of interpreting disease variation between racial and ethnic groups in different places and times. For example, it is difficult to compare coronary heart disease rates in "South Asian" populations across the world because of differences in disease diagnosis and recording. Observations that in many countries rates have been higher among "South Asians" than among the local comparison population have made some interpretation possible.[38] Comparison populations also help researchers interpret changes in disease trends and assess whether the health of minority groups deviates from expectations. Finally, in the context of access to and quality of health care, the comparison population permits assessment of inequities by ethnic or racial group.

Terms

Table 1 summarizes the qualities of most of the terms for nonminority populations in race, ethnicity, and health research in the United States and the United Kingdom.[1,2,8,10-12,16-21] The dictionary-derived meanings shown in the table come mainly from the *Shorter Oxford English Dictionary*.

The term *White* has long served social, political, and everyday life and is embedded in scientific language.[10,11,14-21] The U.S. Constitution institutionalized racial categories by allocating to slaves (Black or mulatto), for the purpose of political representation, the value of three-fifths of a free person and by giving no such value to "Indians not taxed."[39] The categories of *free person, slave,* and *Indians not taxed* were rapidly replaced by the preexisting color-based social classification of White, Black, and Red.[39] The categories *White* and *Black* remain key descriptors of American society today[14,16,39] and are the basis of administrative statistics. The

Table 1. Analysis of Terms Currently in Use to Describe Nonminority Populations

Term	Dictionary-Derived Meaning	Strengths	Weaknesses	Comments and Recommendations
White	Applied to those races (chiefly European or of European extraction) characterized by light complexion.	Used in censuses. Socially recognized and historically lasting concept. Antithesis of the term *Black*.	Used to describe heterogeneous populations. Unrelated to ethnicity. Geographic links are historical rather than contemporary.	Misnomer. In practice refers to people of European origin with pale complexions. Abandon in scientific writing.
Caucasian	Indo-European; Blumenbach's (1800) term for the White race of mankind, which he derived from the Caucasus	Some relation to genetic composition. Defines populations by geographic origin in the distant past.	Used to describe heterogeneous populations. No contemporary geographic link. Unrelated to ethnicity.	Means originating in the Caucasus region and refers to Indo-Europeans. Widely misunderstood. Widely used a synonym for *White*. Abandon.
Occidental	Native or inhabitant of the Occident (West).	Geographically based.	Used to describe heterogeneous populations. Unrelated to ethnicity.	Means belonging to the West (occident is where the sun sets). Abandon.
Western	Of or pertaining to the Western or European countries or races, as distinguished from the Eastern or Oriental.	Refers to a culture and place.	Not geographically specific. Used to describe heterogeneous populations.	Abandon.
European	A native of Europe.	Signifies geographic origin. Purports to describe a culture (though some would dispute its validity).	Used to describe heterogeneous populations. Ancestral origins may be difficult to ascertain.	Comparable in breadth to terms such as *Chinese, South Asian*. Useful for international studies comparing large areas.

Term	Definition	Advantages	Disadvantages	Comments
Europid	Not defined but clearly connotes origins in Europe.	Clear geographic status. New term, no past associations.	Used to describe heterogeneous populations. Ancestral origins may be difficult to ascertain.	Unfamiliar term. Comparable in breadth to terms such as *Chinese, South Asian.* Useful for international studies comparing large areas.
General population	Not defined but epidemiological meaning is everyone in population being studied.	Makes no assumptions about racial/ethnic origin. Truly a whole population.	Inaccurate unless it is a truly representative population.	Excellent term for representative population samples.
Indigenous	Native or belonging naturally to a place. Pertaining to natives, aborigines.	Links to land and birthplace.	Imprecise. Conflates concepts of place of birth, place of residence, and ancestry.	Some in the nonminority groups are not indigenous; some in the minority groups are. Abandon.
Native	One born in a place. One belonging to a non-European and imperfectly civilized or savage race.	Links to land and birthplace.	Historical connotations of being non-European. Conflates concepts of place of birth, place of residence, and ancestry.	Similar to, and used synonymously with, *indigenous.* Abandon except in historical treatises.
Majority	Greater number or part.	Does not presume ethnicity.	Extremely broad and imprecise.	Avoid if possible.
Non-Asian, non-Chinese, etc.	Not defined but implies those not belonging to the group under study.	Logically correct.	Extremely broad and imprecise.	Avoid if possible.
Reference, control, comparison	The standard against which a population being studied can be compared. In science, a standard of comparison used to check inferences deduced from an experiment, by application of the "method of difference." To place together so as to note the similarities and differences of.	Neutral terms Recognize purpose of the nonminority group in the research. Forces writer to describe population and clarify terminology of study or review.	Nature of the reference or control population is not self-evident. Could be misunderstood to mean closer matching than is actually carried out.	Preferred

term *Black* has been debated and changed in everyday and official language, but the term *White* has not. The use of the term *White* in the British 1991 census question on ethnicity has legitimized its use in British epidemiology.

The U.S. Office of Management and Budget's Directive 15 defines a White person as a person having origins in any of the original peoples of Europe, North Africa, or the Middle East.[14] Until recently, persons from India were considered White in the U.S. census,[2] and Middle Eastern people still are. In Britain, Middle Eastern and North African people would not be considered White, and Asian Indians have never been considered so.

The term *White* includes persons of Scottish, New Zealander, Greek, Spanish, English, Canadian, Welsh, Irish, and—in the United States—Iranian and Moroccan descent and has little value in gauging ethnicity or race. It encourages the division of society by skin color, reinforcing racial stereotyping, and hides a remarkable heterogeneity of cultures. In a study carried out in London,[40] of 39 White patients, 7 were Greek or Turkish Cypriot, 5 were Irish, and 9 were of non-British European origin.

The term *Caucasian* categorizes populations on the ill-defined basis of a common origin in the distant past in the Caucasus region of Central Europe. Most populations originating in India, Pakistan, and Bangladesh, for example, are Caucasian. Except as an erroneous euphemism for referring to persons of European descent, the word has little value in race, ethnicity, and health research. Freedman's[8] plea that this term be rejected by science should be accepted.

The words *Occidental* and *Western* have similar meanings and are geographic concepts (meaning belonging to the West). The heterogeneity of such populations is also so great that the words have little value in research. *Occidental* and its opposite, *Oriental* (belonging to the East), are out of vogue. *Western* is commonly used, but with the global spread of "western" populations and cultures its value is being undermined.

European has a geographic meaning and a more general one. In international research comparing, say, World Health Organization health statistics from different regions, *European* has a specific meaning. In practice, the term refers to people of European ancestral origin (e.g., studies in America may refer to persons of European stock) rather than nationality or residence.

Freedman argues the merits of the unfamiliar term *Europid*. It denotes a geographic base, has no alternative meanings, is self-evident, and is a single word. These facts do not resolve the heterogeneity issue: a study from Aberdeen and one from Athens could both use the words *European* and *Europid* to describe the local population. The only attraction of *Europid* is that it would require users to pause and question the label.

General population is a good description if a population is truly representative of that under study, as in the work of Ecob and Williams.[41] In their research the minority population was compared with the whole community (including minorities), an unusual strategy that dilutes variations between groups. The terms *indigenous* and *native* have no exact definitions and have pejorative associations. It is difficult to judge when an individual or population becomes indigenous or native. Terms such as *majority population* and *non-(minority) population* (for example, *non-Asian*) are as broad as the terms above but permit fewer assumptions about the racial/ethnic composition of the population. These terms can be interpreted as referring to the White population.

The terms *reference, control,* and *comparison populations* are grounded in scientific method and lead to no assumptions about race and ethnicity and so mandate a description of the population by the authors, as recommended in recent guidelines to authors.[6,7] They invite the question, What is the composition of the comparison population? They also focus thought on the need to compare like with like and hence on the purposes of research on ethnicity and race. We recommend the use of these terms, provided they are not taken to imply normality, and suggest that *comparison population* be the preferred term.

Conclusion: Toward Guiding Principles

In recent years researchers have followed administrative categories for race and ethnicity, even when these are acknowledged as having no scientific or anthropological validity (see references 14 and 15). This unsatisfactory state of affairs can be remedied only if scientists use the most specific term suitable to the purpose and context of the study and avoid pejorative words. Careful description of the characteristics of each population studied to make clear the basis of racial or ethnic classification (e.g., ancestry, geographic origin, birthplace, language, religion, migration history) is an essential starting point.

In comparative work including a group from the majority population, terms such as *reference, control,* or *comparison population* have advantages compared with terms such as *White* or *European*. They raise fewer expectations and prior assumptions and require the writer to provide detail on the populations studied, including their heterogeneity and origins. Editors and reviewers will find it easier to spot a lack of such information if these terms are used. *Comparison population* avoids the implication of a standard or norm associated with the terms *control* and *reference*; therefore we suggest that this be the preferred term for a White population used for comparison.

This approach will not solve the problem of how populations perceive themselves in society, nor is it a solution to the classification problems in the collection of statistics for social and administrative purposes. It should allow scientists to break free from a nomenclature developed for nonscientific purposes and to participate in conceptualizing the basis of the racial and ethnic groupings they use. Given that scientific use of a social category can be interpreted as an endorsement of its validity,[13] avoidance of loose terminology in research might influence everyday language and counter the predominance of color as a means of grouping populations.

There are problems of poverty and excess disease in subgroups of the White population, which cannot be unearthed and tackled by using the label *White*. For example, the Irish-born and Scottish-born residents of England and Wales have recently been shown to have the highest standardized mortality ratios in England and Wales, higher than those of racial and ethnic minorities born in countries of the Caribbean and South Asia.[42] Clearly, there are subgroups within the White community with special needs. The argument that the focus of race and ethnicity statistics should be on those with adverse health outcomes is a sound one. Clearly, it is not only ethnic groups of color who are in this position.

This essay widens debate on the issue of conceptualizing, categorizing, and naming racial and ethnic groups. This debate has been misperceived as an issue mainly for minority groups. This essay has focused on the terminology used for populations in comparative studies of the health of ethnic and racial minority groups, but there are many aspects that need work by other scholars, such as whether there is international understanding and agreement on the meaning of the term *White* and other commonly used labels; whether such agreement is achievable; the comparative health of population subgroups aggregated within the term *White*; developing a valid nomenclature for that population and its subgroups; and demonstrating that data on subgroups of the White population can be successful in improving the health status of worse-off subgroups. Work is also needed to define whether comparisons of the health of minority populations with that of the majority population are an appropriate foundation for ethnicity, race, and health research. We recognize the scope of these tasks. Their achievement is a long-term goal, but discussion needs to start now.

Notes

1 O'Donnell M. Terminology. In: O'Donnell M. ed. *Race and Ethnicity.* New York, NY: Longman; 1991.

2 Wright L. One drop of blood. *The New Yorker.* July 25, 1994:46–55.

3 Gimenez ME. Latino/"Hispanic"—who needs a name? The case against a standardized terminology. *Int J Health Serv.* 1989; 19:557–571.

4 Hayes-Bautista DE, Chapa J. Latino terminology: conceptual bases for standardized terminology. *Am J Public Health.* 1987; 77:61–68.

5 Bhopal RS, Phillimore P, Kohli HS. Inappropriate use of the term "Asian": an obstacle to ethnicity and health research. *J Public Health Med.* 1991; 13:244–246.

6 McKenzie K, Crowcroft NS. Describing race, ethnicity, and culture in medical research. *BMJ.* 1996; 312:1054.

7 Ethnicity, race, and culture: guidelines for research, audit, and publication. *BMJ.* 1996; 312:1094.

8 Freedman BJ. Caucasian. *BMJ.* 1994; 288:696–698.

9 A note on views and terminology from *Share. Share Newsletter.* 1995; no. 10:16.

10 Smaje C. *Health, "Race" and Ethnicity.* London, England: King's Fund; 1995.

11 Polednak AP. *Racial and Ethnic Differences in Disease.* New York, NY: Oxford University Press; 1989.

12 Papers from the CDC-ATSDR Workshop on the Use of Race and Ethnicity in Public Health Surveillance [special section]. *Public Health Rep.* 1994; 109:4–45.

13 Hahn RA, Stroup DF. Race and ethnicity in public health surveillance: criteria for the scientific use of social categories. *Public Health Rep.* 1994; 109:4–12.

14 *Race and Ethnic Standards for Federal Statistics and Administrative Reporting.* Washington, DC: Office of Management and Budget; 1977. Directive No. 15.

15 *Recommendations from the Interagency Committee for the Review of Federal Measurements of Race and Ethnicity.* Washington, DC: Office of Management and Budget; 1997.

16 Evinger S. How shall we measure our nation's diversity? *Chance* 1995; 8:7–14.

17 Caldwell SH, Popenoe R. Perceptions and misperceptions of skin color. *Ann Intern Med.* 1995; 122:614–617.

18 Williams DR, Lavizzo-Mourey R, Warren RC. The concept of race and health status in America. *Public Health Rep.* 1994; 109:26–41.

19 Williams DR. The concept of race in *Health Services Research:* 1966 to 1990. *Health Serv Res.* 1994; 29:261–274.

20 Jones CP, LaVeist TA, Lillie-Blanton M. "Race" in the epidemiologic literature: an examination of the *American Journal of Epidemiology,* 1921–1990. *Am J Epidemiol.* 1991; 134:1079–1084.

21 Ahdieh L, Hahn RA. Use of the terms "race," "ethnicity," and "national origins": a review of articles in the *American Journal of Public Health,* 1980–1989. *Ethn Health* 1996; 1:95–98.

22   International Committee of Medical Journal Editors. Uniform requirements for manuscripts submitted to biomedical journals. *Ann Intern Med.* 1997; 126:36–47.

23   Kuper L, ed. *Race, Science and Society.* London, England: Allen & Unwin; 1975.

24   Barkan E. *The Retreat of Scientific Racism.* London, England: Cambridge University Press; 1992.

25   Senior PA, Bhopal RS. Ethnicity as a variable in epidemiological research. *BMJ.* 1994; 309:327–330.

26   Hopkinson ND, Doherty M, Powell RJ. Clinical features and race-specific incidence/prevalence rates of systemic lupus erythematosus in a geographically complete cohort of patients. *Ann Rheum Dis.* 1994; 53:675–680.

27   Cruikshank JK, Beevers DG. *Ethnic Factors in Health and Disease.* Oxford, England: Butterworth-Heinemann; 1989.

28   Marmot MG, Adelstein AM, Bulusu L. *Immigrant Mortality in England and Wales 1970–78.* London, England: Her Majesty's Stationery Office; 1984.

29   Balarajan R, Raleigh VS. *Ethnicity and Health in England.* London, England: Her Majesty's Stationery Office; 1995.

30   *On the State of Public Health 1991.* London, England: Her Majesty's Stationery Office; 1992.

31   *Report of the Secretary's Task Force on Black and Minority Health.* Washington, DC: US Dept of Health and Human Services; 1985.

32   Centers for Disease Control and Prevention. *Chronic Disease in Minority Populations.* Atlanta, GA: Centers for Disease Control and Prevention; 1994.

33   Osborne NG, Feit MD. The use of race in medical research. *JAMA* 1992; 267:275–279.

34   Sheldon TA, Parker H. Race and ethnicity in health research. *J Public Health Med.* 1992; 14:104–110.

35   Witzig R. The medicalization of race: scientific legitimization of a flawed social construct. *Ann Intern Med.* 1996; 125:675–679.

36   Cooper R. A note on the biological concept of race and its application in epidemiological research. *Am Heart J.* 1984; 108:715–723.

37   Bhopal RS. Is research on ethnicity and health racist, unsound, or important science? *BMJ.* 1997; 314:1751–1756.

38   McKeigue PM, Miller GJ, Marmot MG. Coronary heart disease in South Asians overseas: a review. *J Clin Epidemiol.* 1989; 42:597–609.

39   Anderson M, Fienberg SE. Black, white, and shades of gray (and brown and yellow). *Chance* 1995; 8:15–18.

40   King M, Coker E, Leavey G, Hoare A, Johnson-Sabine E. Incidence of psychotic illness in London: comparison of ethnic groups. *BMJ.* 1994; 309:1115–1119.

41   Ecob R, Williams R. Sampling Asian minorities to assess health and welfare. *J Epidemiol Community Health* 1991; 45:93–101.

42   Wild S, McKeigue P. Cross sectional analysis of mortality by country of birth in England and Wales, 1970–92. *BMJ.* 1997; 314:705–710.

Racial Profiling in Medical Research
Robert S. Schwartz

Two articles in this issue of the *Journal* deal with the treatment of heart failure in white and black patients. One, concerning carvedilol, reports that the benefit of this beta-blocker is similar in nonblacks and blacks with chronic heart failure.[1] The other contends that enalapril, an angiotensin-converting enzyme inhibitor, is more effective in whites than in blacks with left ventricular dysfunction.[2] The authors of both articles refer to "race," "racial groups," "racial differences," and "ethnic background" but offer no plausible biologic justification for making such distinctions. In a nod to the quandary faced by anyone who tries to explain the complex therapeutic effect of a drug along racial lines, the authors of the enalapril study acknowledge "the difficulty in ascertaining whether racial differences in outcomes are attributable to race or to other factors" and concede that "racial categorization [may be] only a surrogate marker for genetic or other factors." I maintain that attributing differences in a biologic end point to race is not only imprecise but also of no proven value in treating an individual patient.

Race is a social construct, not a scientific classification. In a 1999 position paper, the American Anthropological Association stated the following: "It has become clear that human populations are not unambiguous, clearly demarcated, biologically distinct groups. . . . Throughout history whenever different groups have come into contact, they have interbred. The continued sharing of genetic materials has maintained humankind as a single species. . . . Any attempt to establish lines of division among biological populations is both arbitrary and subjective."[3]

Racial identification does have importance in the formulation of just and impartial public policies. However, recently released data from the 2000 U.S. Census show that even self-identification of race can be problematic. Following the decision by the Office of Management and Budget to allow multiple responses to a question on racial identification in the 2000 Census, almost 7 million people identified themselves as members of more than one race; about 800,000 respondents said they were both white and black.[4] This degree of multiracial identification underscores the heterogeneity of the U.S. population and the futility of using race as a biologic marker.

It is indisputable that social perceptions of what a person is or is not influence the availability, delivery, and outcome of medical care. It is incontrovertible that these perceptions apply with dismaying regularity to black people and other minorities in the United States. And it is undeniable that lifestyle, socioeconomic status, and personal beliefs are powerful influences on health. But these are matters of morality and culture, and we must clearly distinguish them from the biologic aspects of race-based medicine—from the danger of attributing a therapeutic failure to the patient's "race" instead of looking for the real reason.

Sadly, the idea of race remains ingrained in clinical medicine.[5] On ward rounds, it is routine to refer to a patient as "black," "white," or "Hispanic," yet these vague epithets lack medical relevance. A racial designation in the context of medical management not only defies everything we have learned from biology, genetics, and history but also opens the door to inequities in medical care. Recently, the possibility of marketing drugs with the aim of promoting their use in particular races has emerged.[6] But since "race" is biologically meaningless, how will a physician know whether a given patient (who may identify with two races) has the combination of alleles that will ensure the efficacy of the drug? And what effect will racial profiling in the choice of therapy have on the bond of trust between patients and physicians?

Beyond the bedside, race-based medical research is widespread. The pseudoscience of race is well represented in clinical investigations. In March 2001, under the search term "Negroid race," Medline contained 13,592 citations, of which 1,301 appeared in 1999 or 2000. Among these studies are race-based investigations of lipid metabolism, renal function, responses to vasodilators, sexual maturation, drug metabolism, neurodegenerative diseases, and even Dupuytren's contracture. Such research mistakenly assumes an inherent biologic difference between black-skinned and white-skinned people. It falls into error by attributing a complex physiological or clinical phenomenon to arbitrary aspects of external appearance. It is implausible that the few genes that account for such outward characteristics[7] could be meaningfully linked to multigenic diseases such as diabetes mellitus or to the intricacies of the therapeutic effect of a drug.

Some geographically or culturally isolated populations can properly be studied for genetic influences on physiological phenomena or diseases. The Pima Indians, who have unusual susceptibility to non-insulin-dependent diabetes mellitus,[8] and the people of Gambia, in whom polymorphisms in the NRAMPI gene influence susceptibility to tuberculosis,[9] are examples. But even these cases are complex, since nongenetic factors also influence the outcome. Among these many factors is culture: for instance, the germ-line BRCAI mutations that render Ashkenazi women susceptible to breast cancer[10] owe their prevalence in that population to the fact that for countless generations, Jews have married Jews.

After 400 years of social disruption, geographic dispersion, and genetic intermingling, there are no alleles that define the black people of North America as a unique population or race. Nevertheless, the prevalence of certain alleles does vary among populations. In some cases, these variant genes originated as mutations that proved advantageous under particular environmental conditions. In central and western Africa, for example, several independent mutations in the ß-globin gene gave rise to different sickle hemoglobins, each with a distinct geographic distribution and phenotype. These mutations spread through the population because they protect against malaria; they were dispersed in Greece, Saudi Arabia, Turkey, Iran, and elsewhere by migration and slavery.

Similar forces account for the different frequencies of certain blood-group alleles: they reflect geographic origins, not race. For all these reasons, hemoglobin S, susceptibility to breast cancer, blood type, skin color, and other manifestations of allelic variation do not define race in a biologically valid manner. This is not to deny that the frequencies of certain allelic variants or mutant genes among people who share a geographic origin or culture have medical value. Obviously, a screening program to detect sickle hemoglobin should focus on populations of African descent, and screening for Tay-Sachs disease in New York should be confined to Ashkenazi Jews.

The publication of the first draft of the sequence of the human genome[7,11] should force an end to medical research that is arbitrarily based on race. The Human Genome Project now gives us the power to uncover the true origins of genetic variations; linking them to race has become passé. And instead of using polymorphisms to seek racial distinctions, we can spark real progress in clinical research by using genetic variations to track down clinically relevant alleles and pathogenic mutations. In another editorial in this issue of the *Journal*, Wood discusses allelic variations that may influence drug metabolism and the responses to treatment with certain drugs.[12]

Education is also essential. Instruction in medical genetics should emphasize the fallacy of race as a scientific concept and the dangers inherent in practicing race-based medicine. Physicians everywhere must teach the immorality of racial discrimination in clinical practice. As for medical research, any investigation that entails so-called racial distinctions, whether a clinical trial or a laboratory study, should begin with a plausible, clearly defined, and testable hypothesis. Before studying a possible relation between skin color and sodium excretion, for instance, investigators should have a credible reason for believing that such a link could exist and a plan for finding the relevant genetic network. Research to root out social injustice in medical practice needs continued support, but tax-supported trolling of data bases to find racial distinctions in human biology must end.

Nature Genetics now obliges authors to "explain why they make use of particular ethnic groups or populations, and how classification was achieved."[13] The requirement to furnish a scientifically valid definition of the population under study should be adopted by all biomedical journals. It will be difficult to abandon long-held preconceptions, but perhaps the first benefit of the Human Genome Project will be to lead us to the understanding that in medicine, there is only one race—the human race.

Notes

1 Yancy CW, Fowler MB, Colucci WS, et al. Race and the response to adrenergic blockade with carvedilol in patients with chronic heart failure. *N Engl J Med* 2001;344:1358–1365.

2 Exner DV, Dries DL, Domanski MJ, Cohn JN. Lesser response to angiotensin-converting-enzyme inhibitor therapy in black as compared with white patients with left ventricular dysfunction. *N Engl J Med* 2001;344:1351–1357.

3 AAA statement on race. *Am Anthropol* 1998;100:712–3.

4 Schmitt E. For 7 million people in census, one race category isn't enough. *New York Times*. March 13, 2001:1.

5 Witzig R. The medicalization of race: scientific legitimization of a flawed social construct. *Ann Intern Med* 1996;125:675–679.

6 Rosenberg R. Firm to test heart drug for blacks: NitroMed hopes for major impact on high-risk population. *Boston Globe*. March 10, 2001:F1.

7 Venter JC, Adams MD, Myers EW, et al. The sequence of the human genome. *Science* 2001;291:1304–1351.

8 Knowler WC, Saad MF, Pettitt DJ, Nelson RG, Bennett PH. Determinants of diabetes mellitus in the Pima Indians. *Diabetes Care* 1993;16:216–227.

9 Bellamy R, Ruwende C, Corrah T, McAdam KPWJ, Whittle HC, Hill AVS. Variations in the NRAMP1 gene and susceptibility to tuberculosis in West Africans. *N Engl J Med* 1998;338:640–644.

10 Rahman N, Stratton MR. The genetics of breast cancer susceptibility. *Annu Rev Genet* 1998;32:95–121.

11 Lander ES, Linton LM, Birren B, et al. Initial sequencing and analysis of the human genome. *Nature* 2001;409:860–921.

12 Wood AJJ. Racial differences in the response to drugs—pointers to genetic differences. *N Engl J Med* 2001;344:1394–1396.

13 Census, race, and science. *Nat Genet* 2000;24:97–98.

I Am a Racially Profiling Doctor
Sally L. Satel

In practicing medicine, I am not colorblind. I always take note of my patient's race. So do many of my colleagues. We do it because certain diseases and treatment responses cluster by ethnicity. Recognizing these patterns can help us diagnose disease more efficiently and prescribe medications more effectively. When it comes to practicing medicine, stereotyping often works.

But to a growing number of critics, this statement is viewed as a shocking admission of prejudice. After all, shouldn't all patients be treated equally, regardless of the color of their skin? The controversy came to a boil last May in the *New England Journal of Medicine*. The journal published a study revealing that enalapril, a standard treatment for chronic heart failure, was less helpful to blacks than to whites. Researchers found that significantly more black patients treated with enalapril ended up hospitalized. A companion study examined carvedilol, a beta-blocker; the results indicated that the drug was equally beneficial to both races. These clinically important studies were accompanied, however, by an essay titled "Racial Profiling in Medical Research." Robert S. Schwartz, a deputy editor at the journal, wrote that prescribing medication by taking race into account was a form of "race-based medicine" that was both morally and scientifically wrong. "Race is not only imprecise but also of no proven value in treating an individual patient," Schwartz wrote. "Tax-supported trolling . . . to find racial distinctions in human biology must end."

Responding to Schwartz's essay in the *Chronicle of Higher Education*, other doctors voiced their support. "It's not valid science," charged Richard S. Cooper, a hypertension expert at Loyola Medical School. "I challenge any member of our species to show where this kind of analysis has come up with something useful."

But the enalapril researchers were doing something useful. Their study informed thousands of doctors that, when it came to their black patients, one drug was more likely to be effective than another. The study may have saved some lives. What's more useful than that?

Almost every day at the Washington drug clinic where I work as a psychiatrist, race plays a useful diagnostic role. When I prescribe Prozac to a patient who is African American, I start at a lower dose, 5 or 10 milligrams instead of the usual 10–20 milligram dose. I do this in part because clinical experience and pharmacological research show that blacks metabolize antidepressants more slowly than Caucasians and Asians. As a result, levels of the medication can build up and make side effects more likely. To be sure, not every African American is a slow metabolizer of antidepressants; only 40% are. But the risk of provoking side effects like nausea, insomnia, or fuzzy-headedness in a depressed person—someone already terribly demoralized, who may have been reluctant to take medication in the first place—is to worsen the patient's distress and increase the chances that he will flush the pills down the toilet. So I start all black patients with a lower dose, then take it from there.

In my drug treatment clinic, where almost all of the patients use heroin by injection, a substantial number of them have hepatitis C, an infectious blood-borne virus that now accounts for 40% of all chronic liver disease. The standard treatment for active hepatitis C is an antiviral drug combination of alpha interferon and ribavirin. But for some as yet undiscovered reason, African Americans do not respond as well as whites to this regimen. In white patients, the double therapy reduces the amount of virus in the blood by over 90% after six months of treatment. In blacks, the reduction is only 50%. As a result, my black patients with hepatitis C must be given a considerably less reassuring prognosis than my white patients.

Without a doubt, there are many medical situations in which race is irrelevant. In an operation to repair a broken leg, for example, a patient's race doesn't matter. But there are countless situations in which the race factor should be considered. My colleague Ronald W. Dworkin, an anesthesiologist in a Baltimore-area hospital, takes race into account when performing one of his most important activities: intubation, the placement of a breathing tube down a patient's windpipe. During intubation, he says, black patients tend to salivate heavily, which can cause airway complications. As a precautionary measure, Dworkin gives many of his black patients a drying agent. "Not every black person fits this observation," he concedes, "but there is sufficient empirical evidence to make every anesthesiologist keep this danger in the back of his or her mind." The day I spoke with him, Dworkin attended a hysterectomy in a middle-aged Asian woman. "Asians tend to have a greater sensitivity to narcotics," he says, "so we always start with lower doses. They run the risk of apnea"—the cessation of breathing—"if we do not."

Could doctors make a diagnosis for and treat a patient properly if they did not know his race? "Most of the time," says Jerome P. Kassirer, a professor of medicine at Yale and Tufts. "But knowing that detail early on helps me make educated guesses more efficiently."

Kassirer, the former editor of the *New England Journal of Medicine,* is a renowned diagnostician. He is legendary among trainees for what he can tell about a case from just a few facts. He gave an example from a recent morning report, the daily session in which young doctors describe to senior physicians the most vexing cases admitted to the hospital the previous night. During one report, the resident began: "The patient is a 45-year-old Asian male who came to the emergency room complaining of 'feeling weak and wobbly in my legs' after drinking two bottles of beer." Kassirer stopped her right there. "Here's what I infer from that information," he said. "First, we know that sudden weakness can be caused by a low concentration of potassium in the blood, and we know that Asian males have an unusual propensity for a rare condition in which low potassium causes temporary paralysis. We know that these paralytic attacks are sometimes brought on by alcohol."

Of course, the patient could have been suffering from some other muscular or neurological disease, and Kassirer instructed the trainees to consider those as well. But in this case the patient's potassium was low, and the diagnosis was correct—and confirmed within 24 hours by simply observing the patient. Thanks to racial profiling, the Asian patient was spared an uncomfortable and costly work-up—not to mention the worry that he might have something like Lou Gehrig's disease.

"Rather than casting our net broadly, doctors quickly focus on a problem by recognizing patterns that have clinical significance," Kassirer says. "Typically, the clinician generates an initial hypothesis merely from a patient's age, sex, appearance, presenting complaints—and race."

All of these examples fly in the face of what we are increasingly told about race and biology: namely, that the two have nothing to do with each other. When the preliminary sequence of the human genome was announced in June 2000, many felt the verdict was conclusive. Race, it was said, was an arbitrary, nefarious biological fiction. Scholars heralded the finding of the Human Genome Project that 99.9% of the human genetic complement is the same in everyone, regardless of race, as proof that race is biologically meaningless. Some prominent scientists said the same. J. Craig Venter, the geneticist whose company played a key role in mapping the human genome, proclaimed, "There is no basis in the genetic code for race."

What does it really mean, though, to say that 99.9% of our content is the same? In practical terms it means that the DNA of any two people will differ in one out of every 1,000 nucleotides, the building blocks of individual genes. With more than 3 billion nucleotides in the human genome, about three million nucleotides will differ among individuals. This is hardly a small change; after all, mutation of a single one can cause the gene within which it is embedded to produce an altered protein or enzyme. It may seem counterintuitive, but the 0.1% of human genetic variation is a medically meaningful fact.

Not surprisingly, many human genetic variations tend to cluster by racial groups—that is, by people whose ancestors came from a particular geographic region. Skin color itself is not what is at issue—it's the evolutionary history indicated by skin color. In Africa, for example, the genetic variant for sickle cell anemia cropped up at some point in the gene pool and was passed on to descendants; as a result, the disease is more common among blacks than whites. Similarly, Caucasians are far more likely to carry the gene mutations that cause multiple sclerosis and cystic fibrosis.

Admittedly, race is a rough marker. A black American may have dark skin—but her genes may well be a complex mix of ancestors from West Africa, Europe, and Asia. No serious scientist, in fact, believes that genetically pure populations exist. Yet an imprecise clue is better than no clue at all.

Jay N. Cohn, a professor of medicine at the University of Minnesota, explains that skin color and other physical features can be a diagnostic surrogate for the genetic differences that influence disease and response to treatment. "Physical appearance, including skin color, is now the only way to distinguish populations for study," he says. "You'd have to use a blindfold to keep a physician from paying attention to obvious differences that may and should influence diagnosis and treatment!" Lonnie Fuller, a professor emeritus at Morehouse School of Medicine, says: "Drugs can stay in the body longer when their metabolism in the liver is slower. We know this can vary by race, and doctors should keep it in mind."

Recognizing that our one-size-fits-all approach to medicine has serious flaws, some doctors are urging research into the development of racially targeted drugs. In March 2001, the Food and Drug Administration allowed the testing of a drug called BiDil in about 600 black subjects who will participate in the African-American Heart Failure Trial, the largest clinical trial ever to focus exclusively on African Americans.

In previous studies including both white and black patients, BiDil provided a selective benefit for the black subjects. White subjects did no better on average than those given a placebo. The leading explanation for this disparity revolves around the molecule nitric oxide, a chemical messenger that helps regulate the constriction of blood vessels, an important mechanical dynamic in the control of blood pressure. High blood pressure contributes to and worsens heart failure because it makes the heart pump harder to overcome peripheral resistance in the arteries. BiDil acts by dilating blood vessels and replenishing local stores of nitric oxide. For unexplained reasons, blacks are more likely than whites to have nitric oxide insufficiency.

To be sure, a small percentage of blacks with high blood pressure do not have low nitric oxide activity. And the fact that BiDil's intended use relies on a crude predictor of drug response—"a poor man's clue" is how one scientist described race—is something its developers at the University of Minnesota School of Medicine readily acknowledge. Nevertheless, in the sometimes cloudy world of medicine, a poor man's clue is all you've got. Perhaps that's why members of the Congressional Black Caucus voiced support for the clinical trial. So did the Association of Black Cardiologists, which is helping recruit patients for the trial. B. Waine Kong, the organization's head officer, put it simply: "It is in the name of science that we participate."

Doctors look forward to the day when they can, in good conscience, be colorblind. Researchers predict that it will eventually be common practice for doctors to generate a "genomic profile" of every patient—a precise analysis of a person's genetic makeup—so that decisions about therapies can be based on subtle characteristics of the patient's enzyme and receptor biology. At that point, racial profiling by doctors won't be necessary. Until then, however, group identity at least offers a starting point.

A high level of sensitivity about race is understandable in view of eugenics programs in early 20th-century America and ethnic cleansing abroad. The memory of the Tuskegee syphilis study, in which hundreds of rural blacks were never told they had the disease nor offered penicillin for it, still haunts the U.S. Public Health Service, the agency that conducted the study. Other scholars have expressed the worry that genetic differences among races could become the only explanation for the health disparities among them—allowing interest in examining social and economic factors to dwindle.

Indeed, the public seems to have embraced the idea of colorblind medicine. "In the last decade, many Americans have urged that the concept of race be abandoned, purged from our public discourse, rooted out of medicine and exiled from science," writes Troy Duster, a sociologist at N.Y.U.

But in this case, the public is wrong. As rough a biological classification as race may be, doctors must not be blind to its clinical implications. So much of medicine is a guessing game—and race sometimes provides an invaluable clue. As citizens, we can celebrate our genetic similarity as evidence of our spiritual kinship. As doctors and patients, though, we must realize that it is not in patients' best interests to deny the reality of differences.

PART III

Social Relationships and Sickness

"Where Crowded Humanity Suffers and Sickens": The Banes Family and Their Neighborhood
Laurie K. Abraham

Robert Banes sat on the edge of his hospital bed, cradling his queasy stomach. A thin cotton gown hung on him like a sack. At five feet, eleven inches, Robert weighs only 137 pounds.

Robert's kidneys stopped functioning when he was 27. He received a transplant a year later, but his body rejected the new kidney after six years. Since then he has required dialysis treatments three times a week. Dialysis clears his body of the poisonous impurities that healthy people eliminate by urinating, but the treatments cannot completely restore his health, and Robert periodically spends a couple of days in the hospital. This time, he had been admitted to the University of Illinois Hospital because he had been urinating blood for a week, a problem that did not appear terribly serious to doctors but nonetheless had to be checked.

Feeling nauseated, Robert was not paying much attention to the game show that droned from his television. A nurse came in and stuck a thermometer in his mouth. Earlier in the day, Robert had undergone a cystoscopy, a procedure in which doctors put a miniaturized scope into his bladder to look for the source of his bleeding. He had not been told the results of the test, so he asked the nurse when his doctor would be stopping by. He also wanted to know how much longer he would have to stay in the hospital.

"You may have to go to surgery," the nurse said vaguely, flipping through his chart. A cloud passed briefly over Robert's face; the thought of surgery scared him, though he did not admit that to the nurse. Instead, he changed the subject.

Laurie K. Abraham, " 'Where Crowded Humanity Suffers and Sickens': The Banes Family and Their Neighborhood," from *Mama Might Be Better Off Dead: The Failure of Health Care in America.* © 1993. Reprinted by permission of University of Chicago Press and Laurie K. Abraham.

"I guess I don't get dinner today," he said.

"You didn't get dinner?" she asked, surprised.

"I need some before I get sick."

"Don't do that," the nurse muttered as she walked out the door.

A minute later Robert hurried to the bathroom. "I was probably throwing up because I didn't have no food to push it down," he said, referring to the missed dinner. Robert returned to his bed and lay down, curling his knees into his stomach and pulling a blanket over his shivering body.

Four years before his kidneys failed, Robert was diagnosed with focal glomerulosclerosis, a progressive scarring of the kidneys that eventually destroys them. Focal glomerulosclerosis can be slowed though not cured, but Robert's disease went at its own destructive pace because he did not get medical treatment until his kidneys had reached the point of no return. None of Robert's low-paying, short-term jobs had provided health insurance, and he could not wriggle into any of the narrow categories of government-sponsored insurance, which are generally reserved for very poor mothers and children, the elderly, and the permanently disabled. In other words, Robert had not been poor-parent enough, old enough, or sick enough to get care.

The game show gave way to the news and a report about a "summer virus" that was infecting children. Robert frowned. He and his wife, Jackie, have two daughters and a son: eleven-year-old Latrice, four-year-old DeMarest, and one-year-old Brianna. "Don't tell me that," he sighed. That is Robert's typical response to bad news: he prefers to avoid it.

At the moment, however, Robert would not have minded a little bad news about his own condition. Since he had been admitted to the hospital on July 5, he had not been urinating as much blood, which frustrated him and Jackie. They felt he almost had to *prove* to doctors that he was sick.

Through his open door, Robert could see his wife arrive for an early evening visit. At 5 feet, 10 inches, Jackie is only one inch shorter than her husband, but she weighs 20 pounds more than he does. When she smiles, her pretty, heart-shaped face gets full and round, captivating her baby daughter, who pokes at her cheeks and giggles, making Jackie giggle, too.

Jackie was not smiling that day, however. When she is in public, Jackie can look impassive, even defiant, though this vanishes when her curiosity gets the better of her. She walked slowly past the nursing station looking straight ahead, moving almost regally, her muscular thighs curving beneath her slacks. Next to her husband's brittle frame, Jackie stood like an oak.

She pulled up a chair next to the hospital bed, and Robert began to relay the sketchy medical update he had heard from the nurse. Jackie listened silently; then she responded in the way she sometimes does when she feels overwhelmed.

"I'm going away for a while," Jackie said coolly. "What are you all going to do without me?"

Robert did not reply. He knew, as she did, that she wasn't going anywhere; she was just letting off steam. Today had been her day to pay the bills, which she does in person since they are usually past due, and she had ridden the bus for hours in 90-degree heat.

Jackie told her husband to call home and tell Latrice to take some drumsticks out of the freezer for dinner. Jackie's invalid grandmother, with whom the family lives in one of Chicago's poorest neighborhoods, answered the phone, so Robert gave her the instructions instead. But a few minutes later Latrice called back because she was not sure her great-grandmother had heard the message correctly. In the way other children might memorize their parents' work numbers, Latrice had memorized the phone number for the university hospital, as well as for Mount Sinai Hospital Medical Center, where her great-grandmother frequently had been hospitalized. Jackie repeated the dinner instructions and hung up the phone. "I need the bed," she said.

She began to empty the stuffed grocery bag she had carried into the hospital. It contained two new T-shirts, underwear, and socks for Robert, a day-old piece of cake from Brianna's first birthday, which he had missed, a can of Sprite, and a bunch of grapes.

The couple watched part of another game show and talked about a report they had heard about a family found murdered mysteriously on the bottom of a lake. This story came from one of the tabloid news programs, whose bizarre stories the family regularly discusses. Then Jackie called home again to check on the children, who were home with her grandmother. The call was not reassuring: one of them had dropped cake on the rug, the other two had stepped in it, and DeMarest reportedly was taunting his great-grandmother.

"I need you to stay in here over the weekend so I can get things straightened out," Jackie wearily told her husband. When one or the other of her sick family members are hospitalized, Jackie sometimes considers it a chance to regroup, to get things together before she has to start taking care of everyone again.

Before Jackie left, she filled the plastic grocery bag she had emptied earlier. From Robert's belated dinner, she took a wedge of leftover chocolate cake home for DeMarest. She took packets of low-salt French dressing, salt, and sugar that Robert had squirreled away from his meal trays, as well as a roll of medical tape left by a nurse. Jackie carefully folded the foil Brianna's birthday cake had been wrapped in and stashed that in her bag, too.

Then she gave Robert $5.00 to pay for his hospital TV, which cost $3.25 a day. Robert slowly walked Jackie to the elevator, past a dimly lit room where the floor's patients congregated. One of the patients, a man about Robert's age, had earlier informed Robert that he was scheduled for a second transplant the next day. He told Robert that he had rejected his first transplanted kidney because he drank a case of beer in one evening—the kind of story that, true or not, flies back and forth among kidney transplant patients.

"This is my wife, Jackie," Robert said to a middle-aged woman sitting on the edge of the day room, closest to where the couple walked. "Nice to meet you," the woman said. Jackie smiled wanly, heading for the door.

The University of Illinois Hospital is part of what is known as the Illinois Medical Center, a 560-acre area just west of the Loop, Chicago's downtown. The center has the highest concentration of hospital beds in the United States, some 3,000 among its four institutions.[1] In addition to the University of Illinois, there is Cook County Hospital, one of the best-known, last remaining, and, as the ancient edifice continues to crumble, most notorious public hospitals in the country, and Rush-Presbyterian-St. Luke's Medical Center, an institution that caters to those who, unlike Robert and Jackie, are privately insured. The Veterans Administration West Side Medical Center is also located there.

The medical and technological might of the complex contrast dramatically with the area around it. Just past the research buildings and acres of parking lots lie some of the sickest, most medically underserved neighborhoods in the city. Medical wastelands abut abundance in American cities because health care is treated as a commodity available to those who can afford it, rather than a public good, like education. Though public schools invariably are better in prosperous suburbs than in poor city neighborhoods, every state at least provides every child with a school to attend, no matter what her family's income. The country has not even come that far with health care. Medicaid, the state and federal health insurance program intended for the poor, covers less than half of them, and much of the program is left to the states' discretion, so that a southerner, for example, generally has to be poorer to receive Medicaid than a northerner.

Even for those poor who manage to squeeze into Medicaid, the government's commitment to providing health care for them does not approach a commitment to equality. Just as education remains in practice separate and unequal, medical treatment for poor people with Medicaid or even Medicare (the government insurance for the elderly) is, in all but exceptional cases, conducted in a separate, second-rate environment.

The Banes family lives in the shadow of the Illinois Medical Center complex, 25 minutes southwest by way of the number 37 bus, which runs along Ogden Avenue. The street cuts diagonally across the city from the gentrified lakefront neighborhoods just north of the Loop to the bungalow enclaves of white ethnic suburbs that border Chicago on the southwest. Jackie and Robert live in between, on the West Side, the city's newest and poorest ghetto.

The streets were still lit by the late afternoon sun when Jackie climbed onto the bus for her trip home. Settling her bag on her lap, she fretted that doctors were going to release Robert before they figured out what was wrong with him. A person can only get so far with a "green card," she said, using the street name for the cards issued to families covered by Medicaid. "You need Palmer Courtland kind of money to get anywhere," she complained. Palmer Courtland is a self-made millionaire on "All My Children," a soap opera Jackie and Robert watch.

In addition to the hospitals and their services, programs in a clutch of other buildings near Ogden attempt to palliate what are often conditions born of poverty. There is the Illinois State Psychiatric Institute, the West Side Center for Disease Control, the Chicago Lighthouse for the Blind, and a bit further southwest, the Cook County Juvenile Court, which handles crimes by children, and those against them by their parents.

These buildings are strung along the Eisenhower Expressway, which zips from the booming western suburbs into Chicago's downtown, whose dramatic growth in the past two decades has bypassed the West Side. Jackie rarely ventures into the Loop. From her perspective, the eight-lane highway is an escape route for the employees of the various hospitals and social service institutions, for people who do not carry poverty home with them in a plastic bag.

As Ogden turns more sharply to the west, it crosses into Jackie's neighborhood of North Lawndale, a name that carries the same ominous weight in Chicago as the South Bronx or Watts carry nationwide.[2] North Lawndale was the subject of a series in the *Chicago Tribune* in 1985 that examined the lives of the so-called underclass. Many people who work and live in North Lawndale were disturbed by what they thought was a distorted, overly negative picture of their neighborhood; the series' very name, "The American Millstone," is hated because it suggests a neighborhood that is no more than a burden to be cast off.

Jackie had never heard of the *Chicago Tribune* series; she reads the *Chicago Sun-Times,* whose pithy city coverage is preferred by poor Chicago blacks. Yet many of her observations of the neighborhood could have served as grist for the millstone.

"My auntie's building got burnt down," Jackie said matter-of-factly one day, pointing to an empty lot where her Aunt Nancy's apartment building used to stand. "Drug dealers moved in." The narrow lot is two lots away from the stone three-flat where Jackie grew up with her grandmother. The building has survived, though its balcony has disappeared and graffiti circles its porch columns. It is just a half-block away from where the family lives today. Since she was eight, Jackie has only once moved from this block, and that was a short three miles north to live with Robert at his mother's house. Her dreams of a better life are circumscribed by the neighborhood. She talks about getting out, but out means a strip of stone and brick three-flats about four blocks west. "I've always liked it up in that area," she said. "It looks like the middle-class people lives up in there, especially during the summer. All the trees are green and everyone has grass. And the buildings look well kept. You can just tell it's homeowners." Her assessment is accurate—the homes are better tended—but it is hardly out of the neighborhood. The buildings there may be relative castles, but the moat protecting them from the drugs and violence that pervade North Lawndale is narrow enough to step across.

As the bus hissed and groaned up Ogden, it passed Mount Sinai Hospital, which lives the same hand-to-mouth existence as the poor blacks and Hispanics it serves. More than the University of Illinois, Mount Sinai is the Baneses' hospital. It is where Jackie's grandmother, Cora Jackson, had been repeatedly hospitalized because of complications from diabetes that eventually resulted in the amputation of her right leg. It's where Jackie's father was rushed after he suffered a stroke caused by high blood pressure. And on a happier note, it's where Jackie gave birth to Brianna a year ago.

At one time or another, the Baneses and Cora Jackson have sought (and not sought) health care in every way available to the poor. When uninsured—Robert, when his kidneys were deteriorating, and Jackie, when pregnant with Latrice—they delayed care, then went to Cook County Hospital. Later, when Jackie went on welfare, she and the children became eligible for Medicaid.

Meanwhile, some of Mrs. Jackson's medical bills were paid by Medicare, which covers the elderly and disabled, rich and poor alike. Robert also got Medicare but only after his kidneys stopped working. People with renal failure have special status under the program: they are the only group covered on the basis of their diagnosis and regardless of age or disability. Mrs. Jackson had been sporadically eligible for Medicaid, too, which she needed because Medicare does not pay for such important things as medications. Her Medicaid coverage had been fitful because she was enrolled in what is called the "spend-down" program. She qualified for Medicaid only during the months that her medical expenses were so high they forced her income to drop below a "medically needy" level set by the state. Notably, neither Mrs. Jackson, nor anyone else in the family, had ever been covered by private insurance.

Leaving Mount Sinai, the bus cut through Douglas Park, which spreads to the north and south of Ogden. Douglas and two other West Side parks were designed in 1870 as a system of "pleasure grounds" linked together by grand boulevards. Progressive reformers came to envision them as breathing spaces to provide respite from crowded tenements and other urban ills.[3] In its heyday from 1910 until 1930, when North Lawndale was populated by first- and second-generation Jews, bands gave free concerts on weekends, couples paddled rowboats on the lagoon just to the north of Ogden Avenue, and children swam in what was one of the city's first public swimming pools—which, with its baths, was considered as important for public hygiene as it was for recreation.

Except for the players and fans at soccer and baseball games, the park these days is barely dotted with people, a young Hispanic couple walking on a path on the south side of Ogden— the Hispanic side—or several dozen black children splashing in the lagoon to the north—the African American side. Ogden is a dividing line between Hispanics and African Americans in North Lawndale, and the race line holds in the park as firmly as it does anywhere else in the neighborhood.

Though the park's glory has faded, it is the last piece of deliberately open land that Jackie passed on the Ogden bus. The rest of it consisted of a series of vacant lots, some of which run together for a block or more and which residents euphemistically call "prairies." As it was summer, some of the lots were covered with reedy grasses and weeds, frilly Queen Anne's lace, and deep brown stands of dock plant. Others were piled high with refuse—in one case, what looked like enough decaying furniture to fill an office. In another lot, a building had fallen in on itself, likely prey to the brick thieves who complete the destruction started when buildings are abandoned by landlords who can't afford their upkeep, then are stripped of sinks, stoves, and fixtures, and then finally picked apart, brick by brick. In still other lots, large fernlike weeds flourished, creating an urban jungle that suggests what a parish priest in a similar neighborhood in New Jersey called "panther beauty, beauty you don't want to mess with."[4]

As for the brick and stone two-flats, or old three-story apartment buildings still standing, it is often difficult to tell whether they are occupied or not. Rusty steel grates are locked across nearly every door, even those of the ubiquitous churches. Signs are hand painted and peeling, and since plywood is used to cover most street-level windows, even establishments that still do business have a boarded-up look.

Worse yet, dozens of storefronts have been reduced to gaping holes, outlined by shards of glass that form jagged frames for dark rooms of rubble. Only the foolhardy, or a drug addict desperate for a place to get high, would step inside.

The shrouded condition of the neighborhood unnerves Jackie. Even the local drugstore, whose windows are blocked with ugly, prehistoric stone, can seem foreboding. "You used to be able to see *in* the drugstore," Jackie complained. "Shoot, now you wonder if you get in somewhere, are you going to make it out safe?"

At one corner along the bus route, Jackie pointed to a currency exchange where several scraggly men clustered. "That's a hangout for iv-drug users," she observed with disgust, going on to tell about a nearby bar that peddled do-it-yourself packets for free-basing cocaine. Jackie had noticed the drug paraphernalia when she once stopped at the bar to change a dollar bill. "When I saw that, I told the man I'd skip the change," Jackie said proudly, comparing herself to Father George Clements, a local African American priest who mounted a boycott against stores that sold drug-related products.

Currency exchanges, storefront churches, auto parts shops, liquor stores and taverns, hot dog stands, and a beauty shop or two are the only businesses left on Ogden, which used to be one of the city's major commercial streets. The largest establishment in the neighborhood, Lawndale Oldsmobile, closed more than two decades ago. Its windowless, graffitied shell has been a fixture in North Lawndale since Jackie was a child. By the time she and her grandmother moved to Chicago from Tupelo, Mississippi, in the early 1960s, the neighborhood was already in rapid decline. The Eastern European Jews who had settled the area in the early part of the century had virtually vanished by the mid-1950s, replaced by black migrants from the South. Driven by the changing nature of their businesses as well as the deteriorating neighborhood, North Lawndale's major companies fled soon after: Sears Roebuck, International Harvester, and Western Electric either departed or reduced the size of their operations. Today, the bruised and battered buildings along Ogden give sad testimony to North Lawndale's knockout blow: the ravaging riots that followed Martin Luther King Jr.'s assassination in 1968. After that, most remaining middle-class blacks fled.

In 1960, Lawndale's population peaked at 125,000; by 1980, it had plummeted to 62,000; by the end of that decade, it fell to 47,000.[5] Statistics describing the economic status of the people who remain are discouraging: almost one of every two people is on welfare; three of every five potential workers are unemployed;[6] and three of every five families are headed by women,[7] whose earning power is, of course, significantly less than that of two-parent families.

Accompanying this kind of poverty is a shocking level of illness and disability that Jackie and her neighbors merely take for granted. Her husband's kidneys failed before he was 30; her alcoholic father had a stroke because of uncontrolled high blood pressure at 48; her Aunt Nancy, who helped her grandmother raise her, died from kidney failure complicated by cirrhosis when she was 43. Diabetes took her grandmother's leg, and blinded her great-aunt Eldora, who lives down the block.

Chicago's poor neighborhoods have always been its sickest. In 1890, a medical writer graphically described the conditions that were contributing to rampant disease among the city's immigrant industrial workers. "[Their] sole recourse usually is to the tenement where, heaped floor above floor, in a tainted atmosphere, or in low fetid hovels, amidst poverty, hunger and dirt, in foulness, want and crime, crowded humanity suffers, and sickens, and perishes; for the landlord here is also the airlord, the lord of sunlight; lord of all the primary conditions of life and living; and these are doled out for a price, failing which the wretched tenant is turned out to seek a habitation still more miserable."[8]

The diseases that killed in the 19th century lent themselves to such dramatic prose. They were the great epidemics, smallpox, cholera, and typhoid fever. Such bacteria-borne infectious diseases festered because of a water supply periodically tainted by sewage and were easily spread in the crowded living quarters of poor city neighborhoods. With the coming of better sanitation methods, which included reversing the flow of the Chicago River so that the city's sewage would be sent to southern Illinois and Missouri rather than into Lake Michigan, these epidemics were largely conquered, though other age-old communicable diseases such as tuberculosis, sexually transmitted diseases, and, recently, childhood measles, still disproportionately plague Chicago's poor.

One reason infectious diseases retain their foothold among the poor remains substandard housing, which is bad and getting worse in North Lawndale. A recent survey by an economic development group found that only 8% of the neighborhood's 8,937 buildings were in good to very good condition. The rest were abandoned, on the verge of collapse, or in need of repair.[9]

Dr. Arthur Jones has visited many of these decrepit buildings on house calls to patients too sick to make it into his clinic, which is located on Ogden almost directly behind Jackie's apartment. The clinic, Lawndale Christian Health Center, was founded by Dr. Jones and several other urban missionaries in 1984 and has succeeded, by most all accounts, at providing affordable and humane health care.

Dr. Jones told of one woman who was suffering a severe case of hives caused by an allergic reaction to her cat, yet repeatedly refused to get rid of the animal. "I really got kind of angry," Dr. Jones remembered, "and then she told me that if she got rid of the cat, there was nothing to protect her kids against rats." Another woman brought her two-year-old to the clinic with frostbite, so Dr. Jones dispatched his nurse practitioner to visit her home a block away from Jackie's. The nurse discovered icicles in the woman's apartment because the landlord had stopped providing heat. The stories go on, most involving landlords who cannot afford to keep up their buildings and tenants who cannot afford to leave them.

By these standards, the Baneses' apartment is in good shape. They have to contend with an occasional rat and wage a constant battle against roaches, but the landlord has kept the two-flat in decent repair; his sister lives on the first floor.

For the most part, the diseases that Jackie and her family live with are not characterized by sudden outbreaks but long, slow burns. As deadly infectious diseases have largely been eliminated or are easily cured—with the glaring exceptions of AIDS and now drug-resistant tuberculosis—chronic diseases have stepped into their wake, accounting for much of the death and disability among both rich and poor. The difference is that for affluent whites, diabetes, high blood pressure, heart disease, and the like are diseases of aging, while among poor blacks, they are more accurately called diseases of *middle*-aging.

In poor black neighborhoods on the West Side of Chicago, including North Lawndale, well over half of the population dies before the age of 65, compared to a quarter of the residents of middle-class white Chicago neighborhoods.[10] Though they occur more often on the West Side, the three most common causes of premature mortality in the two areas would correspond—heart disease, diabetes, and high blood pressure—were it not for one fatal condition that increasingly is considered a major public health problem: homicide. It ranks sixth in the white neighborhoods but is the number two killer of West Siders under 65.[11] Alcohol and drugs are the poisons that induce many of the West Side's deaths, whether from homicide or heart attack. Thirteen percent of fatalities in that part of the city are directly attributable to alcohol and drugs, four times the rate in white, middle-class neighborhoods.[12]

These statistics are not, of course, unique to Chicago. A study of premature mortality in Harlem showed that black men there were less likely to reach the age of 65 than men in Bangladesh.[13] "When 67 people die in an earthquake in San Francisco, we call it a disaster and the president visits," said Dr. Harold Freeman, one of two Harlem Hospital Center physicians who conducted the study. "But here everyone is ignoring a chronic consistent disaster area, with many more people dying. And there is no question that things are getting worse."[14]

Though genetic differences still are occasionally cited in medical literature in order to explain disproportionate disease among blacks, nearly all health experts put most of the blame on poverty—and the lack of access to care and hardscrabble lifestyles that accompany it. The situation worsened during the mid-1980s when the gap in life expectancy between the two races began to widen for the first time in history. Blacks' life expectancy has been less than whites' for as long as health statistics have been gathered, though since the turn of the century both races have lived a little longer each year. But from 1985 to 1988, blacks' life expectancy declined each year while whites' continued to creep ahead.[15] In 1989, blacks regained some of the time they lost, when their life expectancy rose slightly, but only to the 1984 level of 69.7 years.[16]

The starkest contrast in longevity is between white and black men, largely because of spiraling rates of homicide and AIDS among minorities. DeMarest, who was born in 1985, can be expected to live for 64 years and

10 months, whereas an average white boy born that year will live 8 years longer.[17] Jackie knows her son's chances of living a long life are not good, but she does not spend much time brooding about the dangers that await him. For now, she keeps him close to home and hopes for the best.

When Jackie stepped down from the bus after visiting Robert at the hospital, it was late in the day; the sun was about level with her shoulders. As she waited to cross Ogden, she glanced back toward the city, where the 110-story Sears Tower was silhouetted against the blue sky. The tower had been a beacon to Jackie as a child. "That was one ambition me and my cousin used to have. We wanted to walk to the Sears Tower." They never made it past a local shopping strip.

Jackie proceeded across Ogden toward the back of her own stone and brick two-flat, which, fortunately, is about a half-block removed from the harsh four-lane street. Her second-floor back porch, where her children had been playing earlier, was now empty. They had gone inside, since they are under orders not to venture beyond the 15-square-feet of the porch. To help make sure they don't, Jackie locks a metal gate across the steps.

The day before Robert was hospitalized, the family had gathered on the porch to celebrate the Fourth of July. It was a normal holiday, normal at least for a family that resigns itself to sickness in the same way that other families resign themselves to being polite to an unwelcome guest.

Robert slumped in a chair, next to the grill, spatula propped up on his knee. His eyes were glassy and he looked more drained than usual. Suffering the side effects of whatever was causing him to urinate blood, he had not been eating well. The rest of the family welcomed the light breeze that cooled the porch, but Robert was shivering despite his long-sleeved sweatsuit.

While Robert listlessly tended the grill, Jackie tossed a salad in the kitchen, then mounded uncooked chicken, ribs, and hamburgers into a large aluminum roasting pan. She took the meat out to the porch for her husband to grill, but when she saw how tired he looked, she took over.

Jackie has not worked outside of her home since Latrice was little and does almost all of the cooking for the family. This pattern was established long ago, when Jackie was a young teenager living alone with her grandmother, whom she calls "Mom," or "Mama." By the time Mrs. Jackson got home from her job cooking and waitressing at a truck stop, she wanted no part of the kitchen, so Jackie began making dinner on week nights.

"I became sort of like the Hazel in the family. Mom the hubby that go to work; I was the wife."

Jackie said she rather enjoyed being in charge at home, picking up after her grandmother, chiding her for tossing her bra and girdle over the shower-curtain rod when she came home from work. But Mrs. Jackson, who left for work at 5 A.M., was not moved by her granddaughter's requests to please, please put her clothes in her room. "I lay them where I take them off," Mrs. Jackson would tell Jackie. And that was the end of it.

Mrs. Jackson has never been one to waste words with her family, Jackie said, but as she has grown sicker, she has spoken less and less. The Fourth of July was no exception. While the rest of the family talked and listened to Latrice's portable radio on the back porch, Mrs. Jackson sat quietly in her wheelchair in the front room, eating from a plate Jackie had fixed for her.

Mrs. Jackson's right leg was amputated in late April because of an infection. First, half of her foot had been removed in February, which doctors had hoped would obviate the need for further amputation. But after a month and a half of erratic outpatient care, Mrs. Jackson's condition worsened, and her leg had to be amputated, too. Like many diabetics, Mrs. Jackson suffers from peripheral vascular disease, a chronic illness that causes blood vessels to thicken and restricts the flow of blood so that infections cannot heal.

Though she wasn't saying much, Mrs. Jackson looked fresh and more alert than she had recently. Wearing a red-and-white gingham dress, she sat up almost erect in her wheelchair, and when Brianna scuttled into the room, she watched her quizzically. Mrs. Jackson had to wait for the family's life to parade before her since she refused Jackie's offers to push her to the back porch. Several notes from hospital social workers in Mrs. Jackson's medical chart said the elderly woman worried about being a burden to her granddaughter; and perhaps that was part of the reason she chose to stay inside.

Then, too, getting the wheelchair through the kitchen to the back porch is something of a production. Jackie has to move the kitchen table and chairs, and even then, Mrs. Jackson's wheelchair barely fits through the narrow hallway connecting the living room and kitchen. The five-room apartment does not easily accommodate three children and three adults, especially since Mrs. Jackson began to require extra equipment such as a portable commode, a walker, and, of course, a wheelchair.

Mrs. Jackson's world had shrunk to include her bedroom and the front room that adjoined it. Emblems of her life cluttered her dark wood dresser. There were a dozen or more brown pill bottles, two Bibles, gauze pads and antiseptic spray, an unopened pack of Red Man chewing tobacco (for a habit she had acquired in Mississippi), latex gloves, and a small photo album. A picture of Latrice in first grade was stuck in the dresser's mirror. A black patent leather handbag and two church hats, one a deep red knit with fur trim, the other decorated with large gold sequins, hung on its corner. The hats were getting dusty. Since Mrs. Jackson's leg was amputated, she had not been able to go to the First Baptist Church on Sundays, her favorite activity of the week. The situation was especially sad because she had not been a woman who spent much time at home, according to Jackie. "As long as I know this lady, she's been the get-up-and-go type. She has really been stripped of all her worldly duties." Jackie remembers her grandmother as her conduit to the outside world; she often boasts about Mrs. Jackson's legendary knowledge of bus routes. "Mama used to show me this way, showed me that way; she got around." Though it is hard to imagine somebody being so stoic, Mrs. Jackson never complained about being homebound, Jackie said, or pined for fresh air and sunshine.

Back on the porch, it was relatively quiet, except when two fire trucks screamed out of the station behind the apartment. No trees or bushes grow on the small patch of dirt and weeds in the back yard the Baneses share with the tenant below, but a tree on the lot behind them provides some shield from the constant traffic on Ogden.

Robert perked up when his 20-year-old half-sister Lativa and her boyfriend arrived. "See, he looks a lot better," Jackie said ruefully. "He gets tired of the same old faces."

The couple indeed brought a burst of vitality to the porch. Lativa was home on leave from the Army, and brought birthday presents for Brianna, whose first birthday was two days away, and for DeMarest, who would not turn five until after Lativa returned to her base in North Carolina.

After dinner, Jackie allowed Latrice and DeMarest to walk to a nearby liquor store to get snowcones, a favorite in the neighborhood. On sweltering summer days, adults and children drag folding chairs and coolers out to the curb and settle in. They pump red, blue, or green syrups into paper cones filled with scoops of chipped ice and sell them to passers-by. Latrice cherishes the rituals of holidays, including the trip for snowcones, so she made sure she and her brother honored the Fourth with their choices, blue-raspberry and watermelon flavors for Latrice, blue-raspberry and strawberry for DeMarest.

Munching on their snowcones as they walked home, the two children passed a narrow general store that was closed for the holiday. Its owner, Jim Downing, a tough 60-year-old with the hard body of someone 30 years younger, sells a little bit of everything. Hand-painted signs propped outside his establishment hawk pecans, extermination service (by Mr. Downing, who went to jail for several weeks for using dangerous, illegal chemicals), roach spray, and $39 burglar gates, one of which the Baneses bought and Mr. Downing mounted across their back door. Jackie does laundry in the two washing machines that are crammed into Mr. Downing's store, and Latrice comes here regularly to buy candy, or pick up soda or a gallon of milk for her mom. Mr. Downing tots up her charges on the back of a brown paper sack, testing Latrice's arithmetic as he goes. If the Baneses are running short of cash, he lets them run a tab.

Dessert and dinner finished, the family waited for darkness to fall, then went to the back yard to set off Roman candles and firecrackers that popped when Latrice or DeMarest flung them to the ground. During the night, Robert continued to urinate blood, and the next morning, he reported to the University of Illinois Hospital.

He went home after three days, on a Friday. Doctors told him to return the next Monday for surgery. The medical tests had revealed that the blood was coming from the stump of his rejected kidney, and they wanted to correct the problem. They called late that afternoon and told him they had changed their minds; they would wait to see if the bleeding cleared up on its own. It did.

Notes

1   Chicago and Cook County Health Care Summit, *Chicago and Cook County Health Care Action Plan: System Analysis and Design* (April 1990), ambulatory care chapter, p. 46.

2   Nicholas Lemann, "The Origins of the Underclass," *Atlantic Monthly*, June 1986, p. 36.

3   Chicago Park District and Chicago Public Library, special collections, *A Breath of Fresh Air: Chicago's Neighborhood Parks of the Progressive Reform Era, 1900–1925* (1989), p. 21.

4   The Rev. Michael Doyle's description of depressed South Camden, New Jersey, was included in an article by Wayne King, "Saving an Urban Wasteland," *New York Times*, 16 August 1991, p. B-2.

5   Chicago Department of Planning, *U.S. Census of Chicago: Race and Latino Statistics for Census Tracts Community Areas and City Wards: 1980, 1990* (February 1991), p. 71.

6   *Chicago Tribune* staff, *The American Millstone* (Chicago: Contemporary Books, 1986), p. 96.

7   Personal communication with Marie Bousfield, demographer for the Chicago Department of Planning, 1991. Figure based on calculations from the 1990 U.S. Census.

8   Thomas Bonner, *Medicine in Chicago 1850–1950* (Urbana: University of Illinois Press, 1991), pp. 20–21.

9   *Chicago Tribune* staff, *The American Millstone*, p. 258.

10 Chicago and Cook County Health Care Summit, Chicago and Cook County Health Care Action Plan, draft appendix, communities in need, pp. 1 and 4.

11 Chicago and Cook County Health Care Summit, Chicago and Cook County Health Care Action Plan, draft appendix, pp. 1 and 4.

12 Chicago Department of Health, *Communities Empowered to Prevent Alcohol and Drug Abuse Citywide Needs Assessment Report*, working draft (December 1991), appendix c, p. 71.

13 Colin McCord and Harold P. Freeman, "Excess Mortality in Harlem," *New England Journal of Medicine* 322, no. 3 (18 January 1990): 173–77.

14 Elisabeth Rosenthal, "Health Problems of Inner City Poor Reach Crisis Point," *New York Times*, 24 December 1990, p. 9.

15 Personal communication with Thomas Dunn, National Center for Health Statistics, vital statistics branch, January 1993.

16 Ibid.

17 Personal communication with Robert Armstrong, actuarial advisor, Division of Vital Statistics, National Center for Health Statistics, March 1993.

First-Person Account: Schizophrenia through a Sister's Eyes—The Burden of Invisible Baggage
Ami S. Brodoff

About 10 years ago, when I was a sophomore in college and my older brother Andy was a junior at a school nearby, I went to visit him for an extended holiday weekend. On Friday, we attended a party given by a classmate in his dorm. When it was time to leave, Andy opened a door that appeared to lead outside, but instead found himself stepping gingerly inside a closet. "Some people are coming out of the closet, but I'm going back inside," he stated matter-of-factly. The quip was funny, but in retrospect, it seemed to convey a hidden message, for it was during that weekend that Andy experienced several psychotic episodes and only a short time later that he was diagnosed as schizophrenic.

When I first saw my older brother that weekend, he looked much the same, though perceptibly more troubled and disheveled than usual. His large hazel eyes radiated a gentle green light and had a dash of yellow in the center, subtly changing color depending on what he wore. He was still handsome, but too thin now, unkempt, and a little unsavory. Although he had looked forward to my visit, he had trouble engaging in any sustained conversations and frequently needed to withdraw.

Andy was barely able to sit through the movie he'd chosen for us on Saturday night and jumped up every 10 or 15 minutes "to take a walk." On a trip to the ladies room, I found him in a dark corner of the lobby compulsively pacing back and forth. At meals, he was silent and preoccupied, ignoring his food, choosing instead to suck and chew on a mug full of ice cubes as he stared blankly into space.

His behavior was bizarre and troubling, but it didn't prepare me for

Ami S. Brodoff, "First-Person Account: Schizophrenia through a Sister's Eyes—The Burden of Invisible Baggage," from *Schizophrenia Bulletin*, vol. 14, 29–32. © 1988. Reprinted by permission of author.

what happened on the last evening of my stay, shortly before I planned to return to school. Andy had always loved animals, but he loathed and feared insects, particularly spiders. When I returned to the dorm after doing some shopping, I found him wearing a pair of gloves, frantically brushing at his clothes as though trying to rid himself of a swarm of clinging insects. The sight of a spider had convinced him that a vast colony of insects was quietly weaving *his* web. Black ants, beetles, gnats, and fluttering moths had teemed in, he believed, fastening themselves to the web—a cage that threatened to imprison him.

My brother was hospitalized, the first in a long series of voluntary and involuntary hospitalizations at institutions around the country as our family embarked on the endless quest for care that might ultimately help him. Although my mother, father, younger brother, two uncles, both grandfathers, and several cousins are all physicians, covering the gamut of specialties including psychiatry, we have yet to find medical care that has led to significant or sustained improvement in Andy's condition.

My brother exists in a subterranean world of fantasy a good deal of the time. Yet, when we were young children, it was I who often created and lived inside an imaginary world complete with a rogue's gallery of characters and a colorful assortment of landscapes, while Andy possessed an unusual hypersensitivity to reality, as though he were perceiving the world through a magnifying glass.

I loved to take long solitary walks in the woods near our home, roaming the meadows beyond our backyard, and exploring the mysterious cemetery and garden that lay hidden behind a stone wall at the corner of our street. In these special secret places, I spun a continuous yarn, a novel in which I was both heroine and author. Just as the sidewalk paintings in Mary Poppins were magically transformed into real life worlds, I was able to transform my own world into a storybook, a private pastime I engaged in for amusement or sought as a refuge: whenever my own life seemed especially bleak or chaotic, I could magically invent another.

In contrast to me, Andy didn't transform the world; he perceived life with the painful acuity of one whose mental filtering mechanism has simply melted away, leaving behind only naked nerve fibers. He seemed to have an emotional sixth sense, enabling him to foresee what was going to happen—particularly painful events—long before anyone else was aware of them. When he was only five, he told me with certainty that our parents were going to get a divorce. I dismissed this notion as nonsense, probably because it was too terrifying to contemplate, and besides, I convinced myself, our parents rarely fought. I refused to worry about things that might never happen—that is, until six years later, when Andy's prediction came true: he had perceived the undercurrent of dissonance and detachment in our parents' relationship long before anyone else was willing or able to acknowledge it, even perhaps, our parents themselves.

Despite the differences in the way we perceived and coped with the world, Andy and I were unusually close as children. His presence in my life and mine in his was more constant than that of either of our parents. I adored and emulated my older brother, tagged after him, and vied for his attention; he was my daily companion, my playmate, and so I believed, my protector.

As young children, Andy and I shared a secret language that included a ditty he made up to comfort me when I felt sad or frightened. Whenever I needed consolation, he'd tenderly rub his face against mine and then pat my cheeks with both of his hands while chanting:

> Ah sista goah, I love you and
> the pack. I give you milk and
> candy to make the bad go back.

Although the poem would never win a Pulitzer Prize, it was pretty good for a toddler, and the chant became a ritual between us, offering reassurance that Andy would watch over me, as well as our puppy, two cats, turtles, salamanders, and tropical fish, providing nurturance and keeping us all safe from harm.

However, a recent look at old family photos has given my memories a jolt, and made me question who was really protecting whom. Paradoxically, these snapshots belie my memories of Andy as my caretaker. In each and every one, I stand in the foreground with Andy several paces behind me, even though he is older by a year and a half and there are only two of us in the picture. I am sturdy and smiling; Andy is frail, his handsome features scrunched up into a scowl. He holds his body in an odd, concave position, sucking in the center of his body, with his head pitched awkwardly forward. Thin arms, bent at the elbows, hang lank behind his torso as if he holds onto a set of invisible supporting bars. Occasionally, he smiles, but these pictures are the most disturbing of all: my brother's taut, clenched smile, baring most of his upper and lower front teeth, conveys only great tension and pain: it is a frozen, soundless scream.

As Andy and I grew older, our lives took very different directions, and the honeymoon phase of our relationship came to a halt. As my world broadened, Andy's became increasingly constricted. I enjoyed school and was a conscientious student with a widening circle of friends and a schedule brimming with athletics and extracurricular activities. Andy did poorly in school and was frequently on the verge of flunking several of his classes, even though his IQ was within the genius bracket. With few emotional resources or social outlets, my brother was a quiet loner, often scapegoated by peers and teachers alike.

I watched with alarm as Andy became progressively out of touch with his own body, as if it were an alien object belonging to someone else. He began to wear mismatched, ill-fitting clothing and neglected basic grooming and hygiene. For several years during high school, his body seemed frighteningly metamorphic, expanding to gross obesity in a matter of months, and then shrinking, just as suddenly, to a haggard thinness bordering on emaciation.

Although I didn't understand what ailed my older brother, it seemed clear that he was on a steady downhill course. Out of a deep fear for my own survival that I scarcely understood, I began to draw rigid boundaries between us, arming myself with evidence that we were nothing alike.

My efforts to dissociate myself from Andy were often quite successful: although we attended the same school for many years, few people were aware that we were brother and sister, despite the evidence of the rather unusual last name we shared. When peers or teachers discovered our relationship, I panicked: somehow, I had been found out.

I felt that the part of me that was emotionally fragile, that sensed I didn't quite belong, despite belonging, had magically burst from its boundaries in my inner life and found expression in Andy's illness: what I harbored secretly, he expressed to the outside world. What was to prevent me from deteriorating just like Andy? After all, we shared the same parents, many of the same genes, and the same childhood environment. In his eyes, I saw the disturbing reflection of what I feared I might become, and his presence became a daily reminder that the carefully ordered world I had painstakingly created could easily topple down like an intricate sand castle washed away by a wave.

However, when outsiders recognized that Andy and I were from the same family, I was also painfully reminded of the deep bond I still felt with him. I loved my brother more than I could admit, and my abandonment of him was an abandonment of part of myself. When I witnessed the cruelty Andy endured, I felt the smarting pain of the barbs personally.

Yet, when I attempted to include Andy in my social life, it was an almost predictable fiasco. Envious of my social acceptance and achievements, enraged by my abandonment of him, and humiliated for being included intermittently out of "charity," Andy sabotaged any prospects for an enjoyable time. It was hard to love him when he remained mute and sullen, hurled a boyfriend's hat in front of a passing car, used my silk scarf to clean his ear, or urinated randomly in the park.

As our family privately lurched from one emergency to another involving my brother and the ebb and flow of his moods became the main focus of each day, I began to feel neglected for being healthy. My own concerns were often dwarfed by Andy's larger problems, while my joys and successes seemed even more trivial. I craved more attention and recognition from my parents, but felt guilty about these longings since Andy was obviously so much more needy. In bitter moments, I felt that the only way I could win my parents' affection was by becoming sick too. Yet I knew that mental illness was far too high a price to pay—even for love.

Some months after Andy was first institutionalized, I went to visit him in the hospital. With a shaved head, a jagged front tooth (a relic of his days rootlessly roaming around Times Square), and gestures that had the diffuse, futile energy characteristic of old men, my brother seemed like a homeless vagabond. His eyes were both vacant and haunted with the naked look of a frightened animal frozen by the beam of approaching headlights. He was pathetically docile, parroting back my words and gestures, as though he didn't know where my identity left off and his own began. The deep sadness I felt at seeing him this way was virtually eclipsed by the welling up within me of panic. His mirroring of my words and gestures had triggered the age-old terror that our identities were entwined, that I too might become schizophrenic. When I told Andy that I would have to leave soon, he clutched the scarlet sleeve of my blazer and asked, "Can you see me?"

During these first few years of Andy's illness, the daily rhythms of our family's lives were often turned topsy-turvy, since my brother frequently ran away from the hospital, stopped taking his medicine, and aimlessly wandered around the most dangerous sections of cities like New York and New Haven in a psychotic state. More times than I can remember, we had to stop whatever we were doing and chase after him, bring him home, and convince him to return to the hospital—only to have the same cycle repeated in several months' time. These unpredictable upheavals made my family seem like a fragile vessel whirling about in an overpowering eddy. When I was sucked into these emergencies, they threatened to overwhelm me: I couldn't rescue Andy and defuse my parents' conflicts (about how best to care for Andy and who was to blame for his illness) while carrying on with the demands of my own life. I felt the destructive force of the eddy in which our family swirled and knew that if I didn't get some distance, I'd be drawn into the vortex and drowned. To save myself, I decided to jump ship, separating myself from Andy and the family, resolving first to pull together the pieces of my own life.

It is now about a decade since Andy was first diagnosed as schizophrenic. I no longer feel that my brother and I are shadow-sides of the same person or that our destinies are entwined. On the deepest level where intellect leaves off and gut emotion begins, I know I am not Andy. Today, I can see him without fear, but not without sorrow. The chronic nature of his illness makes it a problem that is never truly resolved, and the sadness I feel about the bleakness of his life is a burden I still carry around like invisible baggage.

Andy now lives at home with my father and stepmother in Connecticut. On my last visit there, he seemed like a sleepwalker existing in a kind of half-life. He sat for hours, apart from the family, rocking himself. In his hand, he held a glass of ice and was absorbed chewing it. He rolled the blocks around in his mouth until they melted to chips. He let the sharp chips bite his tongue and the cool, melted liquid slide back against his throat. When the glass was empty, he sighed and went back into the kitchen for more. Occasionally, his sighs became deep and rhythmic, building to a crescendo like a heartbeat whose pulse has magically become audible to the outside world. Every few minutes, a strange, inappropriate smile passed his lips as if he could hear something. He gave me the feeling he couldn't speak because he didn't want to be interrupted.

That day, many days before it, and many days since, I've missed my older brother with the persistent ache and longing usually reserved for a loved one lost through death. Although grieving for someone who has died is painful, some sense of peace and acceptance is ultimately possible. However, mourning for a loved one who is alive—in your very presence and yet in vital ways inaccessible to you—has a lonely, unreal quality that is extraordinarily painful.

When I remember the closeness Andy and I shared as children, the memory often seems dim, almost illusionary, as though it not only happened in another time, but in another realm, to two other people.

The Loneliness of the Long-Term Care Giver
Carol Levine

I am standing at a bank of phones, desperately punching in codes and numbers. Each time, the line goes dead. "Why can't I get through to anyone?" I think. "I must be doing something wrong."

I wake up. This time it's only a dream. But the dream originated in a real experience. On the icy morning of January 15, 1990, my husband lay comatose in the emergency room of a community hospital after an automobile accident. Uninjured but dazed, I stood at a bank of hospital phones trying to reach people who could help me transfer him to a major medical center. I was unaware that, by a malevolent coincidence, most of the phones in the region were not working.

The dream recurs, and it has now taken on a new meaning. In the nine years since the accident, and especially in the eight years I have struggled to take care of my husband at home, I have frequently despaired: "Why can't I get through to anyone?" Only in the past few years have I realized that I am not doing anything wrong. It is the health care system that is out of order.

Since I have spent 20 years as a professional in the fields of medical ethics and health policy, it is hardly surprising that I should reach such a conclusion. A recent series of articles in the *Journal* made clear the increasing fragmentation and inequities in the current market-driven health care economy.[1] But my personal experience as a family care giver has given me a different perspective. I see the health care system through everyday encounters with physicians, nurses, social workers, receptionists, vendors, ambulette drivers and dispatchers, administrators, home health aides, representatives of my managed-care company, and a host of other "providers." The attitudes, behavior, and decisions of specific individuals make the system work or fail for me.

There are of course critical links between the behavior of individual persons and the system's structural and financial incentives and rewards. Health policy makers and analysts rarely consider the impact of these incentives on the 25 million unpaid, "informal" care givers in the United States, who get little from the system in return for the estimated $196 billion a year in labor they provide.[2] Family care givers are largely invisible, as individuals and as a labor force.

When my journey began, no one told me what to expect. There is no process of informed consent for family care givers. On that unforgettable January day, I knew that I must ask, "Is my husband brain-dead?" And I knew what to do if the answer was yes. "No," said the neurosurgeon at the community hospital, "but he has suffered a severe brain-stem injury. At his age [then 62] it is unlikely that he will survive." The neurosurgeon at the medical center disagreed. "He will walk out of here 100%, but it will take some time." "How long?" I asked. "Weeks," he replied, "maybe months."

My husband did survive, a testament to one of American medicine's major successes—saving the lives of trauma patients. But he will never walk, and he is far from 100%. While he was in a coma, I read to him, played his favorite music, and showed him family pictures. After four months he gradually emerged from the coma, his thinking chaotic. After many more months of relearning basic words and concepts, he recovered many cognitive functions, and there were occasional flashes of his old intelligence and humor. But he is not the same person in any sense.

Although I worried most about his mental functioning, it is his body that has recovered least. He is totally disabled and requires 24-hour care. He is incontinent of bladder and bowel. He is quadriparetic, with mobility limited to the partial use of his left hand. (His right forearm was amputated as a result of an iatrogenic blood clot that failed to respond to surgery and drug treatment.) Even so, the most difficult aspect of his care is his changed personality and extreme emotional lability. Antipsychotic drugs now generally control his violent outbursts, but there are still unpredictable rages and periods of withdrawal.

As a rehabilitation inpatient he had physical therapy, occupational therapy, speech therapy, cognitive therapy, psychological counseling, nerve blocks, injections of botulinum toxin, hydrotherapy, recreational therapy, and therapeutic touch. He benefited to some degree, but nothing restored true function. He has undergone numerous operations, including placement of a shunt after a blood clot formed in his leg, tendon releases in both legs, removal of a kidney stone, and most recently, removal of a pituitary tumor. He has undergone oral surgery and extensive dental work.

During my nine-year odyssey, I stopped being a wife and became a family care giver. In the anxious weeks when my husband was in the intensive care unit, I was still a wife. Doctors and nurses informed me of each day's progress or setbacks and treated me with kindness and concern. At some point, however, when he was no longer in immediate danger of dying, and as the specialists and superspecialists drifted out of the picture, I became invisible. Then, when the devastating and permanent extent of his disabilities became clear to clinicians, I became visible again.

At that point, I was important only as the manager and, it was expected, the hands-on provider of my husband's care. In retrospect, I date my rite of passage into the role of family care giver to the first day of my husband's stay in a rehabilitation facility, a place I now think of as a boot camp for care givers. A nurse stuck my husband's soiled sweat pants under my nose and said, "Take these away. Laundry is your job." A woman whose husband had been at the same facility later told me the same story—different nurse. The nurse's underlying message, reinforced by many others, was that my life from now on would consist of performing an unrelieved series of nasty chores.

The social worker assigned to my husband's case had one goal: discharge. I was labeled a "selfish wife," since I refused to take him home without home care. "Get real," the social worker said. "Nobody will pay for home care. You have to quit your job and 'spend down' to get on Medicaid." Eventually I got the home care I needed—temporarily. Despite a written agreement to pay for it, the insurance company later cut off the benefit retroactively, without informing me, leaving me with an $8,000 bill from a home care agency. The agency, which had failed to monitor its own billing, sued me. We settled for less.

When I brought my husband home, he had undiagnosed severe sleep apnea (which caused nighttime screaming), undiagnosed hearing loss, and poorly treated major depression. The first few months at home were nightmarish. Since the problems had not been diagnosed correctly, much less treated, I did not know where to turn. Yet a single home visit by a psychiatrist and a specially trained home care nurse, arranged by a sympathetic colleague who treats patients with cancer, gave me enough information, advice, and referrals to begin to master the situation.

In addition to holding a full-time job, I manage all my husband's care and daily activities. Being a care manager requires grit and persistence. It took me 10 days of increasingly insistent phone calls to get my managed-care company to replace my husband's dangerously unstable hospital bed. When the new bed finally arrived—without notice, in the evening, when there was no aide available to move him—it turned out to be the cheapest model, unsuitable for a patient in my husband's condition. In these all-too-frequent situations, I feel that I am challenging Goliath with a tiny pebble. More often than not, Goliath just puts me on hold.

Being a care manager also takes money. I now pay for a daytime home care aide and serve as the night nurse myself. My husband's initial hospitalization and rehabilitation were paid for by his employer-based indemnity insurance plan. He is now covered by my employer-based managed-care company, which pays for hospital and doctors' bills and, with a $10 copayment, for prescription medicines. Home care aides, disposable supplies, and most forms of therapy are not covered, because they are "not medically necessary." My husband recently needed a new customized wheelchair, which cost $3,700; the managed-care company paid $500. Medicare, his secondary payer, has so far rejected all claims. No one advocates on my husband's behalf except me; no one advocates on my behalf, not even me.

I feel abandoned by a health care system that commits resources and rewards to rescuing the injured and ill but then consigns such patients and their families to the black hole of chronic "custodial" care. I accept responsibility for my husband's care. Love and devotion are the most powerful motives, but there are legal and financial obligations as well. My income would be counted toward his eligibility for Medicaid, should we ever come to that.

The broader issue of a family's moral responsibility to provide or pay for care is much more complex.[3] Why should families be responsible for providing such demanding, intensive care? Should this be a social responsibility? American society places a high value on personal and family responsibility. The thin veneer of consensus that supported some sense of communal responsibility in the past is cracking. This is not a uniquely American problem, however. Even with national health insurance, Australian, Canadian, and British care givers report similar problems of isolation and unmet financial and other needs.[4] Only the Scandinavian countries assume that the community as a whole is primarily responsible for long-term care. Even so, the Swedish Social Services Act specifies some spousal responsibility.[5]

Widely held concepts of family responsibility derive from religious teachings, cultural traditions, community expectations, emotional bonds, or gratitude for past acts. Care givers rarely sort out their mixed feelings. From a policy perspective, there are historical antecedents and financial realities that encourage looking first to families for care. Perhaps the most important justification is that most families, or some members, want this responsibility. Many derive spiritual or psychological rewards from care giving. Taking care of each other comes with being a family. This is an especially strong value among recent immigrants or tightly knit ethnic communities who distrust the formal system but who often have too few resources to cope on their own.

The problem is not that public policy looks first to families but that it generally looks only to families and fails to support those who accept responsibility. The availability of family care givers does not absolve policy makers of their own responsibility to make sure that their actions assist rather than destroy families. Family members should not be held to a level of moral or legal responsibility that entails jeopardizing their own health or well-being.

Given the complexity of the health care system, what changes would make a difference for family care givers? The automatic answer tends to be: Whatever they are, we can't afford them. Or, whatever we can afford is not worth doing. Many family care givers have serious financial problems. Nevertheless, a single-minded focus on money, based on an unsubstantiated assumption that most care givers want to be replaced by paid help, diverts attention from other critical needs.

The reaction to the Clinton administration's January proposal for assistance for the elderly and family care givers is an instructive example of the differing worldviews of health policy analysts and family care givers. Most professionals focused on the proposed tax credit of $1,000 and found it wanting. The credit would not apply to people who pay no taxes, nor would it make a dent in the heavy costs of full-time paid care. The proposal does not do anything to create a coherent long-term care policy.[6] All these observations are true. On the other hand, family care givers and organizations that represent their interests have been largely positive about the proposal. The tax credit is a tangible benefit that will help many middle-class families. Equally important, the proposal puts family care giving on the national agenda and gives states money and incentives to develop resource centers. These points are also all true.[7]

In my professional role, I know that much more is needed, including a restructuring of Medicare to better meet the long-term needs of the elderly and disabled and the creation of a more flexible range of options for home and community-based care.[8] I also know that change will take a long time and will be determined by the interests of the major players and by political considerations. As a family care giver, I will take whatever help I can get when I need it, and that is right now.

Clinicians as well as policy makers have responsibilities toward family care givers. Care givers say they want better communication with professionals, education and training, emotional support, and advocacy to obtain needed services for their relatives and themselves. They want help in negotiating the impenetrable thicket of financing mechanisms, the frequent denials of services or reimbursements, and the inconsistent interpretations of policies and eligibility. They want respite, too, but through services that they can tailor to their needs. These are modest requests—too modest, perhaps—but unfulfilled nonetheless.

Care givers in the focus groups convened by the United Hospital Fund's Families and Health Care Project reported a lack of basic information about the patient's diagnosis, prognosis, and treatment plan, the side effects of the patient's medication, the symptoms to watch for at home, and whom to call when problems occur.[9] Sometimes care givers reported that they were given conflicting information.

Managed care did not create this problem, but it seems to have exacerbated it. Often, professionals convey information in such a hurried, technical way that anxious care givers cannot absorb it. Hospital staff members may assume, erroneously, that a home care agency will instruct the care giver. There are costs to these lapses. Failures in communication can lead to serious problems with the care of patients, including unnecessary hospital readmissions. Some families, however, become experts on the conditions of their relatives and the specifics of their care. Yet professionals frequently ignore this expertise, because it comes from laypersons.

Family care givers also want to be involved in decision making that affects the patient and themselves. Elsewhere, Connie Zuckerman and I have described some of the reasons clinicians have difficulties with family members, especially with respect to decisions about acute care.[10] In my husband's case, I alone made the only important decision, which was to transfer my husband to a medical center on the day of the accident. After that there were never any clear-cut decisions, no discussions about the goals of care, and certainly no long-term planning. Although I repeatedly asked to attend a team meeting to discuss his prognosis and care, I was never given that opportunity. Nor was there ever any follow-up at home, a common complaint among care givers.

Care givers want education and training that recognizes their emotional attachment to the patient. Professionals seldom appreciate how much fear and anxiety complicate the learning of new tasks. Learning how to operate a feeding tube or change a dressing or inject a medication is hard enough for a layperson; care givers learn how to perform these procedures for the first time on a person they love. Fearful of making a mistake or simply upset by the idea of having to perform unaccustomed and unpleasant tasks, care givers may resist or fail, or persist at great emotional cost.

Months before my husband was ready to go home, a nurse insisted that I learn how to put on my husband's condom catheter. "I don't need to know this yet," I protested, "and besides, maybe he won't need it later." Ignoring our emotional state at the time, she forced me to do it (badly) until both my husband and I burst into tears. Later, when I complained to her supervisor, I was told, "We just wanted to break through your denial."

Families need emotional support. They frequently bring a patient home to a living space transformed by medical equipment and a family life constrained by illness. Privacy is a luxury. Every day must be planned to the minute. The intricate web of carefully organized care can unravel with one phone call from an aide who is ill, an ambulette service that does not show up, a doctor's office that cannot accommodate a wheelchair, an equipment company that does not have an emergency service. There are generally no extra hands to help out in a crisis and no experienced colleagues to ask for advice. Friends and even family members fade away.

Programs that train and support family care givers can be based in hospitals, community agencies, schools and colleges, home care agencies, managed-care companies, or other settings. The United Hospital Fund's Family Caregiving Grant Initiative is funding several such projects.

If family care givers need education, professionals need it just as much. Education for doctors, nurses, and social workers should include understanding the needs of family care givers. Ideally, all professionals should have the experience of seeing firsthand what is really involved in home care. In-service programs can educate health care professionals about family dynamics as well as build communication and negotiating skills.

Family care givers must be supported, because the health care system cannot exist without them. And there is another compelling reason: Care givers are at risk for mental and physical health problems themselves. Exhausted care givers may become care recipients, leading to a further, often preventable, drain on resources. Does my managed-care company realize, for instance, that during the past year it paid more for my stress-related medical problems than for my husband's medical care?

No single intervention will change the system, but small steps taken together can cover a long distance. As I enter my 10th year as a family care giver, it is hard to believe I have come this far. Today is a reasonably good day. But what about tomorrow? And next week? Hello? Is anyone listening?

Notes

1 Angell M. The American health care system revisited—a new series. *N Engl J Med* 1999;340:48.
2 Arno PS, Levine C, Memmott MM. The economic value of informal caregiving. *Health Aff (Millwood)* 1999;18(2):182–8.
3 Levine C. Home sweet hospital: the nature and limits of private responsibilities for home health care. Pp. 169–191 in *New directions in bioethics*. Eds. AW Galston and EG Shurr. Boston: Kluwer, 2001.
4 Schofield H, Booth S, Hermann H, Murphy B, Nankervis J, Singh B. *Family caregivers: disability, illness and aging*. St. Leonards, Australia: Allen & Unwin, 1998.
5 Barusch AS. Programming for family care of elderly dependents: mandates, incentives, and service rationing. *Soc Work* 1995;40:315–22.
6 Graham J. Halfway measures. *Chicago Tribune.* January 17, 1999.
7 Statement by Suzanne Mintz, President, National Family Caregivers Association, Kensington, Md., January 6, 1999.
8 Cassel CK, Besdine RW, Siegel LC. Restructuring Medicare for the next century: what will beneficiaries really need? *Health Aff (Millwood)* 1999;18(1):118–31.
9 Levine C. *Rough crossings: family caregivers' odysseys through the health care system.* New York: United Hospital Fund, 1998.
10 Levine C, Zuckerman C. The trouble with families: toward an ethic of accommodation. *Ann Intern Med* 1999;130:148–52.

What Do Children Owe Elderly Parents?
Daniel Callahan

In the spring of 1983 the Reagan administration announced that states may under Medicaid legally require children to contribute to the support of their elderly parents. At the time a number of states were considering or enacting just such laws. The administration, one spokesman said, was not proposing anything inherently new. It was simply responding to a state request for clarification of the existing Medicaid law, and wanted only to say that state statutes enforcing family responsibility laws were not in conflict with federal policy.[1]

As it turned out, the administration's initiative was a policy shift whose time had not come. While a number of states flirted for a time with new family responsibility policies, only a few (Virginia, Idaho, and Mississippi, for example) actually adopted them, and even fewer seem to be enforcing them. As pressing as the state Medicaid nursing home burden is, it rapidly became clear that there is little general sentiment to force children to provide financially for their elderly parents.[2]

Nonetheless, Reagan's initiative was an important social and policy event and raises significant moral issues. In one form or another, the idea is likely to arise again. Anything that can be done to raise revenue to reduce the Medicaid burden probably will be done. Three questions are thus worth considering. What kind of a moral obligation do children have toward the welfare of their elderly parents? Can it be said that the changed health, longevity, and social circumstances of the elderly justify a shift in traditional moral obligations? Even if children do have some significant

Daniel Callahan, "What Do Children Owe Elderly Parents?," from *The Hastings Center Report*, vol. 15, 32–37. © 1985. Reprinted by permission of The Hastings Center and Daniel Callahan.

duties to parents, is it still legitimate to ask the state to take over much of the direct burden of care?

The first question is of course an old one. Each generation has had to make its own sense of the biblical injunction that we should honor our fathers and mothers. It neither tells us in what "honor" consists nor how far filial obligation should be carried. As a piece of practical advice, however, it once made considerable sense. In most traditional and agricultural societies, parents had considerable power over the lives of their offspring. Children who did not honor their parents risked not only immediate privation, but also the loss of the one inheritance that would enable them to raise and support their own families—land they could call their own.

The advent of industrialization brought about a radical change. It reduced the direct coercive power of parents over their children, setting into motion a trend toward the independence of both parents and children that has been a mark of contemporary society. Though the affective bond between parents and children has so far endured in the face of industrialization and modernity, the combination of actual attachment and potential independence frames the question of the obligation of children toward their elderly parents.

The moral ideal of the parent-child relationship is that of love, nurture, and the mutual seeking for the good of the other. While the weight of the relationship will ordinarily shift according to the age of children and their parents, mutual respect and reciprocity have been a central part of the moral standard. Yet the reality of human lives can stand in the way of the realization of moral ideals. Just as not all children are lovable, neither do all parents give the welfare of their children their serious attention and highest priority. Many children do not find their parents lovable and feel no special sense of duty toward them. Many parents are not happy with the way their children turn out, or with the kind of lives they live, and do not seek to remain intertwined with them.

To what extent, and under what circumstances, flaws and faults of that kind can be said to alter the mutual obligations is obviously an important question. Yet even when the affectional bonds between parent and child are strong, it is still by no means clear what each morally owes to the other. If parents ought to help their children to grow up and flourish, should they go so far as to seriously jeopardize their own future welfare in doing so? If children should honor their elderly parents, how great a sacrifice ought that to entail?

The present relationship between children and their elderly parents is shaped in part by the changing status of the elderly in society. A rising number and increasing proportion of our population are the elderly. The "young old" (65–75) appear to be in better health than ever, but as people live longer, there is also an increasing number of the "old old" (75+) who are frail and dependent. Despite a variety of public programs and considerable improvement in recent decades, a significant proportion of the elderly (about 25 percent in 1980) still live in poverty or near-poverty. A large proportion do not have immediate family or relatives to whom they can turn for either financial or emotional assistance, and many—particularly women—live alone or in institutions. Even so, as Victor Fuchs notes in summarizing available data, rising income has "made it possible for an ever higher percentage [of the elderly] to maintain their own households, health permitting."[3]

Independence, however, need not mean an absence of family ties. Gerontologists take great pleasure in demolishing what they tell us are two prevalent myths, that the caring family has disappeared, and that the elderly are isolated from their children. There has indeed been a decline in the number of elderly who live with their children or other relatives, from three-fifths in 1960 to one-third in 1980,[4] and an equally sharp drop—down to 1 percent—in the number of elderly who depend upon their children for financial support.[5] Yet it still seems to be true, as Ethel Shanas has noted, that "most old people live close to at least one of their children and see at least one child often. Most old people see their siblings and relatives often, and old people, whether bedfast or housebound because of ill health, are twice as likely to be living at home as to be residents in an institution. . . ."[6] In addition, it is estimated that 60–80 percent of all disabled or impaired persons receive significant family help.[7]

One important change involves the proportion of young and old who believe that children should be financially responsible for their elderly parents. This has shifted downward (from about 50 percent in the mid-fifties to 10 percent in the mid-seventies),[8] and a simultaneous reduction in financial assistance has occurred. However, this need not be taken as an indication of a diminished sense of filial responsibility. The advent of Social Security, and the increasing financial strength of the elderly for other reasons, all indicate important social variables that have reduced financial pressure on children to support parents.

Other social changes could eventually alter that situation. The increasing number of divorced families, of small families, and of families where both spouses work, have created the possibility of a reduced sense of obligation in the future, though that has yet clearly to materialize.[9] In his 1981 book *New Rules*, the pollster Daniel Yankelovich wrote that "one of the most far-reaching changes in [moral] norms relates to what parents believe they owe their children and what their children owe them. Nowhere are the changes in the unwritten social contract more significant or agonizing. The overall pattern is clear: today's parents expect to make fewer sacrifices for their children than in the past, but they also demand less from their offspring in the form of future obligations than their parents demanded of them. . . . Sixty-seven percent [of Americans surveyed] believe that 'children do not have an obligation to their parents regardless of what their parents have done for them.' "[10]

To what extent this shift (assuming it is real) will lead to a change in the behavior and attitudes noted earlier remains to be seen. According to other available data and most commentators, children and families remain the principal source of emotional support and companionship for the elderly. At the same time, there is a pronounced distaste, on the side of both children and parents, for burdening children with financial obligations toward their parents. It seems widely assumed that contemporary life requires a different moral standard. A brief look at the present legal situation is useful in that respect; it brings out some of the ambivalence that exists and opens the way for a more direct look at the moral issues.

What the Law Says

Some twenty-six states at present have statutes that can require children to provide financial support for needy parents. Though erratically administered, difficult to implement, and of doubtful financial value, they remain as testimony to an effort dating back to the early seventeenth century to shift from the public to the private sphere the care of poverty-stricken elderly. While such laws had no precedent in either common law or medieval law, they came into being in England with the Elizabethan Poor Law of 1601, representing a culmination of at least three centuries of efforts to cope with the problem of the poor in general. The Poor Law did not concentrate on the children of the elderly, but extended the network of potential support to include the fathers and mothers, and the grandfathers and grandmothers, of the poor. The family, as a unit, was to be responsible for poverty-stricken kinfolk.

When these laws passed over into the American scene, during the seventeenth and eighteenth centuries, the focus was on the responsibility of children toward their elderly parents, though a few states have retained the wider scope.[11] Blackstone's famous *Commentaries* succinctly state the moral basis of such a responsibility: "The duties of children to their parents arise from a principle of natural justice and retribution. For to those who gave us existence we naturally owe subjection and obedience during our minority, and honor and reverence ever after; they who protected the weakness of our infancy are entitled to our protection in the infirmity of their age; they who by sustenance and education have enabled their offspring to prosper ought in return to be supported by that offspring in case they stand in need of assistance."[12]

The American state laws were little invoked during the eighteenth and nineteenth centuries, but they were increasingly turned to during the twentieth century, particularly in the aftermath of the depression and World War II. While there is broad historical agreement that the primary purpose of the laws was to protect the public from the burden of caring for the poor, including the elderly, the laws were buttressed by a variety of moral assumptions.[13]

Martin R. Levy and Sara W. Gross have identified three moral premises that underlie the American laws and developed some cogent criticisms of them. First, "the duty of a child to support his parents is a mirror-image of the parents' responsibility to support a child."[14] They point out the doubtful logic of that position. In procreation parents not only bring a child into the world, but by the same action undertake the moral obligation of sustaining that child, whose existence is entirely dependent upon the parents. As Levy and Gross put it, "In the converse situation of the duty of a child to support a parent, there is no proximate cause, no volitional act, and no rational basis for the demand of support. The child has not acted to bring about the life of the parent. While the father assumes the voluntary status of fatherhood, the child assumes no duty by having been born. His birth is the result of the act of the father and mother, and such a result cannot logically or physically be turned into a proximate cause."[15] While they do not deny that there can be a moral bond of love and affection, "moral duty and gratitude, or lofty ideals, cannot be used as a justification for the taking of property."[16] By focusing on "the taking of property," the authors focus on a relatively narrow point.

The second general moral premise turns on what they call "the relational interest of family status."[17] They mean that the simple fact of a family relationship—creating a special tie between parent and child, both biological and social—may itself engender the basis for a demand made upon children to support their elderly parents. Yet they point out that the relational interests are both too broad and too narrow to serve as a reasonable criterion for determining the duty to provide support. "It is too broad in . . . that not all children love and revere their parents. The status of a child confers no special emotional tie in and of itself."[18] It is too narrow in that, if emotional commitment is the standard, then a child would logically be bound to support everyone to whom he or she is tied by emotional commitment, whether family member or not.[19]

The analogy of a contract provides the third moral premise. Since the child was at one time supported by the parent, does not that create an implicit contract requiring that the child in turn support the parent when that becomes necessary? Levy and Gross point out that no direct contract is negotiated between parent and child when the child is procreated, and that any analogy must thus be based on an implied or quasi-contract. But the analogy of an implied contract does not work: the two parties necessary to the making of a contract did not exist simultaneously. A common standard in the law, moreover, is that neither the carrying out of a duty, nor the promise of rendering a performance already required by duty, is a sufficient condition of a return promise—an obligation to do likewise.[20]

Parents as "Friends"

Although Levy and Gross effectively dispatch the argument that the benefits bestowed by parents upon children automatically entail a duty of the children in return to aid parents, there is considerably more that needs to be said. Are we to hold that the obligation flows in one direction only, that because children were given no choice about being born, they owe nothing whatever to their parents? That seems too extreme. At the least, it fails to explain why in fact many children feel an obligation toward their parents, nor does it sufficiently plumb the moral depths of the family relationship.

The late Jane English also argued that the language of "owing" is mistakenly applied in the circumstances. Children "owe" parents nothing at all—which is not to say that there are not many things that children ought to do for their parents. Instead, she held that "the duties of grown children are those of friends and result from love between them and their parents, rather than being things owed in repayment for the parents' earlier sacrifices."[21] In situations where one person does a favor for another, there may be an obligation to reciprocate, but parents do not do favors for their children in the same sense that strangers or acquaintances may do them for each other. The bond that should unite parents and children is that of friendship, and "friendship ought to be characterized *by mutuality* rather than reciprocity: friends offer what they can give and accept what they need without regard for the total amount of benefits exchanged. And friends are motivated by love rather than by the prospect of repayment. Hence, talk of 'owing' is singularly out of place in friendship."[22] Thus children ought to do things for their parents, but the "ought" is that which follows from friendship; it resists both quantitative measurement and the stricter language of owing something in return for earlier benefits.

While English's argument has some plausibility, it is ultimately unsatisfying. Friendship can certainly exist between parent and child, but it often does not. Quite apart from those circumstances where parents have neglected their children or otherwise alienated their affection, they may have little in common other than their biological origins. Moreover, the nature of the friendship that exists between parent and child can and usually will be different from the kind that exists between and among those who are unrelated. A child might plausibly say that, while he is not a friend of his parents, he nonetheless feels toward them respect and love. To push the same point further, many children actively dislike their parents, find no pleasure in their company, and yet feel they ought to do things for them despite those feelings. In distinguishing between favors and friendship, English says that "another difference between favors and friendships is that after a friendship ends, the duties of friendship end."[23] That may be true enough in the case of nonfamily relationships, but it then raises all the more forcefully the question of whether friendship, however much it may mark a relationship between parent and child, can catch the fullness of the moral bond.

The origin and nature of the parent-child bond—or whatever other relationship may exist—is unique. By the procreation of children parents create a social unit that otherwise would not and could not exist. If children do not select their parents, neither do parents select their individual children (they choose to have *a* child, not *this* child). Even so, the family relationship is not something one can simply take or leave. It is a fundamental and unavoidable part of our social nature as human beings. That psychotherapists can spend a good deal of time untangling problems between parents and children provides at least a clue to the emotional depth of the biological relationship, whether marked by unhappiness or happiness. We can and do drift away from ordinary friendships, but parents stay in our memory and exert their influence even in the face of distance or active hostility. Whether we like it or not, we are in some sense always one with our parents, both because of the unique circumstances by which we came to know them and because of the long period of nurture when we were utterly dependent upon them. The mutual interaction of parents and children, even when friendships exist, cannot then entirely be reduced to the category of friendship. The emotional and biological bond between parent and child gives the relationship a permanent and central place in our lives, quite apart from whether that relationship turns out well or poorly. That cannot be said of friendship in the usual sense of the term.

Capturing Intimacy in Moral Language

Ferdinand Schoeman catches some of this flavor when he argues that the traditional language of morality, that of rights and obligations, does not seem to fit well in describing the bond among family members: "We *share ourselves* with those with whom we are intimate and are aware that they do the same with us. Traditional moral boundaries, which give rigid shape to the self, are transparent to this kind of sharing. This makes for non-abstract moral relationships in which talk about rights of others, respect for others, and even welfare of others is to a certain extent irrelevant."[24] Perhaps Schoeman takes things a bit far, but he tries to make clear that the intimacy of family relationships forces us into revealing and sharing a self that may not be revealed to others on the public stage. While it is often the case that parents do not really know their own child, just as often they do, even when their perceptions differ from those of the child. Whether they understand their child or not, the fact that they shared considerable intimacy when the child was young gives them access to a self that others may never see. For their part, children have unique access to parents, seeing a side of them that may never be revealed to others.

Another powerful candidate for the source of obligation is that of gratitude on the part of children toward their parents. Gratitude would be due, not simply because parents discharged their obligations toward the children, but because in their manner of doing so they went beyond the demands of mere duty, giving voluntarily of themselves in a way neither required nor ordinarily expected of them. As Jeffrey Blustein notes, "Duties of gratitude are owed only to those who have helped or benefited us freely, without thought of personal gain, simply out of a desire to protect or promote our wellbeing. The givers may hope for some return, but they do not give in expectation of it."[25] A consequence of this line of reasoning, however, is that only those parents who did more than was morally required could be said to have a right to the gratitude of their children. And it is by no means obvious that a "debt of gratitude" carries with it a strict obligation to provide like goods or services, that is, to go beyond what is otherwise required.

I am searching here with some difficulty for a way to characterize the ethical nature of the parent-child relationship, a relationship that appears almost but not quite self-evident in its reciprocal moral claims and yet oddly elusive also. We seem to say too much if we try to reduce the relationship to mutual moral duties, rights, and obligations. That implies a rigor and formalism which distorts the moral bond. We say too little if we try to make it a matter of voluntary affection only. Yet we cannot, I suspect, totally dismiss the language of obligation nor would we want to give up the ideal of mutual affection either. If the procreation and physical rearing of a child does not automatically entail reciprocal duties toward the parents when they are needy and dependent, it is certainly possible to imagine a sense of obligation arising when parents have done far more for children than would morally be required of them. My own parents, for example, did not throw me out on my own when I reached eighteen. They sacrificed a good deal to provide me with a higher education, and in fact provided financial support for my graduate education until I was thirty, topping that off by giving my wife and me a down-payment on our first house. They did it out of affection, rather than duty, but I certainly felt I owed them something in return in their old age. There need not be, then, any necessary incompatibility between feeling both affection and a sense of duty. But we lack a moral phrase that catches both notions in one concept; and neither taken separately is quite right.

The Power of Dependence

Another aspect of the relationship between children and their elderly parents bears reflection. Much as young children will have a special dependence upon parents, as those human beings above all others who have a fateful power over their destinies, so many elderly parents can come in dire circumstances similarly to depend upon their children. In a world of strangers or fleeting casual acquaintances, of distant government agencies and a society beyond their control, elderly parents can see in their children their only hope for someone who ought to care for them. Neither parent nor child may want this kind of emotional dependence, and each might wish that there were an alternative. Nonetheless, parents may be forced to throw themselves upon their children simply because there is no other alternative. Who else is likely to care?

Can that sense of utter need, if not for money then only for affection and caring, in and of itself create a moral obligation? It is surely a difficult question whether, as a general matter, a moral obligation is incurred when one human being is rendered by circumstance wholly dependent upon another—whether, that is, the dependency itself creates the obligation, quite apart from any other features of the relationship. A moral claim of that kind will inevitably be controversial, if only because it is (regretfully) common to rest claims of obligation upon implicit or explicit contracts of one kind or another; or upon features of the relationship that can be subjected to utilitarian calculation. It is difficult in this case plausibly to invoke such norms. Still, the power of sheer dependence—whether of newborn child upon parent or elderly, dependent parent upon child—can be potent in its experienced moral demands. The fate of one or more persons rests in the hands of another. The issue, as it presents itself, may be less one of trying to discover the grounds of obligation that would require a response than one of trying to find grounds for ignoring a demand that so patently assaults the sensibilities. It is not so much "must I?" as it is "how can I not?"

Joel Feinberg, commenting on the moral place of gratitude, moves in a similar direction when he writes, "My benefactor once freely offered me his services when I needed them. . . . But now circumstances have arisen in which he needs help, and I am in a position to help him. Surely, I owe him my services now, and he would be entitled to resent my failure to come through."[26] A qualification is in order here: gratitude is ordinarily thought due only when, as noted above, a benefactor has gone beyond ordinary duties. In some cases, parents may have only done their duty, and in such a minimal way that no gratitude seems due them. We are then brought back to the starkest moral situation—in which the dependency only seeks to establish a claim on us.

In trying to unravel the nature of the possible moral obligations, it may be helpful to speak of some specific claims or demands that might be made. Money is by no means the only, or necessarily the most important, benefit that parents can ask of their children. Children can also contribute their time and physical energy, and provide affection and psychological support. On a scale of moral priorities, it would be difficult to persuasively argue that parents have an obligation to deprive their own dependent children of necessary financial support in order to support their elderly parents. By virtue of procreating those children, the latter have a claim upon them that their parents cannot equal. Of course, where a surplus exists after their own children have been taken care of, the financial support of needy parents might become obligatory, particularly if there were no other available sources of support. Ordinarily, however, their principal economic duties will be toward their own children.

The same cannot necessarily be said of providing either physical help or affection to their parents. While the giving of physical help or affection could readily be merged, I think it is useful to distinguish between them. Physical help—such as assistance in moving, cleaning, shopping, and trips to visit friends or doctors—is a somewhat different contribution to the welfare of the elderly than simply talking with them. Parents of young children may not readily be able to adapt their schedules to such demands upon their time or energy. Yet they may be able to provide affection, either by visits at times they find convenient, or through letters and telephone calls. An inability to provide some kinds of care does not exempt children from providing other forms. In fact, the available evidence suggests that affection is most wanted, and it is not difficult to understand why. The uncertainties of old age, the recognition of growing weakness and help-lessness, can above all generate the desire to believe that at least some people in the world care about one's fate, and are willing to empathetically share that burden which few of us would care to bear alone—a recognition that life is gradually coming to an end and that nature is depriving us of our body, our individuality, and our future.[27]

In terms of financial obligations, there is considerable evidence from human experience in general, and from state efforts to impose financial burdens upon children in particular, that enforced legal obligations of children toward parents are mutually destructive. If only from the view-point of promoting family unity and affection, the provision of economic and medical care for the elderly by the government makes considerable sense. Ben Wattenberg quotes someone who nicely catches an important point: "We [older folks] don't like to take money from our kids. We don't want to be a burden. They don't like giving us money, either. We all get angry at each other if we do it that way. So we all sign a political contract to deal with what anthropologists would call the 'intergenerational transfer of wealth.' The young people *give* money to the government. I *get* money from the government. That way we can both get mad at the government and keep on loving each other."[28]

If the burden of economic care of the elderly can be difficult even for the affluent, it can be impossible for the poor. Moreover, adults with elderly parents ought not to be put in the position of trying to balance the moral claims of their own children against those of their parents, or jeopardizing their own old age in order to sustain their parents in their old age. Though such conflicts may at times be inescapable, society ought to be structured in a way that minimizes them. The great increase in life expectancy provides a solid reason, if one was ever needed, for arguing that all of us collectively through the state—rather than the children of the elderly—should supply their basic economic support. Both parents and children legitimately want an appropriate independence, not the kind that sunders their relationship altogether or makes it merely contingent upon active affection. A balance is sought between that independence which enables people to have a sense of controlling their own destinies, and those ties of obligation and affection that render each an indispensable source of solace in the face of a world that has no special reason to care for them.

A minimal duty of any government should be to do nothing to hinder, and if possible do something to protect, the natural moral and filial ties that give families their power to nurture and sustain. To exploit that bond by coercively taxing families is, I believe, to threaten them with great harm. It is an action that presupposes a narrower form of moral obligation of children to parents than can rationally be defended. At the same time it promises to rupture those more delicate moral bonds, as powerful as they are conceptually elusive, that sustain parents and children in their lives together. Such bonds do not necessarily rule out financial incentives for children to care for their aged parents, as some recent legislative proposals suggest.[29] But if such incentives are to receive support, in that case considerable care would be needed to guard against an exploitation of parents by avaricious children. There are, I ruefully note, as many ways to corrupt the parent-child relationship as ways to sustain it.

Notes

1   Statement of James L. Scott, Associate Administrator for Operations, Health Care Financing Administration, before the House Select Committee on Human Services, May 16, 1983.

2   Cf. the overwhelmingly negative responses to the Administration initiative at hearings conducted by the Subcommittee on Human Services on "Medicaid and Family Responsibility: Who Pays?" May 16, 1983.

3   Victor R. Fuchs, *How We Live: An Economic Perspective on Americans from Birth to Death* (Cambridge: Harvard University Press, 1983), p. 201.

4   Stephen Crystal, *America's Old Age Crisis* (New York: Basic Books, 1982), p. 40.

5   Ibid., p. 52.

6   Ethel Shanas, "The Family Relations of Old People," *The National Forum* 62 (Fall 1982), p. 10. As for the motivation behind the visits of children to their parents, Victor Fuchs cites a study purporting to show "that the number of visits was positively related to the parents' bequeathable wealth . . . ," in Victor Fuchs, " 'Though Much Is Taken': Reflections on Aging, Health, and Medical Care," *Milbank Memorial Quarterly* 62:2 (Spring 1984), p. 160.

7   James J. Callahan, Jr., et al., "Responsibilities of Families for Their Severely Disabled Elderly," paper prepared by the Brandeis University Health Policy Consortium, July 1979, p. iii.

8   Crystal, op. cit., pp. 56–57.

9   Cf. Mary Jo Bane, "Is the Welfare State Replacing the Family?" *The Public Interest* (Winter 1983), pp. 91–101.

10 Daniel Yankelovich, *New Rules: Searching for Self-Fulfillment in a World Turned Upside Down* (New York: Random House, 1981), p. 104.

11 For some pertinent analysis of the present state statutes, see, for example, Paul R. Ober, "Pennsylvania's Family Responsibility Statute—Corruption of Blood and Denial of Equal Protection," *Dickinson Law Review* 77 (1972), pp. 331–351; Gregory G. Sarno, "Constitutionality of Statutory Provision Requiring Reimbursement of Public by Child for Financial Assistance to Aged Parents," *American Law Reports Annotation* 75, 3rd (1977), pp. 1159–1178; W. Walton Garrett, "Filial Responsibility Laws," *Journal of Family Law* 18 (1979–80), pp. 793–818; James L. Lopes, "Filial Support and Family Solidarity," *Pacific Law Journal* 6 (July 1975), 508–535.

12 *Commentaries on the Laws of England*, Vol. 1 (Philadelphia: J. B. Lippincott and Co., 1856) book 1, ch. 16, section 1, cited in Jeffrey Blustein, *Parents and Children: The Ethics of the Family* (New York: Oxford University Press, 1982), p. 181. It is worth noting that the People's Republic of China apparently persists in upholding stringent filial obligations. The Constitution of 1982 states that ". . . children who have come of age have the duty to support and assist their parents"; and the Marriage Law of 1980 says that "When children fail to perform the duty of supporting their parents, parents who have lost the ability to work or have difficulties in providing for themselves have the right to demand that their children pay for their support." Cited in Alice and Sidney Goldstein, "The Challenge of an Aging Population in the People's Republic of China." Paper presented at annual meeting of Population Association of America, May 3–5, 1984, Minneapolis.

13 See especially W. Walton Garrett, op. cit., pp. 793–796.

14 Martin R. Levy and Sara W. Gross, "Constitutional Implications of Parental Support Laws," *University of Richmond Law Review* 13 (1979), p. 523.

15 Ibid., p. 524.

16 Ibid., p. 525.

17 Ibid.

18 Ibid., p. 526.

19 Ibid., p. 527.

20 Ibid., pp. 527–528.

21 Jane English, "What Do Grown Children Owe Their Parents?" in Onora O'Neill and William Ruddick, eds., *Having Children: Philosophical and Legal Reflections on Parenthood* (New York: Oxford University Press, 1979), p. 351.

22 Ibid., p. 353.

23 Ibid.

24 Ferdinand Schoeman, "Rights of Children, Rights of Parents, and the Moral Basis of the Family," *Ethics* 91 (October 1980), p. 8.

25 Blustein, op. cit., p. 177.

26 Joel Feinberg, "Duties, Rights, and Claims," *American Philosophical Quarterly* 3 (1966), p. 139; cited in Blustein, ibid., p. 176.

27 For further helpful discussions on the general topic, see Andrew Joseph Christiansen, "Autonomy and Dependence in Old Age," Yale University doctoral dissertation, 1982; Abraham Monk, "Family Supports in Old Age," *Social Work* (November 1979), pp. 533–538; Wilma T. Donahue, "What About Our Responsibility to the Abandoned Elderly?" *The Gerontologist* 18:2 (1978), 102–111; Wayne C. Seelbach, "Correlates of Aged Parents' Filial Responsibility Expectations and Realizations," *The Family Coordinator* (October 1978), pp. 341–350; Stanley J. Brady, et al., "The Family Caring Unit: A Major Consideration in the Long-Term Support System," *The Gerontologist* 18:6 (1978), 16–20; Elizabeth S. Johnson and Barbara J. Bursk, "The Relationship Between the Elderly and Their Adult Children," *The Gerontologist* 17:1 (1977), 90–96; Alvin Schorr, ". . . Thy Father and Thy Mother: A Second Look at Filial Responsibility and Family Policy," U.S. Department of Health and Human Services, SSA Publication No. 13-11953 (Washington DC: Government Printing Office, July 1980); W. Andrew Achenbaum, *Old Age in the New Land* (Baltimore: Johns Hopkins Press, 1978), pp. 75–80; Joanne P. Acford, "Reducing Medicaid Expenditures Through Family Responsibility: Critique of A Recent Proposal," *American Journal of Law and Medicine* 5:1 (Spring 1979), 59–79; "Relative Responsibility," *The Nursing Home Law Letter* (February 1982), pp. 1–8.

28 Quoted by Irving Kristol in a review of Ben Wattenberg's *The Good News Is the Bad News Is Wrong* (New York: Simon and Schuster, 1984), in *The New Republic* (October 29, 1984), p. 37.

29 Representative Mario Biaggi, for instance, introduced a bill in Congress in 1983, H.R. 76, that proposed "to allow a credit against income tax to individuals for maintaining in a household a member of which is a dependent of the taxpayer who has attained age sixty-five." The bill died in committee.

Index to Authors

About the Editors

Larry R. Churchill, PhD, holds the Ann Geddes Stahlman Chair in Medical Ethics, Department of Medicine, Center for Clinical and Research Ethics, Vanderbilt University. He also holds appointments in Vanderbilt's Divinity School and in the Department of Philosophy. From 1988 to 1998 he was chair of the Department of Social Medicine, University of North Carolina at Chapel Hill School of Medicine. His recent research is focused on justice and U.S. health policy, the ethics of research with human subjects, and the relationship between bioethics and ordinary moral experience.

Sue E. Estroff, PhD, is a professor in the Department of Social Medicine and an adjunct professor in the Departments of Anthropology and Psychiatry, School of Medicine and College of Arts and Sciences, University of North Carolina at Chapel Hill. She is the author of numerous cultural analyses of schizophrenia and other severe persistent psychiatric disorders, focusing most recently on the topics of contested identity and conflicting representations between medical and psychiatric formulations and those of people with schizophrenia. Her other current work includes cultural analysis of consent in the context of experimental fetal surgery, exploring moral quandaries in the production of knowledge, and examining the roles of social and cultural factors in violence in the lives of people with schizophrenia.

Gail E. Henderson, PhD, is a professor in the Department of Social Medicine, School of Medicine, and an adjunct professor in the Department of Sociology, College of Arts and Sciences, University of North Carolina at Chapel Hill. Her teaching and research interests include health and inequality, health and health care in China, and research ethics. She has extensive experience with qualitative and quantitative data collection and analysis, as well as with conceptual and empirical cross-disciplinary research and analysis. In China, she has taught social science research methods to clinical epidemiologists, and conducted research ethics training workshops for HIV/AIDS researchers. Her current research focuses on ethical issues in gene transfer clinical trials and cancer genetic epidemiology studies, and understanding how research ethics committees in China and Africa oversee international collaborative research.

Nancy M. P. King, JD, is a professor in the Department of Social Medicine, University of North Carolina at Chapel Hill School of Medicine. Her scholarly interests focus on individual and policy-level decision making in health care and research, and the relationship between bioethics and law. She teaches and advises on human subjects research ethics and health care ethics locally, nationally, and internationally, addressing issues ranging from literature and medicine to end-of-life court decisions to genetic databases. Her current research and most recent publications address informed consent in gene transfer research.

Jonathan Oberlander, PhD, is an associate professor in the Department of Social Medicine at the University of North Carolina at Chapel Hill, where he teaches health policy in the School of Medicine and Department of Political Science. He is a Greenwall Foundation Faculty Scholar in Bioethics and the author of *The Political Life of Medicare* (University of Chicago Press). His research and teaching interests include health politics and policy, Medicare, health care reform, and medical care rationing. Current research focuses on market-based strategies for Medicare reform, the politics of incremental and state-led health reform, and a study of the Oregon Health Plan.

Ronald P. Strauss, DMD, PhD, is a professor in the Department of Social Medicine, School of Medicine, and Dental Friends Distinguished Professor and Chair, Department of Dental Ecology, School of Dentistry, University of North Carolina at Chapel Hill. He is both a sociologist of medicine and a dentist, with a research focus on stigmatization and the social impacts of chronic health problems including craniofacial anomalies and HIV/AIDS. He is the director of the Social and Behavioral Sciences Research Core of the UNC Center for AIDS Research. Current research includes an oral health disparities research project in Hawaii, a study of health promotion in low-income workplaces in eastern North Carolina, a study that examines stigma experience related to TB and HIV in south Thailand, and a multisite project that evaluates quality of life in adolescents with facial differences.

Library of Congress Cataloging-in-Publication Data
The social medicine reader.—2nd ed.
p. ; cm.
Includes bibliographical references and index.
ISBN 0-8223-3555-7 (v. 1 : cloth : alk. paper)
ISBN 0-8223-3568-9 (v. 1 : pbk. : alk. paper)
ISBN 0-8223-3580-8 (v. 2 : cloth : alk. paper)
ISBN 0-8223-3593-X (v. 2 : pbk. : alk. paper)
ISBN 0-8223-3556-5 (v. 3 : cloth : alk. paper)
ISBN 0-8223-3569-7 (v. 3 : pbk. : alk. paper)
1. Social medicine.
[DNLM: 1. Social Medicine—Collected Works.
2. Ethics, Clinical—Collected Works. 3. Health
Policy—Collected Works. 4. Professional-Patient
Relations—Collected Works. 5. Sick Role—Col-
lected Works. 6. Socioeconomic Factors—Collected
Works. 7. Terminal Care—Collected Works.
WA 31 S67803 2005] I. King, Nancy M. P.
RA418.S6424 2005   362.1′042—dc22   2005010301